HEALTH EDUCATION
AND HEALTH PROMOTION

HEALTH EDUCATION AND HEALTH PROMOTION

LEARNER-CENTERED INSTRUCTIONAL STRATEGIES

FIFTH EDITION

JERROLD S. GREENBERG

UNIVERSITY OF MARYLAND

Boston   Burr Ridge, IL   Dubuque, IA   Madison, WI   New York
San Francisco   St. Louis   Bangkok   Bogotá   Caracas   Kuala Lumpur
Lisbon   London   Madrid   Mexico City   Milan   Montreal   New Delhi
Santiago   Seoul   Singapore   Sydney   Taipei   Toronto

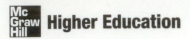

Higher Education

HEALTH EDUCATION AND HEALTH PROMOTION: LEARNER-CENTERED
INSTRUCTIONAL STRATEGIES FIFTH EDITION

Published by McGraw-Hill, a business unit of The McGraw-Hill Companies, Inc., 1221 Avenue
of the Americas, New York, NY 10020. Copyright " 2004 by The McGraw-Hill Companies,
Inc. All rights reserved. Previous edition(s) 1998, 1995, 1992, 1989. All rights reserved. No
part of this publication may be reproduced or distributed in any form or by any means, or stored
in a database or retrieval system, without the prior written consent of The McGraw-Hill
Companies, Inc., including, but not limited to, in any network or other electronic storage or
transmission, or broadcast for distance learning.

Some ancillaries, including electronic and print components, may not be available to customers
outside the United States.

This book is printed on acid-free paper.

Domestic   1 2 3 4 5 6 7 8 9 0 DOC/DOC 0 9 8 7 6 5 4 3

ISBN 0-07-231958-5

Vice president and editor-in-chief: *Thalia Dorwick*
Executive editor: *Vicki Malinee*
Developmental editor: *Gary O'Brien*
Senior marketing manager: *Pamela S. Cooper*
Project manager: *Mary Lee Harms*
Production supervisor: *Enboge Chong*
Associate designer: *George Kokkonas*
Art editor: *Jen DeVere*
Manager, Photo research: *Brian J. Pecko*
Senior supplement producer: *David A. Welsh*
Compositor: *ColorType*
Typeface: *Times*
Printer: *R. R. Donnelley/Crawfordsville, IN*

Library of Congress Cataloging-in-Publication Data

Greenberg, Jerrold S.
    Health education and health promotion: learner-centered instructional strategies / Jerrold S.
 Greenberg. — 5th ed.
      p. cm.
    Previous ed. has title: Health education
    Includes bibliographical references.
    ISBN 0-07-231958-5 (alk. paper)
1. Health education. 2. Health promotion. I. Greenberg, Jerrold S. Health education. II. Title

RA440.5.G74 2004
613′.071 — dc21

                                                                        2003046447

The Internet addresses listed in the text were accurate at the time of publication. The inclusion
of a website does not indicate an endorsement by the authors or McGraw-Hill, and McGraw-Hill
does not guarantee the accuracy of the information presented at these sites.

www.mhhe.com

DEDICATION

This book is dedicated to my son Todd. There is no one I admire more, or of whom I am more proud. It is appropriate that a book about health — as defined broadly — should be dedicated to Todd. Todd is a manifestation of good health. He is physically fit, intelligent, conscientious, sociable, trustworthy, and spiritually grounded. Even his career choice evidences his concern for bettering society through representing the interests of the community as a whole. A parent — this parent — could not have molded a son any better than mine. Thanks, Todd, for being who you are. This dedication is but a small way of expressing my love and admiration for you.

CONTENTS

Preface xiii

PART ONE
HEALTH EDUCATION: THEORY AND PRACTICE

1 Health Education Clarified 3

Definitions 3
   Health 3
   Wellness 7
   Health Education 8
Summary 14

2 The Certified Health Education Specialist 16

Health Education Certification 16
The Certified Health Education Specialist 17
Health Educator Competencies 17
Health Educator Competencies and
   This Book 30
In Conclusion 34
Summary 34

3 A New Form for Health Education 35

The Rationale for Health Education 35
   The Current Emphasis on
      Health Education 35
   Objectives for the Nation 36
   Social Responsibility 39

   Cost Benefit 39
   Recruitment and Retention 40
A Health Communication Model 40
Iatrogenic Health Education Disease 42
Health Education as Freeing 43
   Enslaving Factors 43
   The Objectives of Health Education
      as Freeing 43
   The Evaluation of Health Education
      as Freeing 44
   Research Goals 45
   The Ultimate Goal 45
Health Education Ethics 45
   Ethical Issues 46
   Code of Ethics 47
Summary 47

4 Service-Learning in Health Education 49

The Need 49
   Children 50
   Poverty 51
   Homelessness 54
   Violence 54
   Suicide 55
   Families 56
Civic Disengagement 56
The Health Educator's Responsibilities 57
   The Politics of Small 58
   Examples of Health Education
      Community Service 58

Service-Learning 59
   Examples of Service-Learning 59
   Service-Learning with Adults 60
   The Benefits of Service-Learning 60
   Evidence of a Need for
      Service-Learning 61
How to Conduct Service-Learning 62
In Conclusion 64

5   Conducting Health Education 65

Health Education Settings 65
   The Academic Setting 65
   The Community and Public
      Health Setting 67
   The Medical Care Setting 69
   The Worksite Setting 70
Planning for Health Education 73
   Needs Assessment 73
   Developing Objectives 74
Implementation 75
   Funding 76
   Facilities 76
   Equipment 76
   Scheduling 76
   Marketing 77
Evaluation 78
   Outcome Evaluation 78
   Process Evaluation 78
   Formative and Summative Evaluation 79
   Evaluation of Long-Range Objectives 79
Summary 79

PART TWO

PREREQUISITE INSTRUCTIONAL
STRATEGIES: GROUP PROCESS
AND THE EXPLORATION OF
VALUES AND HEALTH

**6   Instructional Strategies for
Development of Group Process Skills
and the Learning Environment** 82

Various Roles of the Instructor 84
Developing Trust among Program
   Participants 84
   Introduction Skits 84
   Pyramiding for Introductions 85
Developing a Trusting Learning
   Environment 85
   Tell Me Statements 86
   Trust Test 86
   Trust Walk 86
Developing Listening Skills 86
   Paraphrasing 87
   Written Conversations 88
Understanding Roles of Group Members 89
   Fishbowls 89
   Leadership Exercise 90
Teaching Cooperation 93
   Cooperation Puzzle 93
Making Sure All Participate 95
   Baseball Clue Game 95
   Building-upon Exercise 96
Developing Empathy 97
Treating People as Individuals 98
   Filling Needs 98
   Appreciation of Individual Differences 98
Analyzing Frustration 100
Managing Group Disagreement 100
Summary 101

**7   Instructional Strategies for Exploring
the Relationship between Values and
Health** 102

Valuing Exercises 104
   Values Ranking 104
   Values Grid 104

Values Continuum 106
Activities Enjoyed 106
Coat of Arms 107
Values Quadrant 108
Who Should Survive? 108
Value Judgment 110
Proud Statement 110
Fantasy Questions 111
Epitaph 111
Making Lists 112
Values Check 112
-ly Descriptions 112
Role Trading 113
Learning Statements 113
To Follow 114

PART THREE
HEALTH EDUCATION: INSTRUCTIONAL STRATEGIES TO ACTIVATE LEARNERS

---

8   Instructional Strategies for Mental Health Education 117

Introductory Activities 117
Tell Me Statements 117
Conversation Starters 118
You're Like Statements 119
Perceptions Survey 120
Perceptual Set 122
Exploring Feelings 125
Acting Out Feelings 126
Staring 127
Break in the Circle 128
Shouting Names 128
Gracious Receiving 128
Blocking 130
Friends and Enemies 130
How/When Questionnaire 130

Feelings Drawings 131
Activities to Affect Behavior 131
Prescriptions 131
Telegramming 132
Permanent Grouping 132
Justification of Self 133
Self-Concept Activities 133
I Am Statements 133
Self-Portraits 134
Bravissimo 134
Fantasy Play 134
Stress Management Activities 134
Mind Control 135
Stress Emitters 135
Time Pressure Buster 135
The Stress Interview 136
Progressive Relaxation 136
Autogenic Training 138
Mediation 138
Valuing Activities 139
Values Grid 139
Values Continuum 139
Proud Statement 140
Values Ranking 140
Values Sheet 140
Summary 141

9   Instructional Strategies for Substance Abuse 142

The Pimple Theory 142
Peer Group Exercises 143
Reversed Seats 143
Blindfolding 144
Commercial Collaging 144
Commercial Recording 145
Commercial Creating 145
Staged Argument 146
Videotaping Plays 146

Crossword Puzzle 147

Debates 148

Brainstorming Highs 149

Program Visitors 149

Case Study 151

Critical Incident 151

Strength Bombardment 152

Forced Arguing 153

Thermometer 153

Interviews 154

Valuing Activities 154

 Values Ranking 154

 Values Statements 154

 Values Judgment 155

 Values Continuum 155

 Medicine Cabinet Inspection 156

 Learning Statements 156

Summary 156

10 Instructional Strategies for Sexuality and Family Living 157

Need-For Activities 159

 Sexy Collage 159

 Sex as . . . Questionnaire 160

 Hot Line 161

 Question Box 161

Masculine/Feminine Roles 162

 Sex Riddle 162

 Imaginary Mirror 162

 Sex Role Dislikes/Likes 163

 Sex Tasking 163

 Head Tapes 164

Sexual Behavior 164

 Boundary Expanding 165

 Sexual Orientation Grid 165

 Premarital Sexual Intercourse Scale 167

 Processing a Contraception Decision 167

Dating and Intimate Relationships 168

 Computer Dating 168

Mate Recipe 170

Genetic Counseling Center 171

Pregnancy Sympathizer 171

Family Life 172

 Generation Gap 173

 Family Values Continuum 174

 Build a House 174

 Family Photos 174

 Family Drawings 176

 Sibling Sequencing 177

Violence Prevention 178

 Human Graph 178

 How Could You Handle It? 180

Controversy: Abortion and HIV/AIDS Education 181

 Abortion Debate 181

 Safer-Sex Communicating 183

 The HIV/AIDS Millionaire Game 187

Valuing Activities 192

 Values Ranking 192

 Epitaph 193

 Role Trading 193

 Values Statements 194

Summary 194

11 Instructional Strategies for Environmental Health 195

Sensory Awareness 195

 Blindfolded Activities 195

 Mixing Senses 196

 Zoo Tripping 197

 Snow Romping 197

Environmental Study 198

 Litter Police 198

 Planned City 198

 Trash Treasures 198

 Trash-Container Spying 198

 Population Growth Experiment 199

 Tug-of-War 200

Grounds Exploring 200
Solid-Waste Instrument Making 201
List of Questions for
    Environmental Study 203
Correlated Activities 206
Language 206
Art 207
Social Studies 207
Mathematics 208
Music 209
Science 209
Town of Barnard Simulation 209
Current Environmental Threats 214
Warming to Global Warming 214
The Bioterrorism Assay 214
Valuing Activities 215
Baker's Dozen 215
Activities Enjoyed 215
Values Grid 216
Values Quadrant 216
Values Voting 217
Fantasy Questions 217
Coat of Arms 217
Introspective Questions 218
Summary 218

**12 Instructional Strategies
for Nutrition** 219

Sociological Aspects of Food 219
Food History 219
Food Culturing 220
Food Sociogram 220
Hot Dogs and Pheasants 221
Weight Control 223
Alter Egoing 223
Problem Analyzing 224
Problem Analysis Questionnaire 224
Weight Goal Telegramming 226
Body Image and Self-Talk 226

Food Association Recalling 227
Healthful Eating 228
Food Guide Pyramid Centering 228
Food Inspectors 228
Fighting Back/Reading Labels 228
Nutrition Labeling and Finagling 232
Eat Well Day 232
Food Investigating 232
Selecting Lunch 233
Restauranting 233
Infant's Letter 233
Food Coaching 234
Malnutrition Epidemic 234
Eating Disorders/Disordered Eating:
    A Self-Analysis 235
Valuing Activities 235
Values Grid 237
Values Ranking 238
Values List 238
Values Voting 239
Values Questions 239
Summary 240

**13 Instructional Strategies for Aging,
Spirituality, and Death** 241

The Aged and Aging 241
Aged Visitors 241
Adoptions 242
Phone Pal 242
Visits 242
Sensory Deprivation Simulation
    Exercises 242
Keeping the Elderly Active 244
Eldercize 244
Elderly Myths 246
Elder Interviews 246
Retirement Brainstorming 247
Spiritual Health 247
The Spiritual Scavenger Hunt 247

Spiritual Sloganing 247
Spiritual Drawings 248
Death and Dying 250
Musical Perspectives on Death 250
Run for Your Life 251
Death Completions 252
Possessions 253
Living Will 253
Last Will 253
Interruption 254
Euthanasia/Assisted Suicide 254
Valuing Activities 257
Values Ranking 257
Survival 257
Values Listings 258
Values Behavior 259
Values Statements 260
Summary 260

**14 Instructional Strategies for
Personal Health** 261

Communicable Diseases 261
Disease Bag 261
Policy Study 262
Simulated Epidemic 263
Health Inspectors 263
Noncommunicable Diseases 263
Family Tree of Life and Death 263
Risko 265
Cancer Paneling 265
Physical Fitness 265
Harvard Step Test 265
The Agility Run 269
Flexibility Assessment 270
Sleep Study 272
Consumer Health 274
Price Sense 274
Gender Advertising and Appealing 274

Creating Ad Appeals 276
Other Personal Health Content 276
Dental Health 277
Genetic Counseling 278
Playing the Mad Scientist 278
Sense Appreciation 279
Valuing Activities 279
Values Statements 279
Values Voting 280
Consistency Check 280
Values Continuum 281
Values Sheet 281
Filling in Blanks 282
Giving Up 282
The Patient 283
Summary 284

PART FOUR

CONCLUSION

Health Education in Summary 285
Learning Experiences in This Book 286
The Hope for the Future 287
Getting There 287
To the Reader 287
Appendixes
A. Code of Ethics for the
   Health Education Profession 288
B. Toll-Free Numbers for Health Information 292
C. A Health and Health Education
   Internet Directory 310
D. 2003 Federal Health Information Centers and
   Clearinghouses 312
E. Health Education Standards 332
F. 2003 National Health Observances 340
G. Selected Professional Health Education
   Organizations 365
   Bibliography 366

PREFACE

Many valuable and effective health education programs are being conducted in schools, worksites, health care settings, and other community facilities. However, too many other programs are dull, ineffective, and more concerned with *what* is being taught than with *whom* is being taught. The result of these programs that miss the mark is too often the development of an adversarial relationship between health educator and health education learner. Nowhere is this situation more evident than in the public schools.

Have you ever thought how much school is like war? Classes like battles? Free periods like truces? Teachers' lounges and student cafeterias like military camps?

Both sides seem committed to battling for 40 or so minutes, resting, and then resuming battle. During the confrontation, teachers utilize weapons such as grading, motivation, hand raising, and parental visitations, while students employ calling out, passing notes, trips to the lavatory, truancy, and daydreaming.

At long last the class period ends, and the teacher retreats to lick his or her wounds. The retreat invariably ends in the teachers' lounge, where new strategies are conceived. First a cup of coffee to stimulate the body; next, conversation with fellow soldiers to benefit from their experiences; and last, the formulation of new or revised strategies to be employed when the battle resumes. With a pat on the back from compatriots indicative of their unwavering support, the teacher leaves the safety afforded by the camp and once again enters the field of battle.

What is the "other side" doing during the truce? The students often retreat to the school cafeteria where they, too, lick their wounds. First a hamburger, cola, and french fries (with plenty of ketchup on all but the cola); next, conversation with fellow soldiers to learn of their reactions to strategies employed by opposing soldiers and the consequences of such reactions; and last, plans for action when the battle resumes are agreed upon. With a "Right on," the students, upon hearing the bell indicating that the opposing soldiers are refreshed and ready to go, leave their camp bent on not losing the war.

Although a tragic situation for all disciplines, such an adversarial relationship in health education—whether conducted in schools, at places of work, in hospitals, or in facilities of community agencies—is particularly disturbing. Health education and health educators should be seen as having program participants' needs and interests at heart, as working with program participants to help them identify and satisfy their health-related goals and objectives, and as a resource for factual, objective information that is the basis of informed decisions. When, instead, the health educator is perceived as working *on* people rather than *with* them, the program itself becomes ineffective, and neither the health educator's nor the program participants' goals are met.

The goal of this book is to remedy this situation. It is designed to help health educators convert their programs into ones that meet participants' goals and objectives by actively involving them in the learning process. The first five chapters describe traditional and nontraditional health education and offer suggestions for making health education programs more responsive to program participants. The following topics are discussed: the definitions of health and wellness; certification of health educators;

the rationale for health education; the ethics of health education practice; service-learning and community service in health education; the settings in which health education occurs and the advantages and disadvantages of each of these settings; and the planning, implementation, and evaluation of health education programs. Chapters 6 and 7 present instructional activities to help program participants develop the requisite skills concerning group process and values clarification. These skills are used throughout other learning activities presented later in the book. Subsequent chapters describe over 200 instructional strategies that can be used by health educators in various settings to implement the form of health education advocated within this book.

If asked to summarize this book's purpose, I would simply say it is to argue for focusing more attention on the *people* who are enrolled in health education programs and to demonstrate how this attention can actually become a part of these programs by incorporating a learner-centered approach to education.

PART ONE

HEALTH EDUCATION

THEORY AND PRACTICE

This opening section introduces health education. Chapter 1 defines and differentiates the terms *health* and *wellness* and discusses the objectives, type of instruction, means of evaluation, and research goals of traditional forms of health education.

Chapter 2 cites the history of certification for health educators and the competencies Certified Health Education Specialists are expected to possess. The contribution of this book in preparing health educators in developing these competencies is described.

Chapter 3 presents the reasoning behind the recent emphasis on health education. This includes the concern over the rising costs associated with health care and over the spread of Acquired Immunodeficiency Syndrome, and the increasing sense of social responsibility for health education. Additionally, Chapter 3 discusses a proposal for a new form for health education, the concept of Iatrogenic Health Education Disease, and the ethical issues affecting the health educator.

Chapter 4 describes the health needs of select populations and the responsibility of health educators to respond to these needs. In particular, health statistics relative to minorities and underserved populations in the United States are presented. Service-learning is described as one means of involving students in their communities while, at the same time, learning health education content more effectively. The benefits of service-learning and how to conduct service-learning to achieve educational goals are discussed.

Chapter 5 describes the settings in which health education programs are typically conducted and discusses the planning, implementation, and evaluation of these programs. Such concerns as developing objectives, funding and scheduling, and the different types of evaluation are included in this discussion.

CHAPTER ONE

Health Education Clarified

British interviewer David Frost used to ask all of his guests, "What is love?" After years of questioning, the conclusion he drew was that love is defined in different ways by different people; when you are in it, you know it, and when you see it, you can identify it. Not a very exact definition!

The term *health* is similar to the term *love* in that it is defined in many different ways, even by the experts. When you have health, like love, you know it; and when someone else has it, you can usually recognize it.

Before we begin a study of health, health education, and strategies that health educators can employ to facilitate the development and maintenance of health, it seems reasonable to define these terms. In this way we will agree conceptually on the topic being explored.

Definitions

In this section we will define the important variables of health education, beginning with the most important: health.

Health

Shirreffs (1982) defines health as a "quality of life, involving social, mental, and biological fitness on the part of the individual, which results from adaptations to the environment." Though more comprehensive than some others, this definition of health does not include spiritual elements, nor does it address the relationship among the components of health. Others write of health as being more holistic. For example, Horowitz (1985) sees self-awareness as a key component of health but also includes skills development, values awareness, goal setting, positive self-concept, cognition, and willpower development among numerous other variables. Eberst (1985) also conceptualizes health as multidimensional and includes vocational health as well as the more traditional health components. Dever (1980, 10–17) summarizes the varying ways that health can be conceptualized when he describes the ecological, social ecological, World Health Organization, holistic, and high-level wellness models of health. These definitions conceptualize health to be multidimensional, to include many components, and to encompass many different aspects of one's life (for example, vocational, spiritual, and interpersonal).

Components of Health   For our purposes, consider health to be a quality of life that is a function of (Dintiman and Greenberg 1992, 8–9) these components:

1. *Social health* — Ability to interact well with people and the environment; having satisfying interpersonal relationships.

2. *Mental health*—Ability to learn; one's intellectual capabilities.

3. *Emotional health*—Ability to control emotions so that one feels comfortable expressing them when appropriate and does express them appropriately; ability to suppress emotions when it is appropriate to do so.

4. *Spiritual health*—Belief in some unifying force. For some people that will be nature, for others it will be scientific laws, and for others it will be a godlike force.

5. *Physical health*—Ability to perform daily tasks without undue fatigue; biological integrity of the individual.*

To illustrate this conceptualization of health, I would like you to meet Jim and know my thoughts about him (Greenberg 1985, 403):

> I could not help wondering if Jim was healthy. Several years had passed—five to be exact—since we last saw each other, and I was looking forward to catching up on old times. When I asked the standard "How've ya been?" Jim replied that he never had felt better. He took up jogging and now was up to 50 miles a week. As a result, he gave up cigarettes, became a vegetarian, and had more confidence than ever.
>
> In spite of Jim's reply, I needed further assurance. Jim looked like "death warmed over." His face was gaunt, his body emaciated. His clothes were baggy, creating a sloppy appearance. He had an aura of tiredness about him.
>
> "How's Betty?" I asked.
>
> "Fine," Jim replied. "But we're no longer together. Betty just couldn't accept the time I devoted to running, and her disregard for her health was getting on my nerves. She's still somewhat overweight, you know, and I started viewing her differently when I became healthier myself."†

At first glance, most people would agree that Jim appears to be healthier than he was prior to taking up jogging. Jim is unarguably healthier cardiovascularly. His circulatory system and his respiratory system are also vastly improved. He has given up cigarette smoking, lost weight, and begun eating more healthful foods. However, Jim looks terrible, and he no longer is happily married. Let's further assume that Jim is so preoccupied by his new lifestyle that he no longer spends time with friends or reads very much. This is not so far-fetched for some runners, who train for many hours a week preparing for marathons with little time remaining for anything other than making a living. If some time does become available, they are too tired to do anything. In this instance, Jim would be suffering a depletion of his social health, his mental health, and maybe even his spiritual health; all this in spite of an improvement in his physical health. Is he healthier than before? The temptation now is to say no. In fact, he's probably unhealthier than he was before. However, let's postpone our evaluation of Jim's health status until we explore health further.

In spite of intellectually agreeing that health is multifaceted, we too often act as though only physical health existed or mattered. If told that Aunt Mary is unhealthy, do you think to yourself, I wonder if she is experiencing spiritual problems? or I wonder if she is not able to manage her emotions? No.

---

*From George B. Dintiman and Jerrold S. Greenberg, *Exploring Health,* Copyright © 1992, Englewood Cliffs, NJ: Prentice Hall.

†From Greenberg, J. S. "Health and Wellness: A Conceptual Differentiation." *Journal of School Health,* vol. 55, no. 10, December 1985, pp. 403–406. Copyright © 1985. American School Health Association, Kent, OH 44240. Reprinted by permission.

Rather, most of us think that she is physically unwell, that she has cancer, ulcers, heart disease, or some other bodily ailment. The problem with this limited perspective regarding health will soon be made clear. For now, let's agree that we usually emphasize physical health to a greater degree than the other components of health.

Health and Values That we view physical health as more important than other components of health reflects our values. The importance of values in a consideration of health was made evident by Greene (1971) when he described the lifestyle of a hypothetical businessman:

> A businessman might be 15 pounds overweight for no apparent reason other than careless eating habits, or an unawareness of the advantages of trim physique, and ignorance of the basic principles of weight control. This should be classed as a remedial health defect and one important indicator of health status. However, let us compare this case with the case of another businessman, equally overweight, who happens to be a well-informed and enthusiastic amateur gourmet. His library of cookbooks includes directions for preparing many of the most popular dishes of other cultures. He spends many interesting hours in offbeat markets shopping for hard-to-get food items. The meals he prepares constitute focal points of an interesting and satisfying social life. This man realizes he is overweight; he knows how to reduce and control his weight and he may even suspect that his coronary may arrive a year or two ahead of schedule, but he does not care. His overweight condition constitutes a health defect only in the absolute sense. When viewed in relation to his value system, it represents a logical concomitant to his particular pattern of good health.

We can see by this example that it is problematic when someone prescribes for someone else what is healthy. The difficulty arises when the one doing the prescribing does not fully comprehend the values of the other. Who is to say for any other person that chancing a heart attack (physical health) by eating fatty gourmet foods is more unhealthy than quitting the gourmet club and losing some mental health (not learning as much about other cultures' foods) or some social health (giving up the friends and social activities involved in the club)? That decision involves the application of one's values, and it is inappropriate (substitute "undemocratic" or "manipulative" here) for someone to apply his or her values in an attempt to influence someone else's behavior. Yet that is what often takes place. With the best of intentions, health educators, physicians, parents, and others try to get people to behave as the "experts" define health, and that definition usually exaggerates physical health over the other components of health. Yet only the person who will be affected is truly able to decide to give up some of one component of health while acquiring more of another.

Now, back to Jim. Is he healthier? That is a question that cannot easily be answered, especially by anyone other than Jim himself. For only Jim knows whether the improvement in his physical health outweighs the loss of some relationships, the time to read, or the time for spiritual activities. Only Jim knows what he values and how much he values one thing compared to others. For that reason it is inappropriate for someone with a different set of values to observe Jim and to judge him as healthy or unhealthy.

Health and Culture One reason why people's values differ is that they come from different cultures or subcultures. We have already seen how these differing values affect health. Now let's see how culture affects health as well.

Most health experts agree that eating salty foods is unhealthy. And yet Orthodox Jews, following *Kasruth* (dietary) laws, require that their meats be salted to remove all the blood in order for that meat to be acceptable and *kosher.* Are these Jewish people less healthy for eating foods prepared in this fashion, or are they healthier because they consider their spiritual health as important as their physical health?

According to health experts, taking responsibility for one's health is an imperative. Many Hispanic people, however, believe illness results from wrongdoing; it is a *castigo,* or punishment. Therefore, conscious acts to alter divine events, such as taking responsibility for one's health, may be interpreted as interference with the will of God.

Health experts also believe that doing purposeful harm to the body is unhealthy. And yet, traditional Indochinese methods of healing include the practice of *Cao Gio:* involves scraping the skin with a coin at the point of disease. For example, someone with a headache would have the skin of the forehead scraped, until it became discolored. Some Indochinese parents living in the United States have even been investigated for child abuse for conceptualizing health as they do and practicing their cultural form of healing on their children.

Many other examples could be cited as evidence of how culture affects health. Our cultural value of thinness compared with the conceptualization of thinness as unhealthy in some European countries; the definition of political dissidents as mentally ill in the former Soviet Union; and the definition of good health by the Navajo Indians as a matter of mind, body, and spirit working together in balance and harmony are a few of these examples. It is apparent that the effect of culture on health is considerable.

The Health–Illness Continuum   Imagine that health appears on one side of a continuum, and illness on the other (see Figure 1.1). Utilizing this model, it is impossible for someone to be both healthy and ill. Some might object to this conceptualization on the grounds that a person who is ill may have some measure of health. For example, a physically disabled person who participates in the Wheelchair Olympics may be healthier than a person who is outwardly "able" but not physically fit. For now, though, withhold such an objection until the implications of the model become clearer and until the concept of *wellness* is discussed.

Imagine now that the health–illness continuum is placed under a microscope and greatly magnified. Further imagine that this magnification discloses that the continuum is not really a solid line but rather a series of dots (see Figure 1.2).

FIGURE 1.1

The Health–Illness Continuum

| Perfect health | Health | Illness | Death |

FIGURE 1.2

The Magnified Health–Illness Continuum

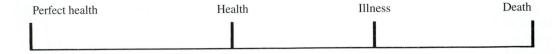

| Perfect health | Health | Illness | Death |

FIGURE 1.3
A Single Health–Illness Continuum Dot

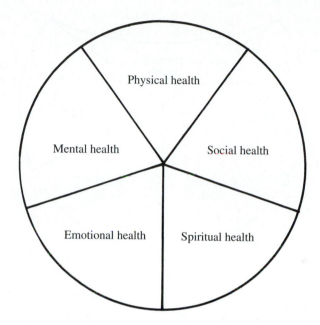

An even more powerful magnification of the dots on the continuum reveals that each dot is circular and consists of the five components of health defined earlier. The dot may appear as shown in Figure 1.3.

Wellness

Using the concept of "health dots," we are now ready to understand how wellness differs from health and how they are related. *Wellness* is the integration of social, mental, emotional, spiritual, and physical health at any level of health or illness. That is, you can be well regardless of whether you are healthy or ill. Because this conceptualization of wellness is different from that which some other health educators use, some elaboration is necessary.

Wellness is always a positive state; illness is always a negative state. How, then, can they coexist? The answer rests on the concept of *potentiality*. Certain illnesses limit the potential for health. Within that limitation, however, there is also a potential for variability. For example, two paraplegics may be defined as ill, but if one becomes depressed, angry, and isolated from other human beings, while the other does not, they surely differ in their degree of social health. When one joins the Wheelchair Olympics and keeps physically active and the other does not, certainly they differ in their degree of physical health. So one paraplegic has obtained more of the potential social health or physical health than the other; therefore, one is more well than the other, although they may be equally disabled. When we combine the five components of health and measure the degree to which each one's potential has been realized, we thereby assess the degree of wellness that has been acquired.

When we view health and illness as being on the *same* continuum, someone who is ill—the paraplegic—cannot also be healthy; but if we conceptualize illness and wellness as being on *different*

FIGURE 1.4

An Out-of-Round Health–Illness Continuum Dot

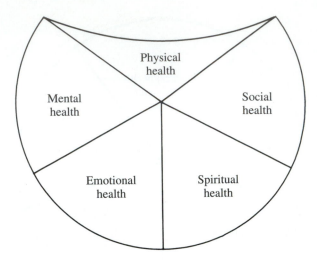

continua, someone can have varying degrees of each concurrently. The point is, the closer we get to our potential of the five components of health, the more well we are, and the more wellness we have achieved.

High-Level Wellness   Recall the health dots made up of the five components of health. Imagine that one of these components is underdeveloped—for example, that you have neglected your physical health by leading a sedentary life. In that instance, your health dot might look like Figure 1.4; that is, it might be out of round.

When a car's tire is out of round, the driver gets a bumpy ride. When your health dot is out of round, you, too, get a bumpy ride. The smoothest automobile ride comes when the tire is perfectly round. The smoothest ride down the road of life comes when your health dot is perfectly round, as depicted in Figure 1.3. Your tire can get out of round if you either neglect a component of health or overemphasize one.

Now back to our friend Jim. Jim neglected his social health by ignoring the need to maintain friendships and his marriage, and he devoted too much time to his physical health by spending inordinate amounts of time jogging. Jim's health dot is depicted in Figure 1.5.

Is Jim healthy? Well, we previously saw the difficulty of answering that question. Is Jim well? Has Jim achieved high-level wellness? The answer to these questions is easier—NO! Jim will have a bumpy ride on his health dots because they are out of round; he has neglected some components of health and has exaggerated others. Jim may or may not be healthy—that is a function of one's values—but he has not achieved a high level of wellness. High-level wellness, then, is the integration and *balance* of the five components of health (Greenberg 1985).

Health Education

Now that we have defined the concepts of health and wellness, we can explore one of the professions devoted to affecting them—health education.

FIGURE 1.5

The Asymmetrical Dot on the Health–Illness Continuum

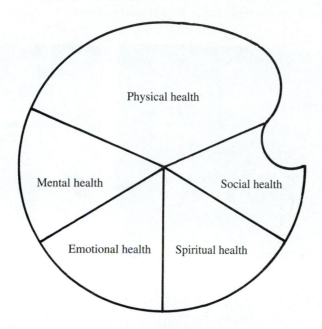

Traditional Health Education   The health education profession has been helping people for a long time now. Rubinson and Alles (1984) trace the history of health education to ancient times. However, in the 1970s, the Role Delineation Project—a national project designed to explore eventual credentialing of health educators—developed a specific description of the roles of health educators. As part of their charge, that national group defined *health education* as "the process of assisting individuals, acting separately and collectively, to make informed decisions on matters affecting individual, family, and community health. Based upon scientific foundations, health education is a field of interest, a discipline, a profession" (Role Delineation Project 1980).

In another frequently used definition, Green et al. (1980) defines health education as "any combination of learning experiences designed to facilitate voluntary adaptations of behavior conducive to health."

The 2000 Joint Committee on Health Education and Promotion Terminology's (2001) definition of health education recognizes that health education is based on well-researched theories and can be conducted at the individual, group, or community levels. The committee defines health education as "any combination of planned learning experiences based on sound theories that provide individuals, groups, and communities the opportunity to acquire information and skills needed to make quality health decisions."

Still another definition pertains to school curricula. *Comprehensive school health education* is defined as that provided from the time of entrance into the school system, with planned, systematic, and ongoing learning opportunities designed to maximize the prospect that each student will be able to make health-enhancing decisions that promote growth throughout life (Seffrin 1990).

These athletes have not let their disabilities prevent them from reaching their physical health potentials. Given that they are as motivated relative to the other health components, it is likely that, in spite of their physical limitations, they have reached a status of high-level wellness.

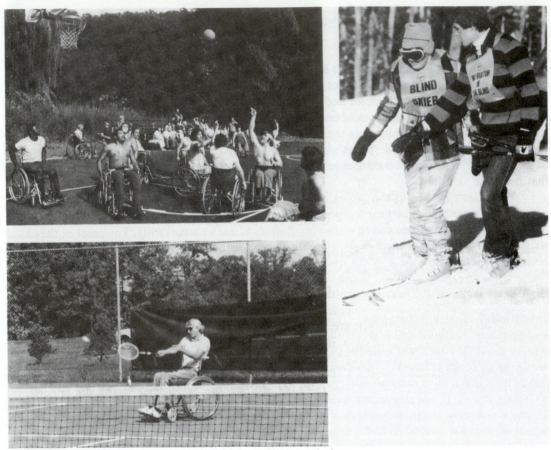

Source: National Handicapped Sports and Recreation Association

These concepts of health education are seen in operation during formal professional activities in educational settings. For example, health educators develop learning *objectives,* designate the *content* they will teach to achieve these objectives, design *learning activities* they will use to teach this content, identify whatever *instructional aids* they will use during these learning activities, and prepare an *evaluation* of the effectiveness of the health education experience by determining to what extent the objectives have been achieved.

These professional activities are conducted in several ways. Either they are taught individually by health educators, or they are offered in groups (for example, at a curriculum development workshop or in a program made available through a community agency like the local heart association). At other times, already existing curricula may be adopted wholly or in part. Rarely, however, are the recipients of health education — students, patients, or other members of the community — ever involved in these professional activities. In other words, health education is, as described by Breckon et al. (1985, 4), planned change — that is, planned by the health educator.

The nature of this traditional form of health education is elucidated here as we consider health education objectives, the type of instruction typical of many health education programs, evaluation of health education, and research goals usually associated with health education.

1. *Objectives.* Health educators value healthful behavior and select objectives that will lead to the adoption of such behavior. That is why health education for schoolchildren includes such objectives as refraining from smoking cigarettes, eating well-balanced meals, and buckling seat belts when driving in an automobile. That is also why health education in the workplace includes such objectives as managing stress, drinking alcohol responsibly (if at all), and obeying safety rules.

   The purpose of the instruction, then, is usually to achieve the objective of behavioral change, or at least adherence to a recommended set of behaviors. The learning of knowledge and the development of healthy attitudes (for example, that one can do things to affect one's health or, more specifically, that wearing seat belts is a valuable and safe behavior) are merely steps necessary for behavior change. Although the acquisition of knowledge, the improvement of attitudes, and the development of certain skills are written into health education curricula as objectives, many health educators argue that unless there is a demonstrable change in health-related behavior — and, ultimately, an improvement in health status — the educational program has not been a success. They argue that knowledge for knowledge's sake is useless, that knowledge must be *used* — that is, result in a change of behavior — in order for people's health to improve. That is why some school-based sexuality education programs are sometimes more concerned with decreasing the number of births to unmarried mothers or the incidence of sexually transmitted infections than they are with enhancing the sexuality of their students. That is why some patient education programs are more concerned with patients' adherence to physicians' recommendations than they are with patients understanding their medical condition. Health educators seek compliance with their professional advice and codify this goal into objectives.

2. *Type of instruction.* Rarely, if ever, are students, workers, patients, or other community members involved in determining the methods used during the instructional process. That is the prerogative of the health educator, the specialist in pedagogy. The people *to whom the health education is being applied* are mostly passive recipients, receptacles for the depositing of health-related information.

   Methods of instruction are selected with an eye on best achieving the objectives of behavior change that we just discussed, or at least that is what we would like to think. However, given that we know people learn best by being actively involved in the learning process (learning by doing) and that instruction involving learners is the most effective in achieving behavioral change, we can see that too often the methods selected are those that are easiest for the health educator to use rather than the best in terms of achieving the instructional objectives. Walk into any school, work site, or patient health education class, and chances are that you will see the health educator lecturing or showing a film or in some other way being active, while the students, workers, or patients sit passively, like sponges waiting to expand with the "waters of knowledge." The type of instruction that actively involves participants often requires different

Evaluation of health education has too often concentrated on rote memory or on unobtainable or unrealistic objectives. Furthermore, the objectives being evaluated are usually established by the health educator with little, if any, input by program participants.

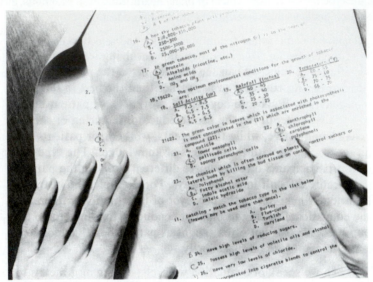

Source: The Diamondback, University of Maryland

skills on the part of the health educator and is more difficult in several ways. For example, the instructor is not the center of attention or necessarily the conveyor of information; rather, the instructor organizes the educational setting to make it conducive for students to learn. That requires a set of group-process skills not often taught as part of health education professional preparation programs. More on this shortly.

3. *Evaluation.* When we speak of evaluation, we are discussing a means to determine whether the educational objectives have been achieved at the conclusion of the session or program. If the objective of the educational process is to effect behavioral change or adherence to behaviors predetermined to be healthful, then that is what needs to be evaluated. If the objective is to decrease the number of births to unmarried teens, then that is what needs to be evaluated. If the objective is to decrease the incidence of HIV, then that is what needs to be evaluated.

The problem with this type of evaluation relates to the causes of these unhealthful behaviors in the first place. To think that some education conducted over a few weeks or even months will have a dramatic effect on behaviors that have taken years to develop is unrealistic. To ignore the many other variables that affect these behaviors and to expect that they will no longer be operative is naive. Health educators, however, get themselves into an "evaluation trap" by initially accepting imposed goals in order to get the programs accepted. For example, when a business organization institutes an occupational health education program in order to reduce absenteeism, improve worker productivity, and decrease health insurance premiums, health educators "buy into" these goals because they believe that is the only way to get the program started. The trap comes later when the organization's management asks for an evaluation of the program, expecting to find certain changes. Left out of the evaluation, however, may be the organization's long history of worker–management relationships that have resulted in poor morale, or the nature of the work (is increased productivity a realistic goal or is the work so well organized that any increase can only be minimal?), or the fact that the health education program has never provided the necessary facilities, equipment, or time needed to be effective.

Some health educators may recognize this potential trap but say, No need to worry. I just won't evaluate the program at all. For example, many school health education programs are not evaluated. The rationale typically offered is that health education's effect upon health behaviors may be some years down the road. That is, the seeds may be laid during the school years only to take effect during the years after school. Therefore, some school health educators argue, this delayed effect cannot be evaluated, so let's not even bother to try. Furthermore, school health educators continue, other educational disciplines don't have to prove that they effect behavioral change. History teachers don't need to show that more students who took history classes vote as adults than those who did not take history, and math teachers don't have to demonstrate that students who took geometry think any more logically than those who didn't. Occupational health educators can be heard to say that even if their health education program doesn't result in an identifiable cost benefit, the intangibles it brings — for example, its value in recruiting new workers — are well worth maintaining the program.

It would be far better to make these points initially rather than allow false and unrealistic expectations to develop and then attempt to reeducate management. For example, management should be told that changes in health knowledge and health attitudes will be easier to achieve than will be changes in health behavior; that changes that occur in health behavior need periodic reinforcement to be maintained; and that postponement of illness and disease does not necessarily mean cost savings because these illnesses and diseases may still develop sometime later on.

4. *Research goals.* Because the major objective of health education is to encourage (some would pejoratively substitute the term *manipulate)* participants to adopt behaviors predetermined to be healthful, research is directed at the best way to effect that change. Consequently, many research studies conducted in health education settings attempt to measure the amount of behavioral change in the participants as compared to a control group of subjects who have not experienced the program. For example, the lecture approach to drug education might be conducted with one group of students and compared to the discussion approach conducted with another group of students and a control group of students who receive no drug education at all. The most effective method for encouraging students to change their drug-related behavior will be sought so it might be used in other drug education programs that also have behavioral change as an objective. However, since behavioral change depends on several other variables — such as health knowledge, attitudes, intentions, and skills — these, too, are measured. Health educators have found it relatively easy to effect changes in health knowledge and skills, somewhat more difficult to effect changes in health attitudes, and extremely difficult to get people to change their health-related behaviors (Connell et al. 1985; Kirby et al. 1979).

When changes in health behaviors have occurred, it is not unusual to find that participants revert to past behaviors shortly after the program's completion. A study of a stress education program for college students is a case in point (Greenberg et al. 1986). The program consisted of five learning stations and included videotapes, slide/tapes, an audiotape, and numerous handouts. This program did not require a trained professional health educator to be present. Instead, all that was needed was a facility in which instructional materials could be set up and students moved through the learning stations. When compared to similar college students who did not experience that stress management program, participants knew more about stress, believed they were better able to manage the stress in their lives, and even practiced more stress management techniques. However, the difference between program participants and nonparticipants was greatest just as the program ended. When these variables were measured 30 days later, this difference, though still statistically significant, was less than at the immediate completion of the program. Further measurements were not feasible given the time and financial limitations of the study, but it would be no surprise to find little if any difference between the two groups on subsequent measurements. That is because behavior changed by educational programs often reverts to what it was prior to the program when further reinforcement is not provided.

The point is that typical or traditional health education is concerned with behavioral change and the variables that affect that change. Research investigations are, therefore, designed to determine the best — most effective, most cost efficient, or most feasible — way to reach this end.

Summary

1. Health is a quality of life that is a function of social, mental, emotional, spiritual, and physical health. Usually physical health is emphasized while the other components of health are forgotten or ignored.

2. It is inappropriate to describe someone else as healthy or unhealthy, because that is a function of a person's values, and people's values differ. Each person must decide whether it is right (for himself or herself) to give up some of one component of health to achieve more of another component of health. That decision is a matter of value; for example, one might ask whether social health is more valuable than, say, mental health to that person at that particular time.

3. Wellness is always a positive state; it is the degree to which a person has reached his or her *potential* regarding each of the components of health. Wellness is the integration of social, mental, emotional, spiritual, and physical health at any level of health or illness.

4. People cannot be both healthy and ill at the same time, but they may be either healthy *or* ill while still having achieved a high level of wellness.

5. High-level wellness is the integration and *balance* of the five components of health; no one component of health is exaggerated, and no one component is neglected.

6. Health education has been traditionally defined as the process of assisting individuals, acting separately and collectively, to make informed decisions on matters affecting individual, family, and community health. Based upon scientific foundations, health education is a field of interest, a discipline, and a profession.

7. The role of health educators is to develop learning objectives, determine the content of programs, design learning activities, identify instructional aids, and evaluate the effects of health instruction. It is unusual for program participants to be involved in these processes.

8. The primary objective of traditional health education has been to effect behavioral change — that is, to encourage program participants either to adopt behaviors health scientists tell us are healthful or to maintain behaviors presently engaged in that are defined as healthful.

9. To achieve health education objectives, subordinate objectives are often focused upon: for example, acquiring health *knowledge,* improving health-related *attitudes,* and learning health-related *skills.* Evaluation of health education programs determines how well the behavioral objectives of health education have been achieved, and the goal of health education research is to identify the most effective, the most cost efficient, and the most feasible way of achieving these objectives.

CHAPTER TWO

The Certified Health Education Specialist

Carmen recently returned from her doctor. Finding her blood pressure high, her doctor told her not to take things so seriously. Carmen agreed with that goal, but had no idea how she was to achieve it.

Frank's doctor was appalled that he still smoked cigarettes after being told during his last office visit that smoking threatened his health. Frank wanted to quit but did not know how.

Beth was overly stressed. She worked full-time outside the home, was raising two children as a single parent, and was very active in her church. To treat the muscle tension and stomach problems she was having, Beth's doctor told her to relax more. Beth knew her doctor was right, but had no clue how she could relax given her lifestyle.

These stories may seem fictional, but they are too often descriptive of physician–patient interactions. In fact, at a conference I attended I heard a physician bemoan the fact that his patients did not listen to him. He told them not to drink, not to smoke, not to engage in sex, and to exercise regularly — all to no avail. In particular, he said, his teenage patients disregarded his advice. Little did he know that just telling people what is "good" for them (as if anyone could really know that for anyone else — more on this in the next chapter) is not enough to get them to change their behavior. If it were, there would not be a need for a whole profession — health education — and professional preparation programs to give people the skills to educate others about their health and lifestyle. There is an abundance of research demonstrating that even though people may have a good deal of health knowledge, that does not mean they will adopt healthful lifestyles.

Health Education Certification

Health is a popular topic. It is so popular that books, videotapes, workshops, and other profit-making vehicles have been used to "market" it. Sarah Ferguson (Princess Fergie) presents herself as a health educator with expertise in nutrition. Jane Fonda presents herself as a health educator with an expertise in physical fitness. Actress Kelly McGillis presents herself as a health educator with expertise on acquaintance rape. One might argue that these celebrities may offer valuable services; they may have researched their topics well and learned about methods of instruction so that they motivate people toward more healthful behavior. And yet, the fact that Sarah Ferguson was once obese does not qualify her as a health educator. Nor do the facts that Jane Fonda is exceptionally fit and Kelly McGillis was once raped qualify them as health educators. In addition to these celebrities are people who are less well-versed in the health topic about which they profess to be experts. In fact, they may be so misinformed that they convey information that, if followed, may actually present a danger to one's health. For example, they may advocate unhealthful diets, or exceptionally high levels of physical activity, or such anxiety about lifestyle and health that one's mental health is harmed.

In an attempt to protect the public from incompetent and potentially harmful instructors of health education, professional health educators started a process many years ago that resulted in the certification of health educators. This certification attests to the educational preparation of and the health education skills acquired by competent health educators, regardless of the health education setting in which they apply these skills.

The Certified Health Education Specialist

The *National Task Force on the Professional Preparation and Practice of Health Education* was charged with identifying the roles common (generic) to health education and to verify those roles with practicing health educators. Once these roles were identified, it was necessary to specify what competencies health educators would need to fulfill these roles. In 1985 the *National Task Force on the Professional Preparation and Practice of Health Education* announced these competencies in a publication entitled "A Framework for the Development of Competency-Based Curricula for Entry-Level Health Educators." In 1997 competencies for graduate-level health educators were published. At that time it became possible to distinguish between entry-level health educators and those with higher-level health education competencies. These competencies appear in their entirety in Table 2.1.

The National Task Force on the Professional Preparation and Practice of Health Education evolved into the *National Commission for Health Education Credentialing,* which now tests graduates of health education professional preparation programs and declares them qualified to conduct health education. Those certified are given the title of "Certified Health Education Specialist" (CHES), which many use after their names and degrees to let others know they have been certified as competent. For example, I might have a business card that lists my name as Jerrold S. Greenberg, B.S., M.S., Ed. D., CHES or Jerrold S. Greenberg, ED.D., CHES. If you are interested in learning more about becoming certified as a health educator, or if you are interested in applying for certification, contact the National Commission for Health Education Credentialing at 944 Marcon Boulevard, Suite 310, Allentown, PA 18103; or telephone the commission at (888) 673-5445.

Health Educator Competencies

The responsibilities required of health educators refer to their being able to

    I. Assess individual and community needs for health education.
   II. Plan effective health education programs.
  III. Implement health education programs.
  IV. Evaluate the effectiveness of health education programs.
   V. Coordinate provision of health education services.
  VI. Act as a resource person in health education.
 VII. Communicate health and health education needs, concerns, and resources.
VIII. Apply appropriate research principles and methods in health education.
  IX. Administer health education programs.
   X. Advance the profession of health education.

TABLE 2.1
Responsibilities and Competencies for Entry-Level and Graduate-Level Health Educators*

(Graduate-level responsibilities and competencies are printed in uppercase and italicized.)

RESPONSIBILITY I—ASSESSING INDIVIDUAL AND COMMUNITY NEEDS FOR HEALTH EDUCATION

Competency A: Obtain health-related data about social and cultural environments, growth, and development factors, needs, and interests.

Subcompetencies:

1. Select valid sources of information about health needs and interests.
2. Utilize computerized sources of health-related information.
3. Employ or develop appropriate data-gathering instruments.
4. Apply survey techniques to acquire health data.
5. *CONDUCT HEALTH-RELATED NEEDS ASSESSMENT IN COMMUNITIES.*

Competency B: Distinguish between behaviors that foster, and those that hinder well-being.

Subcompetencies:

1. Investigate physical, social, emotional, and intellectual factors influencing health behaviors.
2. Identify behaviors that tend to promote or compromise health.
3. Recognize the role of learning and affective experience in shaping patterns of health behavior.
4. *ANALYZE SOCIAL, CULTURAL, ECONOMIC, AND POLITICAL FACTORS THAT INFLUENCE HEALTH.*

Competency C: Infer needs for health education on the basis of obtained data.

Subcompetencies:

1. Analyze needs assessment data.
2. Determine priority areas of need for health education.

COMPETENCY D: DETERMINE FACTORS THAT INFLUENCE LEARNING AND DEVELOPMENT.

Subcompetencies:

1. *ASSESS INDIVIDUAL LEARNING STYLES.*
2. *ASSESS INDIVIDUAL LITERACY.*
3. *ASSESS THE LEARNING ENVIRONMENT.*

Competency A: Recruit community organizations, resource people, and potential participants for support and assistance in program planning.

Subcompetencies:

1. Communicate need for the program to those who will be involved.
2. Obtain commitments from personnel and decision makers who will be involved in the program.
3. Seek ideas and opinions of those who will affect or be affected by the program.
4. Incorporate feasible ideas and recommendations into the planning process.
5. *APPLY PRINCIPLES OF COMMUNITY ORGANIZATION IN PLANNING PROGRAMS.*

Competency B: Develop a logical scope and sequence plan for a health education program.

Subcompetencies:

1. Determine the range of health information requisite to a given program of instruction.
2. Organize the subject areas comprising the scope of a program in logical sequence.
3. *REVIEW PHILOSOPHICAL AND THEORY-BASED FOUNDATIONS IN PLANNING HEALTH EDUCATION PROGRAMS.*
4. *ANALYZE THE PROCESS FOR INTEGRATING HEALTH EDUCATION AS PART OF A BROADER HEALTH CARE OR EDUCATION PROGRAM.*
5. *DEVELOP A THEORY-BASED FRAMEWORK FOR HEALTH EDUCATION PROGRAMS.*

Competency C: Formulate appropriate and measurable program objectives.

Subcompetencies:

1. Infer educational objectives facilitative of achievement of specified competencies.
2. Develop a framework of broadly stated, operational objectives relevant to a proposed health education program.

Competency D: Design educational programs consistent with specified program objectives.

Subcompetencies:

1. Match proposed learning activities with those implicit in the stated objectives.
2. Formulate a wide variety of alternative educational methods.

(continued)

3. Select strategies best suited to implementation of educational objectives in a given setting.

4. Plan a sequence of learning opportunities building upon and reinforcing mastery of preceding objectives.

5. *SELECT APPROPRIATE THEORY-BASED STRATEGIES IN HEALTH PROGRAM PLANNING.*

6. *PLAN TRAINING AND INSTRUCTIONAL PROGRAMS FOR HEALTH PROFESSIONALS.*

COMPETENCY E: DEVELOP HEALTH EDUCATION PROGRAMS USING SOCIAL MARKETING PRINCIPLES.

Subcompetencies:

1. *IDENTIFY POPULATIONS FOR HEALTH EDUCATION PROGRAMS.*

2. *INVOLVE PARTICIPANTS IN PLANNING HEALTH EDUCATION PROGRAMS.*

3. *DESIGN A MARKETING PLAN TO PROMOTE HEALTH EDUCATION.*

RESPONSIBILITY III—IMPLEMENTING HEALTH EDUCATION PROGRAMS

Competency A: Exhibit competence in carrying out planned educational programs.

Subcompetencies:

1. Employ a wide range of educational methods and techniques.

2. Apply individual or group process methods as appropriate to given learning situations.

3. Utilize instructional equipment and other instructional media effectively.

4. Select methods that best facilitate practice of program objectives.

5. *ASSESS, SELECT, AND APPLY TECHNOLOGIES THAT WILL CONTRIBUTE TO PROGRAM OBJECTIVES.*

6. *DEVELOP, DEMONSTRATE, AND MODEL IMPLEMENTATION STRATEGIES.*

7. *DELIVER EDUCATIONAL PROGRAMS FOR HEALTH PROFESSIONALS.*

8. *USE COMMUNITY ORGANIZATION PRINCIPLES TO GUIDE AND FACILITATE COMMUNITY DEVELOPMENT.*

Competency B: Infer enabling objectives as needed to implement instructional programs in specified settings.

Subcompetencies:

1. Pretest learners to ascertain present abilities and knowledge relative to proposed program objectives.

2. Develop subordinate measurable objectives as needed for instruction.

Competency C: Select methods and media best suited to implement program plans for specific learners.

Subcompetencies:

1. Analyze learner characteristics, legal aspects, feasibility, and other considerations influencing choices among methods.

2. Evaluate the efficacy of alternative methods and techniques capable of facilitating program objectives.

3. Determine the availability of information, personnel, time, and equipment needed to implement the program for a given audience.

4. *CRITICALLY ANALYZE TECHNOLOGIES, METHODS, AND MEDIA FOR THEIR ACCEPTABILITY TO DIVERSE GROUPS.*

5. *APPLY THEORETICAL AND CONCEPTUAL MODELS FROM HEALTH EDUCATION AND RELATED DISCIPLINES TO IMPROVE PROGRAM DELIVERY.*

Competency D: Monitor educational programs and adjust objectives and activities as necessary.

Subcompetencies:

1. Compare actual program activities with the stated objectives.

2. Assess the relevance of existing program objectives to current needs.

3. Revise program activities and objectives as necessitated by changes in learner needs.

4. Appraise applicability of resources and materials relative to given educational objectives.

RESPONSIBILITY IV—EVALUATING EFFECTIVENESS OF HEALTH EDUCATION PROGRAMS

Competency A: Develop plans to assess achievement of program objectives.

Subcompetencies:

1. Determine standards of performance to be applied as criteria of effectiveness.

2. Establish a realistic scope of evaluation efforts.

3. Develop an inventory of existing valid and reliable tests and survey instruments.

4. Select appropriate methods for evaluating program effectiveness.

5. *IDENTIFY EXISTING SOURCES OF HEALTH-RELATED DATABASES.*

6. *EVALUATE EXISTING DATA-GATHERING INSTRUMENTS AND PROCESSES.*

7. *SELECT APPROPRIATE QUALITATIVE AND/OR QUANTITATIVE EVALUATION DESIGN.*

8. *DEVELOP VALID AND RELIABLE EVALUATION INSTRUMENTS.*

(continued)

Competency B: Carry out evaluation plans.

Subcompetencies:

1. Facilitate administration of the tests and activities specified in the plan.

2. Utilize data-collecting methods appropriate to the objectives.

3. Analyze resulting evaluation data.

4. *IMPLEMENT APPROPRIATE QUALITATIVE AND QUANTITATIVE EVALUATION TECHNIQUES.*

5. *APPLY EVALUATION TECHNOLOGY AS APPROPRIATE.*

Competency C: Interpret results of program evaluation.

Subcompetencies:

1. Apply criteria of effectiveness to obtained results of a program.

2. Translate evaluation results into terms easily understood by others.

3. Report effectiveness of educational programs in achieving proposed objectives.

4. *IMPLEMENT STRATEGIES TO ANALYZE DATA FROM EVALUATION ASSESSMENTS.*

5. *COMPARE EVALUATION RESULTS TO OTHER FINDINGS.*

6. *MAKE RECOMMENDATIONS FROM EVALUATION RESULTS.*

Competency D: Infer implications from findings for future program planning.

Subcompetencies:

1. Explore possible explanations for important evaluation findings.

2. Recommend strategies for implementing results of evaluation.

3. *APPLY FINDINGS TO REFINE AND MAINTAIN PROGRAMS.*

4. *USE EVALUATION FINDINGS IN POLICY ANALYSIS AND DEVELOPMENT.*

RESPONSIBILITY V—COORDINATING PROVISION OF HEALTH EDUCATION SERVICES

Competency A: Develop a plan for coordinating health education services.

Subcompetencies:

1. Determine the extent of available health education services.

2. Match health education services to proposed program activities.

3. Identify gaps and overlaps in the provision of collaborative health services.

Competency B: Facilitate cooperation between and among levels of program personnel.

Subcompetencies:

1. Promote cooperation and feedback among personnel related to the program.
2. Apply various methods of conflict reduction as needed.
3. Analyze the role of health educator as liaison between program staff and outside groups and organizations.

Competency C: Formulate practical modes of collaboration among health agencies and organizations.

Subcompetencies:

1. Stimulate development of cooperation among personnel responsible for community health education programs.
2. Suggest approaches for integrating health education within existing health programs.
3. Develop plans for promoting collaborative efforts among health agencies and organizations with mutual interests.
4. *ORGANIZE AND FACILITATE GROUPS, COALITIONS, AND PARTNERSHIPS.*

Competency D: Organize in-service training programs for teachers, volunteers, and other interested personnel.

Subcompetencies:

1. Plan an operational, competency-oriented training program.
2. Utilize instructional resources that meet a variety of in-service training needs.
3. Develop plans for promoting collaborative efforts among health agencies and organizations with mutual interests.
4. *FACILITATE COLLABORATIVE TRAINING EFFORTS AMONG HEALTH AGENCIES AND ORGANIZATIONS.*

RESPONSIBILITY VI—ACTING AS A RESOURCE PERSON IN HEALTH EDUCATION

Competency A: Utilize computerized health information retrieval systems effectively.

Subcompetencies:

1. Match an information need with the appropriate retrieval system.
2. Access principal online and other database health information resources.
3. *SELECT A DATA SYSTEM COMMENSURATE WITH PROGRAM NEEDS.*

(continued)

4. *DETERMINE RELEVANCE OF VARIOUS COMPUTERIZED HEALTH INFORMATION RESOURCES.*

5. *ASSIST IN ESTABLISHING AND MONITORING POLICIES FOR USE OF DATA-GATHERING PRACTICES.*

Competency B: Establish effective consultative relationships with those requesting assistance in solving health-related problems.

Subcompetencies:

1. Analyze parameters of effective consultative relationships.
2. Describe special skills and abilities needed by health educators for consultation activities.
3. Formulate a plan for providing consultation to other health professionals.
4. Explain the process of marketing health education consultative services.
5. *APPLY NETWORKING SKILLS TO DEVELOP AND MAINTAIN CONSULTATIVE RELATIONSHIPS.*

Competency C: Interpret and respond to requests for health information.

Subcompetencies:

1. Analyze general processes for identifying the information needed to satisfy a request.
2. Employ a wide range of approaches in referring requesters to valid resources of health information.

Competency D: Select effective educational resource materials for dissemination.

Subcompetencies:

1. Assemble educational material of value to the health of individuals and community groups.
2. Evaluate the worth and applicability of resource materials for given audiences.
3. Apply various processes in the acquisition of resource materials.
4. Compare different methods for distributing educational materials.
5. *APPLY COMMUNICATION THEORY AND PRINCIPLES IN THE DEVELOPMENT OF HEALTH EDUCATION MATERIALS.*

RESPONSIBILITY VII—COMMUNICATING HEALTH AND HEALTH EDUCATION NEEDS, CONCERNS, AND RESOURCES

Competency A: Interpret concepts, purposes, and theories of health education.

Subcompetencies:

1. Evaluate the state of the art of health education.
2. Analyze the foundations of the discipline of health education.
3. Describe major responsibilities of the health educator in the practice of health education.
4. *ARTICULATE THE HISTORICAL AND PHILOSOPHICAL BASES OF HEALTH EDUCATION.*

Competency B: Predict the impact of societal value systems on health education programs.

Subcompetencies:

1. Investigate social forces causing opposing viewpoints regarding health education needs and concerns.
2. Employ a wide range of strategies for dealing with controversial health issues.
3. *ANALYZE SOCIAL, CULTURAL, DEMOGRAPHIC, AND POLITICAL FACTORS THAT INFLUENCE DECISION MAKERS.*
4. *PREDICT FUTURE HEALTH EDUCATION NEEDS BASED UPON SOCIETAL CHANGES.*
5. *RESPOND TO CHALLENGES TO HEALTH EDUCATION PROGRAMS.*

Competency C: Select a variety of communication methods and techniques in providing health information.

Subcompetencies:

1. Utilize a wide range of techniques for communicating health and health education information.
2. Demonstrate proficiency in communicating health information and health education needs.
3. *DEMONSTRATE BOTH PROFICIENCY AND ACCURACY IN ORAL AND WRITTEN PRESENTATIONS.*
4. *USE CULTURALLY SENSITIVE COMMUNICATION METHODS AND TECHNIQUES.*

Competency D: Foster communication between health care providers and consumers.

Subcompetencies:

1. Interpret the significance and implications of health care providers' messages to consumers.
2. Act as liaison between consumer groups and individuals and health care provider organizations.

(continued)

RESPONSIBILITY VIII—APPLY APPROPRIATE RESEARCH PRINCIPLES AND METHODS IN HEALTH EDUCATION

COMPETENCY A: CONDUCT THOROUGH REVIEWS OF LITERATURE.

Subcompetencies:

1. *EMPLOY ELECTRONIC TECHNOLOGY FOR RETRIEVING REFERENCES.*
2. *ANALYZE REFERENCES TO IDENTIFY THOSE PERTINENT TO SELECTED HEALTH EDUCATION ISSUES OR PROGRAMS.*
3. *SELECT AND CRITIQUE SOURCES OF HEALTH INFORMATION.*
4. *EVALUATE THE RESEARCH DESIGN, METHODOLOGY, AND FINDINGS FROM THE LITERATURE.*
5. *SYNTHESIZE KEY INFORMATION FROM THE LITERATURE.*

COMPETENCY B: USE APPROPRIATE QUALITATIVE AND QUANTITATIVE RESEARCH METHODS.

Subcompetencies:

1. *ASSESS THE MERITS AND LIMITATIONS OF QUALITATIVE AND QUANTITATIVE RESEARCH METHODS.*
2. *APPLY QUALITATIVE AND/OR QUANTITATIVE RESEARCH METHODS IN RESEARCH DESIGNS.*

COMPETENCY C: APPLY RESEARCH TO HEALTH EDUCATION PRACTICE.

Subcompetencies:

1. *USE APPROPRIATE RESEARCH METHODS AND DESIGNS IN ASSESSING NEEDS.*
2. *USE INFORMATION DERIVED FROM RESEARCH FOR PROGRAM PLANNING.*
3. *SELECT IMPLEMENTATION STRATEGIES BASED UPON RESEARCH RESULTS.*
4. *EMPLOY RESEARCH DESIGN, METHODS, AND ANALYSIS IN PROGRAM EVALUATION.*
5. *DESCRIBE HOW RESEARCH RESULTS INFORM HEALTH POLICY DEVELOPMENT.*
6. *USE RESEARCH RESULTS TO INFORM HEALTH POLICY DEVELOPMENT.*
7. *USE PROTOCOL FOR DISSEMINATION OF RESEARCH FINDINGS.*

RESPONSIBILITY IX: ADMINISTERING HEALTH EDUCATION PROGRAMS

COMPETENCY A: DEVELOP AND MANAGE FISCAL RESOURCES.

Subcompetencies:

1. *PREPARE PROPOSALS TO OBTAIN FISCAL RESOURCES THROUGH GRANTS, CONTRACTS, AND OTHER INTERNAL AND EXTERNAL SOURCES.*

2. *DEVELOP AND MANAGE REALISTIC BUDGETS TO SUPPORT PROGRAM REQUIREMENTS.*

COMPETENCY B: DEVELOP AND MANAGE HUMAN RESOURCES.

Subcompetencies:

1. *ASSESS AND COMMUNICATE QUALIFICATIONS OF PERSONNEL NEEDED FOR PROGRAMS.*
2. *RECRUIT, EMPLOY, AND EVALUATE STAFF MEMBERS.*
3. *PROVIDE STAFF DEVELOPMENT.*
4. *DEMONSTRATE LEADERSHIP IN MANAGING HUMAN RESOURCES.*
5. *APPLY HUMAN RESOURCE POLICIES CONSISTENT WITH RELEVANT LAWS AND REGULATIONS.*

COMPETENCY C: EXERCISE ORGANIZATION LEADERSHIP.

Subcompetencies:

1. *ANALYZE THE ORGANIZATION'S CULTURE IN RELATIONSHIP TO PROGRAM GOALS.*
2. *ASSESS THE POLITICAL CLIMATE OF THE ORGANIZATION, COMMUNITY, STATE, AND NATION REGARDING CONDITIONS THAT ADVANCE OR INHIBIT THE GOALS OF THE PROGRAM.*
3. *CONDUCT LONG-RANGE AND STRATEGIC PLANNING.*
4. *DEVELOP STRATEGIES TO REINFORCE OR CHANGE ORGANIZATIONAL CULTURE TO ACHIEVE PROGRAM GOALS.*
5. *DEVELOP STRATEGIES TO INFLUENCE PUBLIC POLICY.*

COMPETENCY D: OBTAIN ACCEPTANCE AND SUPPORT FOR PROGRAMS.

Subcompetencies:

1. *APPLY SOCIAL MARKETING PRINCIPLES AND TECHNIQUES TO ACHIEVE PROGRAM GOALS.*
2. *EMPLOY CONCEPTS AND THEORIES OF PUBLIC RELATIONS AND COMMUNICATIONS TO OBTAIN PROGRAM SUPPORT.*
3. *INCORPORATE DEMOGRAPHICALLY AND CULTURALLY SENSITIVE TECHNIQUES TO PROMOTE PROGRAMS.*
4. *USE NEEDS ASSESSMENT INFORMATION TO ADVOCATE FOR HEALTH EDUCATION PROGRAMS.*

(continued)

TABLE 2.1   *(continued)*
Responsibilities and Competencies for Entry-Level and Graduate-Level Health Educators*

RESPONSIBILITY X: ADVANCING THE PROFESSION OF HEALTH EDUCATION.

COMPETENCY A: PROVIDE A CRITICAL ANALYSIS OF CURRENT AND FUTURE NEEDS IN HEALTH EDUCATION.

Subcompetencies:

1. *RELATE HEALTH EDUCATION ISSUES TO LARGER SOCIAL ISSUES.*
2. *ARTICULATE HEALTH EDUCATION'S ROLE IN POLICY FORMATION AT VARIOUS ORGANIZATIONAL AND COMMUNITY LEVELS.*

COMPETENCY B: ASSUME RESPONSIBILITY FOR ADVANCING THE PROFESSION.

Subcompetencies:

1. *ANALYZE THE ROLE OF THE HEALTH EDUCATION ASSOCIATIONS IN ADVANCING THE PROFESSION.*
2. *PARTICIPATE IN PROFESSIONAL ORGANIZATIONS.*
3. *DEVELOP A PERSONAL PLAN FOR PROFESSIONAL GROWTH.*

COMPETENCY C: APPLY ETHICAL PRINCIPLES AS THEY RELATE TO THE PRACTICE OF HEALTH EDUCATION.

Subcompetencies:

1. *ANALYZE THE INTERRELATIONSHIPS AMONG ETHICS, VALUES, AND BEHAVIOR.*
2. *RELATE THE IMPORTANCE OF A CODE OF ETHICS TO PROFESSIONAL PRACTICE.*
3. *SUBSCRIBE TO A PROFESSIONALLY RECOGNIZED HEALTH EDUCATION CODE OF ETHICS.*

---

*From the National Task Force on the Preparation and Practice of Health Educators. *A Framework for the Development of Competency-Based Curricula for Entry-Level Health Educators.* New York: National Task Force on the Preparation and Practice of Health Educators, 1985. Reprinted by permission of the National Commission for Health Education Credentialing, Inc. Also from "Standards for the Preparation of Graduate Level Health Educators," *Journal of Health Education* 28 (1997): 69–73.

Years ago it was the country doctor that dispensed health education, along with medications and treatments. Today a professional cadre of health educators has formed, with competencies designed to increase the effectiveness of health education.

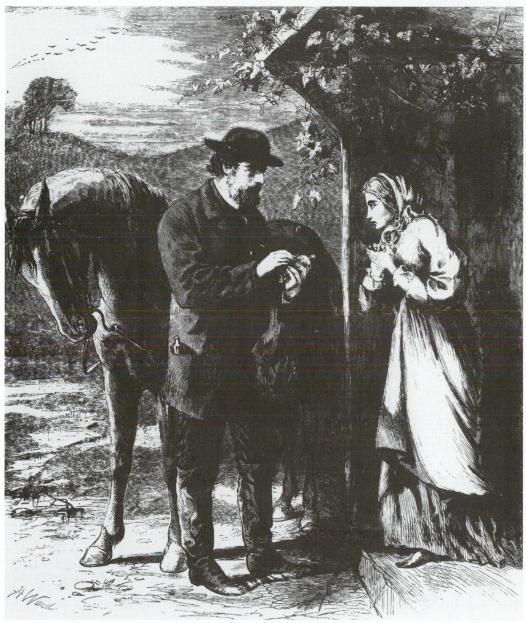

Source: The Library of Congress

The first seven areas of responsibility are common to all health educators. The latter three areas are specific to graduate-level health educators and were added in 1997 (Standards for the Preparation of Graduate Level Health Educators 1997).

For each *responsibility* cited by the National Task Force, *competencies* and *subcompetencies* necessary to meet that responsibility were listed. For example, under the responsibility of "Planning effective health education programs" is the competency "Formulate appropriate and measurable program objectives." And one subcompetency under "Formulate appropriate and measurable program objectives" is to be able to "Develop a framework of broadly stated operational objectives relevant to a proposed health education program."

Health Educator Competencies and This Book

Several areas of responsibility and competencies employed in the health education certification process are not specifically related to this book, whereas others are. For example, we are less concerned here with evaluation of health education than with its implementation. The competency "Exhibit competence in carrying out planned educational programs" and its subcompetency, "Employ a wide range of educational methods and techniques," are directly addressed in this book. Evaluation of health education programs is a different, though related, topic about which other books have been written.

The competencies and subcompetencies to which this book is directed are discussed next.

Responsibility I, Competency B: Distinguish between behaviors that foster, and those that hinder, well-being.

Subcompetency 1: Investigate physical, social, emotional, and intellectual factors influencing health behaviors. This competency is addressed in several chapters. For example, Chapters 6 and 7 present instructional strategies related to social (group process) and emotional (values) factors. Chapter 14 concerns itself with physical health factors.

Subcompetency 3: Recognize the role of learning and affective experience in shaping patterns of behavior. This material is discussed throughout much of this book since affective experience is described as vital for meaningful learning to occur. Particularly, affective instructional strategies are presented in Chapters 5, 6, 7, and 8.

Responsibility II, Competency C: Formulate appropriate and measurable program objectives.

Subcompetency 1: Infer educational objectives facilitative of achievement of specified competencies.

Subcompetency 2: Develop a framework of broadly stated, operational objectives relevant to a proposed health education program.

Both of these subcompetencies are specifically addressed in Chapter 5, as well as being discussed in Chapters 1 and 3.

Responsibility II, Competency D: Design educational programs consistent with specified program objectives.

Subcompetency 1: Match proposed learning activities with those implicit in the stated objectives.

Subcompetency 2: Formulate a wide variety of alternative educational methods.

Subcompetency 3: Select strategies best suited to implementation of educational objectives in a given setting.

These objectives are the major focus of this book. Within various chapters, alternative instructional strategies are presented to help meet specified educational objectives. In particular, these strategies are presented in Chapters 6 through 14.

Responsibility III, Competency A: Exhibit competence in carrying out planned educational programs.

Subcompetency 1: Employ a wide range of educational methods and techniques. This competency is discussed throughout this book as various instructional strategies and methods are presented.

Subcompetency 2: Apply individual or group process methods appropriate to given learning situations. Chapter 5 is devoted to the development of group process skills.

Subcompetency 2: Select methods that best facilitate practice of program objectives. This competency is addressed in various chapters. More specifically, Chapters 6 through 14 present methods appropriate to various health content.

Responsibility III, Competency C: Select methods and media best suited to implement program plans for specific learners.

Subcompetency 1: Evaluate the efficacy of alternative methods and techniques capable of facilitating program objectives. This competency is discussed throughout this book as numerous alternative methods and instructional strategies are presented.

Responsibility III, Competency D: Monitor educational programs, adjusting objectives and activities as necessary.

Subcompetency 1: Compare actual program activities with the stated objectives.

Subcompetency 2: Assess the relevance of existing program objectives to current needs.

Subcompetency 3: Revise program activities and objectives as necessitated by changes in learner needs.

These competencies are considered in the discussion in Chapter 5 regarding educational objectives, and throughout the text when instructional strategies are associated with specific instructional objectives.

Responsibility V, Competency A: Develop a plan for coordinating health education services.

Subcompetency 1: Match health education services to proposed program activities.

Responsibility V, Competency B: Facilitate cooperation between and among levels of program personnel.

Subcompetency 1: Promote cooperation and feedback among personnel related to the program.

Responsibility V, Competency C: Formulate practical modes of collaboration among health agencies and organizations.

Subcompetency 1: Stimulate development of cooperation among personnel responsible for community health education programs.

Subcompetency 2: Suggest approaches for integrating health education within existing health programs.

Subcompetency 3: Develop plans for promoting collaborative efforts among health agencies and organizations with mutual interests.

Responsibility V, Competencies A, B, and C, are incorporated throughout this text. For example, cooperation between the organization's nutritionists and health educators is recommended when nutrition education is discussed in Chapter 12; involvement of community organizations and personnel is encouraged when instructional strategies pertaining to aging and death education are presented in Chapter 13; and Chapter 14 describes how physical education/fitness experts and medical personnel (physicians, nurses) can be employed in health education for personal health. In addition, Chapter 6 presents numerous methods of cooperating, communicating, and resolving conflict among group members.

Responsibility V, Competency D: Organize in-service training programs for teachers, volunteers, and other interested personnel.

Subcompetency 2: Utilize instructional resources that meet a variety of in-service training needs.

Subcompetency 3: Demonstrate a wide range of strategies for conducting in-service training programs.

The instructional strategies presented in Chapters 6 through 14 can be adapted to in-service training programs. They can be used to teach health *content* (about safety, nutrition, drugs, sexuality, and so on) to those being trained during in-service training programs, or to teach various methodologies (the *process* of health education).

Responsibility VII, Competency A: Interpret concepts, purposes, and theories of health education.

Subcompetency 1: Evaluate the state of the art of health education.

Subcompetency 2: Analyze the foundation of the discipline of health education.

Subcompetency 3: Describe major responsibilities of the health educator in the practice of health education.

These competencies are discussed in detail in Chapters 1, 3, and 5. These chapters present an introduction to health education; define certain terminology; present several theories associated with health and health education; discuss the settings in which health education occurs and the advantages and disadvantages of each of those settings; and consider the major ethical issues in the practice of health education.

Responsibility VII, Competency B: Predict the impact of societal value systems on health education programs.

Subcompetency 2: Employ a wide range of strategies for dealing with controversial health issues.

Values are discussed in detail in Chapter 7, and instructional strategies are presented in various sections of this book concerned with controversial health issues. For example, ethical issues are discussed in Chapter 3, sexuality issues (such as abortion and homosexuality) are discussed in Chapter 10, and death and dying issues (such as euthanasia) are discussed in Chapter 13.

Certified Health Education Specialists must acquire sufficient course work in health education at colleges and universities in order to be eligible to take the certification examination.

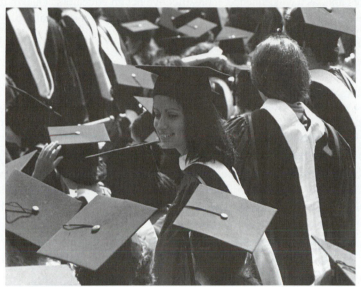

Source: Sanford Weinstein

Responsibility VII, Competency C: Select a variety of communication methods and techniques in providing health information.

Subcompetency 1: Utilize a wide range of techniques for communicating health and health education information.

Subcompetency 2: Demonstrate a proficiency in communicating health information and health education needs.

Responsibility VII, Competency D: Foster communication between health care providers and consumers.

Subcompetency 1: Interpret the significance and implications of health care providers' messages to consumers.

Subcompetency 2: Act as a liaison between consumer groups and individuals and health care provider organizations.

The numerous instructional methods and strategies presented throughout this book can be adapted to communicate health and health education information to various constituencies (students, the public, administrators, and other decision makers). In this way, health educators will be prepared with Responsibility VII, Competencies C and D.

In Conclusion

It is expected that health education certification will result in better professional preparation programs for health educators and, as a consequence, more effective health educators. This, in turn, should translate into a more health-informed and conscious public that behaves in more healthful ways and becomes healthier.

Summary

1. Just because someone is either popular or a celebrity does not mean that person is an expert on health issues. To prevent harm that might result from misinformation being conveyed by unqualified celebrities and others seeking to make a "quick buck," the National Task Force on the Professional Preparation and Practice of Health Education was formed.

2. The National Task Force on the Professional Preparation and Practice of Health Education evolved into the National Commission for Health Education Credentialing, which now tests graduates of health education professional preparation programs and declares them qualified to conduct health education.

3. The Certified Health Education Specialist (CHES) graduates from college with sufficient coursework qualifying him or her to take a competency test in health education. Upon passing that test, that person is a certified health educator.

4. A CHES is able to meet the following responsibilities: assess individual and community needs for health education; plan effective health education programs; implement health education programs; evaluate the effectiveness of health education programs; coordinate provisions for health education services; act as a resource person in health education; and communicate health and health education needs, concerns, and resources. In addition, graduate-level responsibilities have been added to the original set of entry-level responsibilities. These additional areas of responsibility specify that, in addition to the entry-level areas of responsibility, graduate-level health educators are able to apply appropriate research principles and methods in health education, administer health education programs, and advance the profession of health education.

5. For each responsibility health educators are expected to meet, the National Task Force lists competencies and subcompetencies required to meet these responsibilities. These competencies and subcompetencies are assessed on the test for certification in health education.

CHAPTER THREE

A New Form for Health Education

At the start of a new school year, a principal sent the following notice around to all of his teachers:

Dear Teacher:
    I am a survivor of a concentration camp. My eyes saw what no man should witness:
        Gas chambers built by learned engineers. Children poisoned by educated physicians. Infants killed by trained nurses. Women and babies shot and burned by high school and college graduates.
    So, I am suspicious of education.
    My request is: Help your students become human. Your efforts must never produce learned monsters, skilled psychopaths, educated Eichmanns. Reading, writing, arithmetic are important only if they serve to make our children more humane.

The principal's concern relates to all educational disciplines, including health education, which has the potential to be undemocratic, authoritative, unethical, and, what's more, ineffective. I draw this conclusion after many years spent as a health educator, a profession I value immensely. It is because of my affinity for a profession I have decided to devote my life to that I feel an obligation to be constructively critical, to help that profession become even more responsive to the needs of the people it educates. I will elaborate on some of these potential problems in this chapter after I present the rationale for health education. An understanding of this rationale is important because any criticism of or decision regarding appropriate professional practice in health education must relate to this rationale in order to be responsible.

The Rationale for Health Education

Health education has been used by various segments of society for various purposes—for example, in public service campaigns by the federal government or by schools to respond to the concern for unintended pregnancies. Consequently, many rationales have been offered for instituting health education programs. Some of these rationales are discussed here.

The Current Emphasis on Health Education

Health education has recently been receiving a great deal of emphasis. The primary impetus behind this emphasis relates to two situations: the escalating cost of health care and the spread of HIV. In addition, the disclosure of drug abuse by athletes, the concern for increasing teen suicide and pregnancy rates, and the degree to which people have taken an interest in physical fitness have contributed to this interest in health education.

The Cost of Health Care   The cost of health care in the United States has been increasing at alarming rates. Many people fear that either much of the population will not be able to afford or obtain health care when they need it, or the tax rate will have to be significantly increased so the federal government can provide funds for this health care. This dilemma has existed for some time, and many solutions have been debated. One solution offered is a system of national health insurance that will cover major health care expenses (termed *catastrophic* health insurance coverage). Another solution is to place a lid on the rate of increase in the cost of health care by grouping certain medical conditions together (called Diagnostic Related Groups or DRGs), identifying potential treatments for these conditions and a reasonable cost of those treatments, and then reimbursing health care providers for only that set fee. The reasoning is that since hospitals and physicians can make more money by treating people expeditiously and by holding down the cost of treatment—for example, by discharging patients from the hospital earlier and by being more selective in recommending diagnostic procedures such as Xrays—they will be more efficient and more cost conscious in their medical decisions. Health maintenance organizations (HMOs) and other managed care plans have been growing by leaps and bounds based on a rationale similar to the adoption of DRGs. Since these plans are prepayment plans—that is, the subscriber pays an annual health insurance fee that covers all but a small amount of his or her care—it is in the interest of managed care plans to limit the use of medical services. Consequently, preventing illness and disease becomes a priority. Others are concerned that the quality of health care will suffer from the interference of containment measures and their inability to respond flexibly to economic and humanistic issues. Another solution suggested for the escalating cost of health care is to help people prevent conditions needing care—that is, provide them with health education so they understand the consequences of their behavior and obtain the knowledge and skills necessary to behave more healthfully. The implications and ramifications of this suggestion are discussed in this chapter.

AIDS   A second societal concern that has led to an increased emphasis on health education is the fear of the spread of human immunodeficiency virus (HIV). We now know that HIV is spread among any population that engages in high-risk behavior. HIV is contracted by newborns if their mothers are HIV-positive. Heterosexuals engaging in high-risk behaviors with HIV-positive sexual partners can contract the virus. Approximately 25 percent of HIV in the United States is first contracted during the teenage years, and the fastest-growing segment of new HIV cases is among women. HIV was thought to inevitably result in acquired immune deficiency syndrome (AIDS), which would lead to death within a few years. That fear of contracting a lethal disease, one without a cure, was enough to mobilize various segments of our society into action. As a result, private foundations, voluntary agencies, and the federal and state governments either engaged in sexuality education campaigns or funded such campaigns. The thinking was that because HIV/AIDS could not be treated, the best approach would be to educate people to avoid high-risk behaviors (such as coitus or anal sexual intercourse without a condom). Today medications appear to have delayed, or in some people, prevented HIV from developing into AIDS. The result is that for some people, HIV infection is considered a chronic disease that can be managed for years without the symptoms of AIDS. Health educators have benefited from this concern with HIV/AIDS by receiving many of the funds that have been directed toward HIV/AIDS education.

Objectives for the Nation

Several years before the federal government became anxious about HIV/AIDS, its commitment to and regard for health education was made evident by the development of health goals for the nation (U.S.

Department of Health and Human Services, *Healthy People,* 1979). Here are some examples of these goals:

1. For infants, a 25 percent lower death rate, from 14.1 deaths per 1,000 in 1977 to fewer than 9 per 1,000 in 1990.

2. For children ages 1–14, a 20 percent lower death rate; that is, a death rate of 34 deaths per 100,000 by 1990 (the 1977 death rate for this age group was 43 per 100,000).

3. For adolescents and young adults aged 15–24, a 20 percent lower death rate, from 117 per 100,000 in 1977 to fewer than 93 per 100,000 in 1990.

4. For adults aged 25–64, a 25 percent lower death rate, from 540 per 100,000 in 1977 to fewer than 400 per 100,000 in 1990.

5. For adults aged 65 and over, a 20 percent reduction in days of restricted activity, to fewer than 30 such days a year.

These goals were converted into specific health objectives in 1981 (U.S. Department of Health and Human Services, *Promoting Health/Preventing Disease,* 1981). The government then committed itself to achieving these objectives in 10 years via a coordinated nationwide approach to health promotion and disease prevention. Health educators were a key professional group involved in this effort. For example, school health educators were viewed as necessary to help Americans develop healthy attitudes and adopt healthful behaviors early in their lives so they would pursue healthful lifestyles as adults. Occupational health educators were considered a necessary ingredient in encouraging healthy workers to remain healthy by eliminating unhealthful behaviors (for example, cigarette smoking) and by adopting healthful behaviors (for example, exercising regularly). Health educators in health care settings were viewed as important in disease prevention by providing services both to prevent illness and disease (for example, immunizations) and to help prevent illnesses and diseases from becoming worse (for example, early diagnosis). Community health educators were encouraged to provide widespread health education to members in their locales about healthful lifestyles and the early detection of illness or disease and did so through some innovative media campaigns and other health education activities.

Many of the national health objectives were achieved by 1990; many were not. However, the coordination among health professionals was considered so positive, the nationally focused effort toward better health so valuable, and the commitment so impressive that objectives have been developed for the year 2000. In 1987 a steering committee was formed in the U.S. Public Health Service to oversee the process of developing these national health objectives. Hearings were held around the country in which health professionals from various settings—medical care, community health departments, schools, work sites—testified regarding what the health priorities ought to be. In September 1989 a draft of the Year 2000 National Health Objectives was published for comment by other health experts (U.S. Department of Health and Human Services, *Promoting Health/Preventing Disease,* 1989). One year later, in September 1990, the Year 2000 National Health Objectives were released (U.S. Department of Health and Human Services, *Healthy People 2000: National Health Promotion and Disease Prevention Objectives,* 1990).

A third set of national health objectives has been developed with a significant shift in emphasis (U.S. Department of Health and Human Services 2000). Year 2010 national health objectives have two goals, one of which is not unexpected: to increase quality and years of healthy life. The shift here is related to quality of life rather than length of life. An even more dramatic shift in emphasis is expressed by the second goal: to eliminate health disparities. Previous health objectives recognized the differences in health status between diverse populations and sought to diminish these gaps. However, Year 2010 national health objectives seek to eliminate these gaps altogether. To encourage the achievement of these goals, Healthy People 2010 was organized around 467 objectives in 28 focus areas. Table 3.1 lists these 28 focus areas.

TABLE 3.1
Healthy People 2010 Focus Areas

1. Access to quality health services
2. Arthritis, osteoporosis, and chronic back conditions
3. Cancer
4. Chronic kidney disease
5. Diabetes
6. Disability and secondary conditions
7. Educational and community-based programs
8. Environmental health
9. Family planning
10. Food safety
11. Health communication
12. Heart disease and stroke
13. HIV
14. Immunization and infectious diseases
15. Injury and violence prevention
16. Maternal, infant, and child health
17. Medical product safety
18. Mental health and mental disorders
19. Nutrition and overweight
20. Occupational safety and health
21. Oral health
22. Physical activity and fitness
23. Public health infrastructure
24. Respiratory diseases
25. Sexually transmitted diseases
26. Substance abuse
27. Tobacco use
28. Vision and hearing

Social Responsibility

One rationale given for health education is that social agents have a responsibility to provide people — in whatever setting — with the information they need to make healthful decisions. To do otherwise, some would argue, would be to act immorally. When children are allowed to grow and develop devoid of health education and later behave in ways that are unhealthful and contrary to their best interests, their society has failed them. When workers are exposed to unsafe practices because they are not instructed about the safe way to perform their work, the company is irresponsible — and legally liable. Successful lawsuits have been brought against companies that create stress for their employees but do not teach them how best to manage this stress (Ivancevich et al. 1985). If community diseases such as influenza pose a threat and the public is not educated regarding ways in which they can protect themselves, community health departments are derelict. When medical practitioners do not educate those with whom they come into contact about their unhealthful behaviors — even if the contact is precipitated by some unrelated condition — they have missed a unique opportunity to best serve their community.

This demonstration of social responsibility — health education in schools, places of work, the community, and medical care settings — does not come without sacrifice. It is costly to provide professional personnel, adequate facilities, and the needed equipment to conduct effective health education. Tax dollars that might have gone elsewhere — for example, national defense — need to be designated for health education. Schools, businesses, communities, and medical facilities demonstrate how they value health by the amount of money, time, and effort they are willing to devote to health education. Of course, other factors come into play — for example, the tax base in the community, the size of the business, other community problems that need attention, or past experience with health education. However, it is hard to imagine a more important societal responsibility or a more important goal than the achievement and maintenance of health.

Cost Benefit

One of the more persuasive and yet more elusive rationales for health education is that it saves money in the long run. This is termed the *cost benefit* of health education. The argument goes that some money invested now to educate people about good health will pay dividends later in several ways. As stated by two leading health educators, "When cost–benefit ratios can be computed comparably for health education and alternative intervention or control mechanisms such as surgery, long-term medication, and hospitalization we will be compelled to budget accordingly" (Rubinson and Alles 1984, 206).

To really appreciate the potential of a cost–benefit analysis of health education, let's look more closely at worksite health promotion programs and their rationale. U.S. businesses pay billions of dollars in health insurance premiums per year, more than they pay their stockholders in dividends! Imagine how excited U.S. businesses would be to learn there is a program that can reduce the amount of illness their workers experience and, therefore, their use of company health insurance. As workers need health insurance less, the premiums paid by their employers are reduced, thereby saving these companies many thousands of dollars each year. These savings have actually occurred in some companies. For example, Mass Mutual reported that its blood pressure program saved the company $245,000 over three years; Campbell Soup Company reported a savings of $245,000 over a 10-year period as a result of its colon/rectal screening program; and, although not reporting actual dollar amounts, Kimberly-Clark Corporation reported a 43 percent reduction in absenteeism and a 70 percent reduction in accidents yearly as a result of its drug and alcohol abuse program (Cooper 1984).

In a review of the major studies that have elucidated health promotion's financial impact, Golaszewski (2001) found several benefits of health promotion worth citing. Golaszewski reports on a company that found for every day of the week that employees engaged in exercise, health care costs decreased from the median by 4.7 percent; and for every body mass index (BMI) increment as a result of poor diets, health care costs increased from the median by 1.9 percent. Another company found that stress cost $6.2 million, tobacco use $4.5 million, overweight $3.2 million, and other unhealthy practices cost millions more (Anderson et al. 2000). Given these financial benefits and cost savings in the worksite, it is not surprising that health education/promotion has been given greater emphasis and been more widely expanded in recent years. The federal government also recognizes the value of worksite health promotion programs. One of the Year 2010 national health objectives is to "increase the proportion of worksites that offer a comprehensive employee health promotion program to their employees" (U.S. Department of Health and Human Services 2000).

These cost benefits of health education programs are, in many instances, readily recognized. However, even when no such cost benefits are found, they likely exist anyhow. It stands to reason, for instance, that with reduced absenteeism more workers are available. This increased productivity has to be making money for the company. When fewer workers are operating under the influence of alcohol, their decisions are probably better, thereby saving the company money that would have been lost due to mistakes or miscalculations. With fewer workers out for extended illnesses—such as recovery from heart attacks—there will be less need to train backup workers to take over their functions. The problem here, though, is that these costs are not easily quantifiable; we can't put dollar amounts on them. Therefore, it is more difficult to make the case for the cost benefit of health education in these instances than in the others previously described. However, that does not mean the cost benefit does not exist.

Recruitment and Retention

The difficulty of defining the cost savings of health education is particularly evident when it comes to the recruitment and retention of workers in a business or of people living in a community. These benefits are real and contribute to the rationale for health education. For instance, how many competent workers have been attracted to work for IBM because of the fitness facilities available to its workers? How many workers have elected to stay at Johnson and Johnson because of its health promotion program, which helps them maintain their health by adjusting their lifestyle? How many people have chosen to remain living in their communities partly due to the availability of community health programs and services? The answers to these questions cannot be made with a great deal of confidence. Yet any reasonable person would assume there was some impact, at the very least, of these variables on recruitment and retention of employees. It is for these beneficial but intangible reasons that companies, schools, community health departments, and medical care facilities offer health education programs in spite of not being able to specifically identify the cost benefit of these programs.

A Health Communication Model

The rationale for health education was presented so we can appreciate the problems associated with traditional forms of health education. One of these problems relates to the perception of how health matters are communicated. Communication can be described by the following model:

SENDER---------------MESSAGE---------------MEDIUM---------------RECEIVER

That is, someone (the *sender*) sends a *message* through some *medium* (for example, a lecture) to some-one else (the *receiver*). The way most health educators would like to view themselves in this model is as the sender of the message (for example, that it is unhealthful to smoke cigarettes). They send this message through various classroom activities (lectures, discussions, films). The message is directed at the students or patients or workers (the receivers). The problem is that more often than not the sender in this model is society — not the teacher — and society's message is sent through the medium — the health educator. A sender is afforded more respect and attention than is the conduit through which mes-sages flow. Furthermore, serving as the medium for someone else's messages sets health educators up for failure. That is because students will understand that educators are trying to get them to behave in certain ways that society has defined as healthful and will be suspicious regarding anyone or anything directed at changing them in ways in which they haven't agreed to be changed. This suspicion interferes with learning and prevents the adoption of the behavior as well. Rather than convey society's message as their own, health educators would be better advised to admit it is society's message, adding, "And now let's analyze that message to determine if it makes any sense or if it is misguided." Health educa-tors should work *with* their programs' participants, not *on* them.

Additionally, the messages educators are expected to convey may themselves be inappropriate. For example, educators tell people that they would be healthier if they exercised strenuously, in spite of the fact that many injuries result from such exercise. That is not to say that aerobic exercise is not good for people, only that there are two points of view on this matter. It would be more appropriate to educate health education program participants about this controversy, to help them to objectively analyze it and then to make their own decisions about how and whether they will exercise.

There are plenty of other behaviors that are taken for granted as being healthful without sufficient justification. For example, is it really healthful to develop a style of disclosure in one's communication with others? Many a marriage or other relationship has been dissolved because one individual told too much about his or her thoughts, fantasies, or past that would probably have been better off closely guarded as a secret. Is it really better to eat margarine than butter, or is one just more prone to lead to cancer and the other to heart disease?

Perhaps the best example of the questionable behavior that we have classified as healthful is the in-oculation against swine flu that was recommended in the early 1970s. Health educators were used to develop campaigns to encourage people to get inoculated, not to encourage people to consider inocula-tion with all of the available evidence at hand. Subsequently it was learned that not only was swine flu not a threat but the inoculation itself led to a form of paralysis in many people and death in others.

Today's knowledge too often becomes tomorrow's misinformation. Health educators need to com-municate to people the *process* of making health-related decisions rather than telling them what their decisions ought to be. This approach would certainly be more democratic than programming people like computers to behave in ways predetermined to be healthful and then evaluating them on whether they adhered to the recommendations. Furthermore, as discussed in Chapter 1, when most people say *healthy* they are referring to physical health. To determine what is really healthy for someone requires that per-son to judge the worth of the behavior using his or her value system and comparing the benefits and dis-advantages of the behavior relative to all five components of health: social, mental, emotional, spiritual, and physical health. If we really can't tell others what is healthy for them (because we do not have the same values as they do), how can we conduct health education that has as its goal predefined healthful behaviors? The alternative to this traditional form of health education will soon be presented. First, though, let's consider some other problems associated with traditional health education.

Iatrogenic Health Education Disease

Another side effect of traditional health education (where objectives are predetermined for students) involves what I have elsewhere termed *iatrogenic health education disease* (Greenberg 1985). IHED is disease caused or exacerbated by health education. How many times, for example, have you heard someone complain that everything causes cancer? People have been taught that all of the fun things—whether eating good-tasting foods or enjoying some sexual activity—are bad for them. They then decide that maintaining good health is not worth it, and they start (or continue) to adopt unhealthful behaviors. These people are suffering from iatrogenic health education disease; they have been taught by health educators that maintaining good health is hard work, is not enjoyable, and involves self-sacrifice. In a sense, health education has led these people to be more unhealthy than they might have been otherwise.

Other IHED signs and symptoms can also be recognized. When people are programmed to behave in ways predetermined by health educators to be healthful, they might adopt behaviors they don't value or those for which they don't fully understand the rationale. How can people who can be controlled by other people be called healthy? By definition, these controlled people are, in fact, unhealthy—albeit in ways other than physically. They are likely to be conformists and easily swayed by others toward unhealthful behaviors, just as they are easily swayed by health educators toward healthful behaviors. Being able to be controlled by others, then, is a side effect of traditional health education, a sign of IHED. It is not a purposeful outcome of health education—that is, health educators don't intentionally go about trying to get people to become conformists—but an outcome nonetheless.

Still another side effect of IHED is blaming oneself for one's illness when that blame is misplaced. *Locus of control* refers to the perception of the amount of control one has regarding the events that affect one's life. People can have an external locus of control; that is, they believe events that affect their lives are the result of fate, chance, luck, or powerful others (such as the doctor or the professor). Likewise, people can possess an internal locus of control; they believe events that affect their lives are a result of things they do, that they are in control of these events and their outcomes. And they may have a locus of control somewhere between external and internal. Health education programs are often designed to increase participants' internality. Health educators value an internal locus of control, believing that people who feel they can control events in their lives will be more apt to adopt healthful behaviors; they believe that what they do about their health will pay dividends, not that illness or disease is a result of being unlucky.

However, let's consider a woman who has experienced a *successful* health education program and now believes she is in control of events that affect her life. One night, after working late, she leaves the office to get into her car in a dark parking lot. Out of the dark a rapist appears, and the woman is attacked. *Blaming the victim,* in this case herself, the woman believes she is responsible for allowing herself to be raped by walking through that parking lot, unescorted, late at night. Nonsense! The fault was the rapist's! The woman may have been careless or not cautious enough, but blaming herself for being raped causes undue anguish and guilt, and that is unhealthy. In this case, a little externality—believing that fate and poor luck played a part in the rape—would serve this woman better than internality.

The truth about locus of control is that we cocreate, with external events over which we have very little influence, our futures. That is, we meet situations that we can't control, although we can control, to some degree, how we deal with or react to these events. Blaming oneself for one's illness or disease is an unfortunate potential side effect of traditional health education, a side effect evidencing iatrogenic health education disease.

Health Education as Freeing

To be critical of traditional forms of health education without suggesting an alternative form would be irresponsible. To avoid that charge, we present in this section an alternative called *Health Education as Freeing.* First we provide a definition of *health education* as used in this alternative form. Consider health education to be "a process in which the goal is to free people so that they may make health-related decisions based upon their needs and interests as long as these decisions do not adversely affect others" (Greenberg 1978, 20).

Enslaving Factors

Though at first glance this definition of health education appears not much different from others, its application certainly is. One implication of health education as a freeing process is the assumption that people enrolled in health education programs are not initially free. These program participants are *enslaved.* The enslaving factors affecting them may be low self-esteem; high levels of alienation; feelings of inferiority, hostility, guilt, and anger; an inability to be assertive; difficulty in communicating with others; loneliness; and so on. For example, people who don't think well of themselves—have poor self-esteem—cannot be expected to have confidence in their own decisions and can, therefore, be expected to be unduly influenced by others. This conformist behavior enslaves them by preventing them from making decisions more consistent with their own interests and values. People who are socially isolated might make choices to alleviate their feeling of loneliness rather than choices more consistent with their natures.

Additional factors that may enslave people are a sense of powerlessness, values confusion, an excessively internal or external locus of control, a lack of problem-solving skills, fear of medical situations, and two that deserve special attention: poor health-related knowledge and poor health-related skills. These last two factors, health-related knowledge and skills, are *necessary but not sufficient* to free people so they are able to make their own decisions. That is, it is necessary to have health knowledge and the skill to apply that knowledge, but study after study demonstrates these two factors are not enough to effect behavioral change—the adoption of healthful behaviors. Just because people know that brushing and flossing their teeth help prevent tooth decay and periodontal disease and have the skills of brushing and flossing down pat doesn't mean they will regularly brush and floss. Unfortunately, numerous enslaving factors intervene between what people know is good for them and how they behave.

The Objectives of Health Education as Freeing

Health education, then, should be designed to remove these enslaving factors so people can make health decisions consistent with their own values, interests, and needs. This means that health education should be directed toward teaching health knowledge and health skills as they presently do, but not at the expense of educating program participants about the enslaving factors and helping them free themselves. Health education programs should be designed to make participants feel less alienated, be less socially isolated, understand the motivations behind their behavior more, feel better about themselves, clarify

Health education that is limited to the instructor standing in front of the group and the program participants seated in relatively passive modes can be expected to be ineffective. Program participants will learn best when they are encouraged to be active learners.

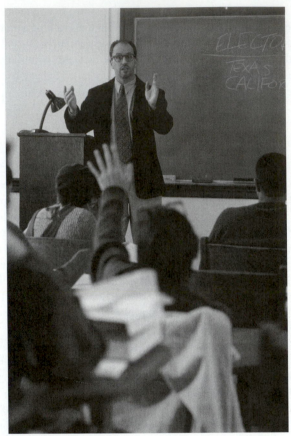

Source: Doug Menuez/Getty Images/PhotoDisc

their values, and in other ways eliminate or diminish the effect of the enslaving factors on their health-related decisions.

The Evaluation of Health Education as Freeing

Evaluating this form of health education requires a different perspective than evaluating more traditional forms of health education. Rather than being concerned with how program participants behave, the focus is on how participants arrived at their decision to behave a particular way. In other words, the decision-making process becomes more important than the decision. If one agrees with the earlier discussion regarding the difficulty and the inappropriateness of deciding whether someone else is healthy—especially when not fully appreciative of their values—then one will be more comfortable with the lack of concern for behavioral change than if one disagreed with that earlier discussion. However, even if concerned with changing program participants' behaviors, paying attention to the enslaving factors will probably facilitate that objective as well.

The following questions illustrate those that might serve as the focus of evaluation for freeing health education programs:

1. Has a decision by program participants been made after thought?
2. Have alternative courses of action been considered by program participants?
3. Have the implications and ramifications of those alternatives been considered by program participants?
4. Have the decisions by the program participants been made freely, without coercion from others?
5. Have program participants' levels of self-esteem improved?
6. Have program participants' levels of alienation decreased?
7. Have program participants' health knowledge and health skills increased?
8. Are program participants now able to act assertively if they choose?
9. Can program participants now develop social support networks?
10. Are program participants' values clearer to them now than before the program?

Research Goals

As the evaluation of freeing health education differs from that of traditional health education, so do its research goals. The goals of research in freeing health education relate to the best ways — most effective, most cost efficient, and most feasible — to free people from the enslaving factors, rather than the best ways to get people to adopt healthful lifestyles. Consequently, how to best improve people's self-esteem, decrease their level of alienation, improve their social support, and the like are the questions investigators seek to answer. How best to encourage people to employ appropriate decision-making strategies and problem-solving skills are also foci of research in freeing health education. In addition, theorizing about adoption of healthful lifestyles, definitions of health, and the ethics and morality of health education practices are also fair game for freeing health education researchers. Again, the focus is away from specific health behaviors or decisions and instead on the way in which those behaviors or decisions are made — on process rather than on outcome.

The Ultimate Goal

Someone once said, "Give me a fish and I eat today; teach me to fish and I eat for all time." Giving fish in health education — telling people how to behave — is not freeing people. Teaching them to fish for themselves — instructing them on decision-making and problem-solving skills — is.

Health Education Ethics

One can't help but consider ethical professional practice when one discusses iatrogenic health education disease and health education as freeing. However, the frustrating aspect of such a discussion for many people is the inexactitude with which it must be approached. That is, there are few answers, and certainly few with which everyone will agree. The best that can be done here is to identify the issues to consider when determining what is and what is not ethical in the health education profession.

Health education should be seen as a way to help people achieve their health-related objectives—a resource people can use—rather than a means of manipulating people to behave in ways predetermined to be healthful.

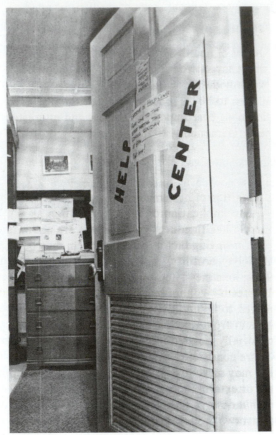

Source: The Diamondback, University of Maryland

Ethical Issues

The issue that jumps out at us from our previous discussions is whether it is ethical to predetermine which behaviors are healthful and then to organize learning experiences to encourage (facilitate? manipulate?) the adoption of these behaviors. This issue becomes more complicated when we consider that some health education program participants (for example, schoolchildren) are not attending voluntarily. Is there a difference between the resolution of this issue for these populations and the resolution for people who are there because they want to be there? Is the fact that the health educator is acting with the best interest of the participants in mind a consideration? Does the age of the participants matter in how you decide this issue? Take a moment to jot down how you would decide the ethics of this issue.

Another ethical issue for health educators is deciding what to do when confronted with other health educators' unethical behavior. For example, what should you do if you find out that another health educator has misrepresented his or her professional qualifications or experience? Should a supervisor be informed? Should the student or patient be informed? Is it appropriate to misrepresent qualifications if that misrepresentation results in the program participants' increased confidence in the health educator, thereby facilitating the adoption of the program's objectives and the improvement of the health status of the participant? In other words, do the ends in this instance justify the means?

What if the health educator misinforms people who are being solicited to participate in a research investigation? If the goal of the research is to discover information that could significantly affect the health of a great number of people, does that change your answer? What if the purpose of the study cannot be accomplished with full disclosure? What should another health educator who sees a lack of full disclosure to potential research subjects do? Write your answers to these questions on a separate sheet of paper.

What are your obligations as a professional health educator when you observe discriminatory practices on the part of another health educator? What if these are unintentional practices — such as expecting less from students from particular ethnic or cultural groups, thinking this to be in their best interest? Whom, if anyone, should be told?

When a health education colleague does not keep current with the latest health information, what is your professional and ethical responsibility? When a health education colleague does not keep current with the latest knowledge regarding the most effective manner in which to plan, implement, and evaluate health education programs, what is your professional and ethical responsibility?

Should health educators in training — for example, student teachers or field-work students in community health education — be allowed to plan, implement, and evaluate health education programs by themselves? Is it ethical to allow these health educators in training to practice on unsuspecting program participants? Is it ethical even if the participants are informed? These are some of the perplexing ethical issues inherent in the professional practice of health education.

Code of Ethics

Several codes of ethics for health educators have been developed over the years. In 1976 the Society for Public Health Education (SOPHE) developed a code of ethics to guide professional behaviors. The American College Health Association (ACHA) also adopted a code of ethics in the 1980s. In 1993 the Association for the Advancement of Health Education (AAHE) adopted still another code of ethics to guide its members. Recognizing the need to develop one professionwide code of ethics rather than separate ones for different professional organizations, the Coalition of National Health Education Organizations (CNHEO) got together and developed a code of ethics that was adopted in 1999. This Code of Ethics for the Health Education Profession (Greenberg, 2001) now guides all health educators regardless of setting or population with whom they work. The Code of Ethics for the Health Education Profession appears at the end of this book in Appendix A.

Summary

1. The current emphasis on health education is due to many factors, of which the escalating costs of health care and the spread of HIV are but two.

2. It is expected that health education can save money in the long term by helping people prevent or postpone illnesses and diseases and detect illnesses and diseases at an earlier stage.

3. The federal government developed health goals for the United States in 1979 and transposed these into health objectives for the nation in 1981, and again in 2000. Currently, Year 2010 National Health Objectives govern national health priorities.

4. One rationale for health education is that social agents have a responsibility to provide people — in whatever setting — with the information they need to make healthful decisions.

5. One of the most persuasive rationales for health education is that it provides a cost benefit; that is, the investment in the program will save money in the long term by decreasing the costs of health care over time. However, since much of the benefit of health education cannot be quantified, determining its cost benefit is very difficult.

6. Health education can help businesses and communities recruit new members and retain the present ones.

7. Health educators prefer to think of themselves as senders of healthful messages. However, sometimes they become the conduits through which society sends its messages. In these instances, health educators are apt to lose the respect and trust of their programs' participants, with the result being difficulty in achieving the programs' objectives.

8. It is more important to teach program participants the process of making health-related decisions than it is to encourage any particular decisions or convey any particular information.

9. Iatrogenic health education disease (IHED) is disease caused or exacerbated by health education. Signs of such disease are conformist behavior, believing that maintaining one's health is an unpleasant activity, and blaming oneself for one's illnesses or diseases.

10. Freeing health education is a new form of health education that begins with the assumption that people are enslaved by such factors as low self-esteem, high alienation, poor decision-making skills, and a lack of social support. Health education, then, is defined as a process to free people to make health-related decisions based on their needs and interests as long as these decisions do not adversely affect others.

11. Professional health educators need to come to grips with many ethical issues. The Code of Ethics for the Health Education Profession is the first professionwide code to provide guidance on these ethical issues.

CHAPTER FOUR

Service-Learning in Health Education*

An exciting new development in education that has important implications for health education is termed *service-learning*. Service-learning is a means of having learners apply what they have learned by participating in community service activities. This creates a win–win situation in which students derive a great deal of learning they might not have derived otherwise, while the community benefits from the service provided. The first section of this chapter describes community health needs in an attempt to foster the attitude that serving the community through service-learning is worth the time and effort required on the part of health educators and participants in the programs they conduct.

The Need

The 1990 Nobel Laureate and Mexican poet Octavio Paz writes of his search for the present. Paz describes his world as a child growing up in Mexico City where his garden and the library were the center of his childhood experience. Then one day Paz was shown a photograph of soldiers returning from war and he first realized that somewhere far away a war had been fought as he was growing up—"in another time and in another place, not here and now." Paz felt dislodged from the present—expelled from his garden—at least the present he thought had existed. That day Octavio Paz began his lifelong search for the present—the real present.

Although the present exists all around us, all too often we are blinded by it, or at least to segments of it. An example is what happened in relation to the O. J. Simpson trial. Generally, whites could not fathom that Simpson was acquitted, whereas blacks rejoiced. The reason for this difference probably lies in the differences between experiences, and consequently the perceptions, of America's black and white citizens. However, this ethnic gap was not widely acknowledged, so it was not a part of our reality—our present. The trial helped us go searching for our present, and we did not like what we found.

---

*This information is reprinted with permission from the *Journal of Health Education,* vol. 26, no. 4, 1995, pp. 214–223. The *Journal of Health Education* is a publication of the American Alliance for Health, Physical Education, Recreation and Dance, 1900 Association Drive, Reston, Virginia 22091. Tables and statistics have been updated.

Children

One perception of our present that stands in stark contrast to the present we acknowledge relates to life in the United States and to the daily existence of many Americans. In the United States, the most advanced country in the world, too many American children experience a life of turmoil and trauma. Tables 4.1 and 4.2 list some of the daily experiences of American children as reported by the Children's Defense Fund (1999).

African American children (Table 4.2), face an even bleaker picture (Black Community Crusade, 1993).

Children living in poverty face an even greater risk for a range of health problems than do other children (Federal Interagency Forum on Child and Family Statistics 2001). As depicted in Table 4.3, the effects of poverty on these children's health are devastating.

TABLE 4.1

Every Day in America for All Children

2	young persons under 25 die from HIV infection.
6	children and youths under 20 commit suicide.
11	children and youths under 20 are homicide victims.
13	children and youths under 20 die from firearms.
36	children and youths under 20 die from accidents.
78	babies die.
146	babies are born at very low birthweight (less than 3 lbs., 4 oz.).
237	children are arrested for violent crimes.
415	babies are born to women who had late or no prenatal care.
420	children are arrested for drug abuse.
787	babies are born at low birthweight (less than 5 lbs., 8 oz.).
1,353	babies are born without health insurance.
1,377	babies are born to teen mothers.
2,162	babies are born into poverty.
2,356	babies are born to mothers who are not high school graduates.
2,658	public school students are corporally punished.
2,789	high school students drop out.
3,453	babies are born to unmarried mothers.
5,388	children are arrested.
17,152	public school students are suspended.

Source: © 1999 Children's Defense Fund. From *The State of America's Children: Yearbook 1999.* All rights reserved.

TABLE 4.2
African American Children's Disadvantage

If black children faced the same odds as white children, each year	
3,011,000	fewer black children would live in poverty.
300,000	fewer black infants would be born to unmarried mothers.
151,000	fewer black teenage women would get pregnant.
92,500	fewer black teenage women would give birth.
61,000	more black high school graduates would start college.
38,200	fewer black teens would become sexually active.
7,114	fewer black infants would die.
1,298	fewer black 20- to 24-year-olds would be killed by guns.
877	fewer black 15- to 19-year-olds would be killed by guns.

And to make matters worse, with the highest standard of living in the world, American children are more likely to live in poverty than are children from many other countries. American children are twice as likely to live in poverty as are Canadian children, 3 times as likely as British children, 4 times as likely as French children, and 7–13 times as likely as German, Dutch, and Swedish children (Arloc 1994).

And in this country, too many of our infants die. We still have an unacceptable infant mortality rate, in particular when compared with other countries. The infant mortality rate for blacks is twice that of whites (see Table 4.4).

What's more, although the infant mortality rate has steadily declined, the disparity in rates between whites and blacks has remained the same. In 1980 the infant mortality rate for blacks was 2 times that of whites, as it was in 1999. There are many explanations for these data, one of which relates to prenatal care. Approximately 6 to 7 percent of black and Hispanic mothers do not obtain prenatal care at all or, if they do, they wait until the last trimester (National Center for Health Statistics 2000).

When we look more closely at these births, we see that 69 percent of African American mothers and almost 42 percent of Hispanic mothers are unmarried, and 9 percent of African American mothers and 7 percent of Hispanic mothers are under 18 years of age (see Table 4.5).

Poverty

Certainly poverty is a major reason that our country's minorities experience these and other health defects. "Poverty." What does that mean? The federal government has a definition that may surprise you.

In 2000, a family of three earning more than $13,738 was *not* classified as living in poverty (see Table 4.6). A family of four could not earn more than $17,603. Given these ridiculously low allowable incomes, it does not take much to realize that many Americans not classified as living in poverty, actually are.

TABLE 4.3
Children's Health Conditions by Family Income

	Poverty Children's Higher Risk
Death during infancy	1.3 times
Death during childhood	3 times
Low birthweight	1.2 to 2.2 times
Stunted growth	2 to 3 times
Partly or completely deaf	1.5 to 2 times
Partly or completely blind	1.2 to 1.8 times
Physical or mental disabilities	About 2 times
Mild mental retardation	More likely
Overall injuries	No more likely
Days in bed because of injuries	1.8 times
Hospitalization for injuries	At least 3 times
Fatal accidental injuries	2 to 3 times
Hospitalization for poisoning	5 times
Fair or poor health	3 times
Iron deficiency in preschool years	3 to 4 times
Frequent diarrhea or colitis	1.5 times
Pneumonia	1.6 times
Repeated tonsillitis	1.1 times
Overall asthma	More likely
Severe asthma	About 2 times
Decayed, missing, or filled teeth	More likely
School days missed due to acute and chronic health conditions	1.4 times

Source: Wasting America's Future by Children's Defense Fund. © 1994 by Children's Defense Fund. Used by permission of Beacon Press, Boston.

TABLE 4.4
Infant Mortality Rates*

Overall infant mortality rate	=	7.2
White infant mortality rate	=	6.0
Black infant mortality rate	=	14.3
*per 1,000 live births		

Source: U.S. Census Bureau. *Statistical Abstracts of the United States: 2001.* Washington, D.C.: U.S. Government Printing Office, 2001.

TABLE 4.5
Birth Statistics

I. Mother less than 18 years of age (% live births):	
All mothers	4.6
White mothers	3.9
African American mothers	8.9
Hispanic mothers	6.9
II. Unmarried mothers (% live births)	
All mothers	32.8
White mothers	26.3
African American mothers	69.1
Hispanic mothers	41.6

Source: National Center for Health Statistics. *Health, United States, 2000.* Hyattsville, MD: Public Health Service, 2000.

TABLE 4.6
Poverty Guidelines

One person	$ 8,794
Two people	$11,239
Three people	$13,738
Four people	$17,603
Five people	$20,819

Source: U.S. Census Bureau, 2000.

   With these guidelines in mind, consider that in this great country, this country with the highest standard of living in the world, over 34 million Americans — that is, 12.7 percent — live in poverty, including 18 percent of young Americans under 18 years of age and over 6 million families (U.S. Census Bureau, 2001).

   Although more whites live in poverty than others, minorities are disproportionately represented among the poor. Over 30 percent of our black and Hispanic neighbors live in poverty. Even more alarming is the realization that over one-third of America's black and Hispanic children under 18 years of age live in poverty (see Table 4.7).

   To exacerbate the problem, the situation regarding health care is getting worse rather than better. In 1980, 12.5 percent of Americans under 65 years of age had no health care insurance coverage, whereas in 1998, 16.3 percent were uninsured (National Center for Health Statistics 2000). And, not surprisingly, blacks and Hispanics are disproportionately represented among the uninsured.

TABLE 4.7
Poverty Rates

All persons:		
All races	=	12.7%
White	=	10.5%
Black	=	26.1%
Hispanic	=	25.6%
Children under 18 years of age:		
All races	=	18.3%
White	=	14.4%
Black	=	36.4%
Hispanic	=	33.6%

Source: National Center for Health Statistics. *Health, United States, 2000.* Hyattsville, MD.: Public Health Service, 2000.

Here, again, income comes into play, with only 8.3 percent of families earning $50,000 or more uninsured, whereas over 35 percent of families earning less than $25,000 do not have health care coverage. And, in this great country, with the highest standard of living in the world, 14 percent of our children under 18 years of age do not have health care coverage (U.S. Census Bureau, 2001).

Where is the outcry? What are we doing, and encouraging participants in our health education programs to do, to express our outrage over this atrocity? Will we remain silent as too many did in Nazi Germany, or during apartheid in South Africa, or as tribal killing was occurring in Rwanda, or during the ethnic cleansing in Bosnia?

Homelessness

In addition, in this great country, this country with the highest standard of living in the world, 100,000 children are homeless each day, comprising an estimated 30 percent of all homeless people seeking shelter (National Academy of Sciences 1988; United States Conference of Mayors 1993). This is inexcusable!

As you can imagine, homelessness has a profound effect on children. Only one example of this effect is the far greater developmental lags experienced by homeless children compared to housed children, as shown in Table 4.8.

Violence

Add to this reality the violence encountered by many children—violence or the threat of violence encountered almost daily—and the lives of far too many American children can be seen as even more troubling. James Darby is an example of this reality. Nine-year-old James Darby wrote President Clinton in 1994 that he was afraid of the violence on the streets of America. "Please," he implored the President, "stop the killing . . . I'm asking you nicely . . . I know you can do it." Should our children

TABLE 4.8

A Comparison Between Homeless and Housed Children

Test Result	Percentage of Homeless Children	Percentage of Housed Children
At least one lag	54	16
Type of lag		
Language	42	13
Gross motor	17	4
Fine motor	15	1
Personal/social	42	3

Source: Reproduced by permission of *Pediatrics,* vol. 85, pp. 257–261, copyright 1990.

TABLE 4.9

Suicide and High School Students

Percentage who seriously considered suicide	19.3%
Percentage who made a specific plan	14.5%
Percentage who attempted suicide	8.3%

Source: Youth Risk Behavior Surveillance System (YRBSS), 1999.

have to live like this? Should they have to fear walking out of their homes, or attending a school dance, or rooting for their school team? Nine days after Darby wrote to President Clinton, while Darby walked home from a Mother's Day picnic with his mother, an angry young man fired a gun into a crowd — and James Darby was shot in the head and killed.

Suicide

Many of our youngsters are deciding not to take it any longer. In a national survey, approximately 20 percent of our country's high school students reported that they seriously considered killing themselves sometime during the preceding 12 months. Almost 15 percent made a specific plan to take their own lives. And 8 percent actually attempted suicide (see Table 4.9).

Even schools are failing to respond to these alarming statistics. In a study of our nation's schools, the School Health Policies and Programs Study, only 38 percent of *states* reported requiring that suicide prevention be taught, only two-thirds of school *districts* required it, and just a little over half of the *schools* actually taught suicide prevention (Collins et al. 1995). Although teachers want to be trained in suicide prevention, they are not receiving adequate training. When suicide prevention is taught, only 29 percent of health education teachers and only 7 percent of other classroom teachers devote more than one class period to the topic.

Families

Well, in spite of this dire picture, at least we live in a country that places a value on the family. At least we *hear* a lot about family values. Let's look at this assumption a little more closely, in our search for the present.

Table 4.10 presents the maternal leave policies of several Western developed countries. As can be noted, many countries allow significantly more time for leave and subsidize that leave with a significant portion of the employee's salary. The policy in the United States is much less supportive of families.

As you may recall, the U.S. policy (known as the Family and Medical Leave Act), as restrictive as it is, was vetoed several times by then President George Bush before finally being signed into law by President Clinton. Furthermore, the U.S. policy applies only to businesses that employ more than 50,000 workers, thereby excluding the myriad workers employed by small businesses.

Civic Disengagement

At the very time when Americans ought to be appalled at the conditions in which too many of their fellow citizens live, we are detaching ourselves from societal institutions that would make our society a better place. Perhaps this detachment is best represented by the research of sociologist Robert Putnam

TABLE 4.10
Paid Maternal Leave in Selected Western Countries

Country	Duration of Leave	Percentage of Wage
Sweden	12 months	90
Finland	11 months	80
Denmark	24 weeks	90
Italy	5 months	80
Norway	18 weeks	100
Austria	16 weeks	100
France	16 weeks	90
Canada	15 weeks	60
Germany	14 weeks	100
Belgium	14 weeks	100
Ireland	14 weeks	80
Portugal	3 months	100
Israel	12 weeks	75
Greece	12 weeks	60
Netherlands	12 weeks	100
United States	12 weeks	0

Source: S. B. Kamerman. "Childcare Policies and Programs: An International Overview," *Journal of Social Issues* 47: 179–196, 1991. Reprinted by permission.

(1995, 2000). Putnam's studies of "civic engagement" noted that between 1960 and 1990, voter turnout declined by 25 percent, attendance at public meetings concerned with town or school affairs declined by 33 percent, daily newspaper readership declined by 25 percent, and membership in groups requiring face-to-face contact declined significantly. For example, PTA membership fell from 12 million in 1964 to 7 million in 1994, membership in the League of Women Voters declined by 42 percent, volunteers for the Boy Scouts declined by 26 percent, and volunteers for the Red Cross were 61 percent fewer. In fact, in 1994 only 60 percent of Americans reported socializing with their neighbors at least once a year, whereas in 1974, 72 percent reported doing so. Add to these data the technological developments that allow us to bank, shop, and perform library searches isolated from others at home with our computers; that allow us to entertain ourselves with virtual reality gizmos or Walkman radios and CD and tape players rather than needing anyone else with whom to interact; and that more people seem to be watching talk shows nowadays than talking: civic disengagement becomes obvious.

The Health Educator's Responsibilities

Health educators have a responsibility to develop programs that improve the lives of people: not only the lives of program participants, but also the lives of the larger community. The way to accomplish this goal is through service-learning described here. However, before launching into this description, I am reminded of a poem by Margaret Sangster that I would like to share with you:

It isn't the thing you do, dear,
It's the thing you leave undone
That gives you a bit of a heartache
At the setting of the sun.
The tender word forgotten,
The letter you did not write,
The flowers you did not send, dear,
Are your haunting ghosts at night.

The stone you might have lifted
Out of a brother's way;
The bit of heartsome counsel
You were hurried too much to say;
The loving touch of the hand, dear,
The gentle, winning tone
Which you had no time nor thought for
With troubles enough of your own.

Those little acts of kindness
So easily out of mind,
Those chances to be angels
Which we poor mortals find—
They come in night and silence,
Each sad, reproachful wraith,
When hope is faint and flagging,
And a chill has fallen on faith.

For life is all too short, dear,
And sorrow is all too great,
To suffer our slow compassion

That tarries until too late;
And it isn't the thing you do, dear,
It's the thing you leave undone
Which gives you a bit of a heartache
At the setting of the sun.

It is long overdue for health educators to adopt the attitude that never again, in this great country, with the highest standard of living in the world, will they stand idly by as children die from poverty or neglect; as black babies are born at too low a birthweight to thrive; as Americans have to search through garbage cans to find food to eat; or as teenagers become pregnant and wrestle with the accompanying social, emotional, financial, and spiritual implications of giving birth or arranging for an abortion.

The Politics of Small

And yet, where do we begin? Each of us would love to be able to eliminate poverty and illness and disease. We cannot. Thinking we can will result in activities that are too grandiose and, therefore, doomed to failure. On the other hand, realizing we cannot have major impact on these severe and debilitating conditions can result in paralysis — that is, doing nothing because we do not believe anything we do will be meaningful. What we can do is make one person's life a little bit better, or maybe two or three. Kim Chernin (1993) calls this the "politics of small." Rather than working on major changes that are unlikely to occur, Chernin suggests we devote our efforts to smaller goals that we can accomplish.

It doesn't take much to make a difference. Chaos theory states that chaotic phenomena occur when complex systems encounter slight, unpredictable variations. For example, although the stock market is governed by rules such as rising when company profits rise, it can be thrown into tumult by unanticipated rumors or the raising of interest rates by the Federal Reserve. Similarly, when the heart goes into fibrillation, its beats go from a regular rhythm to a chaotic one.

Chaos can be controlled, however, with small nudges (such as mild electrical charges for atrial fibrillation). Imagine balancing a pencil on the tip of your finger. All that is required are small adjustments to keep it balanced, but without those adjustments you have chaos.

As with the pencil, the health of too many of our fellow citizens is precariously out of balance. The good news is that small nudges can right the situation. That is, instead of trying to change the world without the resources to do so, health educators can change something in the immediate environment. Feed one homeless person, provide clothing for a poor family, spend time with a child to discuss his or her feelings of anger or frustration, volunteer at a community health clinic. Make a small nudge in the chaotic health of people to whom you have access.

Examples of Health Education Community Service

In spite of the civic disengagement just described, there are still many examples of community service by health educators and others each and every day in this country. I share with you one that I have experienced not because it is the most significant, but because it is the one with which I am most familiar.

I conducted monthly stress management workshops for parents residing at the Ronald McDonald House in Washington, D.C. Participants' children are seriously ill — often terminally ill — and, while their children are being treated at local hospitals, parents reside at the Ronald House. If it were only in my power to make their children well, I would jump at the chance. But in this regard I am helpless. As Forrest Gump said when his girlfriend revisited the home in which she was sexually abused as a child and began throwing rocks in anger, and in vain: "Sometimes there aren't enough rocks to throw." However, I was able to help them manage some of the stress they experienced. Was it enough? Not by a long stretch. Did it help? You bet! When asked, "As a result of attending this workshop do you feel you can manage stress better?" all but one of the approximately 100 parents who participated answered, "Yes." This is an example of what was earlier referred to as the "politics of small"—doing what we can do, even though it is not all we would wish we could do.

Many professional associations also offer pro bono community service, and their members are involved in improving the lives of underserved populations through their professional organizations. For example, the Association for the Advancement of Health Education (AAHE) and the American School Health Association (ASHA) recognize that the annual gathering of nationally and internationally renowned experts that attend their conventions each year should do more than just march into town, meet in cloistered rooms, spend some money, and leave without having contributed to the health and welfare of their hosts—the citizens of the convention city. Consequently, each city in which these associations hold their conventions receives pro bono health education services designed to improve the lives of the residents of those cities. To date, AAHE members have offered free services to residents of San Francisco; Indianapolis; Washington, D.C.; Denver; Portland; and Atlanta; and in Houston in 1994, the American School Health Association provided similar service.

Other professionals have responded in kind. Physicians' spouses have developed antiviolence programs, and trauma surgeons—frustrated with having to treat victims of violence and family abuse—have promoted conflict resolution skills among youth in their communities. A unique project is Volunteers in Medicine. Retired physicians, nurses, and other health care providers in Hilton Head, South Carolina, decided to volunteer their time, energy, and skills to provide free health care to the island's poor population. This project was so successful that it is serving as a national model for other communities.

These may seem like small contributions, and they are, given the enormity of the problem. "Sometimes there aren't enough rocks to throw." But these health professionals have determined it is better to throw some than to be inattentive to the needs of their fellow Americans.

Service-Learning

Colleges and universities have also responded to community needs with expanding service-learning programs. The National and Community Service Act of 1990 defined *service-learning* as "a method by which young people learn and develop through active participation in thoughtfully organized service experiences" (Alliance for Service-Learning in Education Reform, undated, 1). These experiences result in a service to the community and its residents, and enhance the learning of the students participating in the service-learning activity.

Examples of Service-Learning

An engineering professor heard of a young quadriplegic who bemoaned the fact that he could not travel around with his friends as they scooted off on their bikes. The professor organized the engineering class around a project: develop some way for this young quadriplegic to participate with his friends. The result was a vehicle that could be operated by the youngster's mouth as he scooted around with the other young boys. A real service was provided, while the students learned engineering. And I would guess that more learning than usual occurred because the course content was immediately put to use in a real problem-solving situation. Here is a quintessential win–win scenario.

One elementary school developed a service-learning project to feed the homeless. Grades 3 and 4 organized the project. They agreed on the menu to be served in the school cafeteria (thereby using home economic and health education content); they wrote letters to local merchants soliciting supplies (thereby using what they learned in English class); and they determined how much bread and other food they needed based on how many people they expected to feed (thereby using their math skills). For this project, the whole school came together. The first and second grades made place mats (using their art class skills); the kitchen staff mixed the tuna that was served; and the school custodian set up the lunch-room tables.

Another school adopted the school's cook's son as a pen pal. He was in the Marines and went to Kuwait during the Desert Storm war. Through the usual subject areas, students learned about the Middle East in preparation for the letters they wrote to this young soldier. When the cook's son returned home, he spoke with the students at an auditorium presentation. You can imagine how the students felt when the young Marine told them how much comfort he received from their letters.

Service-Learning with Adults

Service-learning can also be organized with adult learners. In an undergraduate course I teach called "Controlling Stress and Tension," students are required to form groups of four members each and provide four hours of direct contact with people in the community to help them better manage stress. They have worked with many different community groups. Some helped students in local schools manage the stress associated with moving from one level of schooling to another (for example, moving from middle school to senior high school). Others worked with cancer patients, helping them to manage the stress associated with their illness. Still others worked with staff of a local nursery school helping them to manage the stress accompanying their jobs as well as the stress they experienced outside of work. Minimal class time is needed to prepare students because they are taking what they learn in class and merely translating that content into something useful for the community group. Still, students develop outlines that are approved in advance of their being reviewed by the community contact person. The community contact person also completes an evaluation of the students, which is mailed directly to me to assure its anonymity. It is encouraging to read these evaluations. They express an appreciation for the service provided and offer a welcome mat for future contact. Again, a win–win situation for everyone.

My graduate students—already working as professionals during the day while taking classes in the late afternoons and evenings—also left their "antiseptic" classrooms to provide service using what they learned in class. A small group of students in a "Foundations of Health Education" class developed a health fair for a local Jewish community center, while another group provided nutrition education for Hispanic parents in a housing development. Still another group of students conducted a needs assessment relative to a planned "Health and Wellness Seminar Series" to be offered at a local hospital.

The Benefits of Service-Learning

As Ralph Waldo Emerson wrote, "It is one of the most beautiful compensations of this life that no man can sincerely try to help another without helping himself." Service-learning is a good example of Emerson's observation. Service-learning has been found to

1. Increase math and reading achievement scores for tutors as well as for those being tutored (Conrad and Hedin 1991; Hedin 1987).

2. Result in no less knowledge than traditional college courses when the same course final examination is administered (Conrad and Hedin 1991). (Therefore, it is as effective as traditional instruction in conveying knowledge.)

3. Develop open-mindedness (Wilson 1974).

4. Increase problem-solving ability (Conrad and Hedin 1982).

5. Increase social and personal responsibility (Giles and Eyler 1994; Conrad and Hedin 1982).

6. Increase self-efficacy (Giles and Eyler 1994) and self-esteem (Boss 1994; Hedin 1989; Luchs 1981), and decrease alienation and isolation (Calabrese and Schumer 1986).

7. Result in fewer discipline problems (Calabrese and Schumer 1986), better communication, and gains in moral and ego development (Cognetta and Sprinthall 1978) and moral reasoning (Boss 1994).

8. Increase empathy (Conrad and Hedin 1991).

In addition, students participating in service-learning differ from students in traditional classes in that they are more likely to value the following (Markus, Howard, and King 1993):

1. Working toward equal opportunity for all in the United States.

2. Volunteering time helping people in need.

3. Finding a career that provides the opportunity to help others in need.

4. Giving to charitable causes.

And they are more apt to believe they can make a difference in people's lives (Markus, Howard, and King 1993).

Evidence of a Need for Service-Learning

One reason college students need to be involved in service-learning is that they are not now engaged in sufficient amounts of community service. Astin (1990) reported only 9.8 percent of college students volunteered frequently, and another 37.7 percent only occasionally (see Tables 4.11 and 4.12). Over half never volunteered at all. In addition, note the decrease in volunteerism as students get older. Only 21 percent of high schoolers did not participate in volunteer activities, whereas, as just mentioned, over half of college students did not participate at all. Furthermore, only 16.5 percent of college students who volunteered frequently while in high school volunteered frequently while in college; and over half of students who volunteered occasionally in high school never volunteered at all in college.

TABLE 4.11

Rates of Volunteer Participation

	PERCENT IN	
Level of Participation	**High School**	**College**
Frequent	21.0	9.8
Occasional	54.0	37.7
Not at all	21.0	32.4

Source: Alexander W. Astin. *Student Involvement in Community Service: Institutional Commitment and the Campus Compact.* Presented to the meeting of the Campus Compact, Royce Hall, UCLA Campus, December 6, 1990. Reprinted by permission.

TABLE 4.12

Consistency in Volunteerism Over Time

Level of High School Participation	LEVEL OF COLLEGE PARTICIPATION (%)			
	N	Not at All	Occasional	Frequent
Frequent	1,033	39.0	44.5	16.5
Occasional	2,645	50.3	40.7	9.0
Not at all	1,227	68.3	25.8	5.9

Source: Alexander W. Astin. *Student Involvement in Community Service: Institutional Commitment and the Campus Compact.* Presented to the meeting of the Campus Compact, Royce Hall, UCLA Campus, December 6, 1990. Reprinted by permission.

How to Conduct Service-Learning

Service-learning incorporates four phases: planning, action, reflection, and evaluation. The planning phase should involve all parties: health educators, program participants, and members of the communities to be served. Often a needs assessment is conducted to determine just what the community needs are, how those needs match with the expertise of the program participants, the key informants that need to be consulted, and the best means of reaching the target population.*

The action phase involves actually conducting the service-learning activity. This may be more complicated than one might first imagine. Access to the community may be limited. If small groups rather than individual program participants are providing the service, their schedules may not coincide, thereby making working together difficult. Transportation must be considered: each group might want to assure themselves that someone has an automobile or that public transportation is readily available. The safety of the program participants may be a concern depending on where and when the service is to be provided. In such an instance, preparations can be made to travel in a group, to provide the service during daytime hours, and to assure that parking is available on the site.

The reflection phase involves activities designed to make sense—to draw meaning—from the service provided. Experience without meaning is just meaningless experience. The best reflective activities (National Center for Service Learning in Early Adolescence 1991, 5)

1. Help people make a real contribution to individuals they are serving.
2. Help meet genuine needs of program participants, and allow for a certain amount of ego development.
3. Challenge students to stretch and to perform at higher levels.
4. Encourage students to participate actively in their own learning.

---

*National Center for Service Learning in Early Adolescence. *Reflection: The Key to Service Learning.* New York: National Helpers Network. Inc., 1991, p. 5. Reprinted by permission.

5. Relate theory to practice and determine what more needs to be learned.

6. Develop a sense of community.

7. Demonstrate a partnership between program participants, the sponsoring agency, and the community.

8. Are both structured and flexible; have a clear sense of direction, yet are responsive to new situations.

9. Promote genuine maturity in both what is reflected on and the roles participants assume.

10. Involve decision making on what will be considered and in what way.

11. Have real consequences: the outcomes make a difference.

Examples of reflective activities include

1. Writing a daily journal:

    What was experienced?

    What new skill was learned?

    What skill was missing or needs to be learned?

    What happened to make you feel uncomfortable? Proud?

    What are some of the things you wanted to say but didn't?

2. Individual conferences with school and agency supervisors.

3. Conversations with other students: large group, small group, partners.

4. Maintaining a portfolio.

5. Individual assessment.

6. An open letter to the supervisor.

7. How I've changed: then and now.

8. Discussing case studies and critical incidents.

Here are some examples of questions that can be asked to help students draw meaning from their service experiences:

1. What was the most meaningful experience associated with your community service?

2. What was your most frustrating experience? Why was this so frustrating to you? What could have been done to prevent or alleviate this feeling of frustration?

3. How successful do you think you were in helping the people to whom you provided community service? What difference did you make?

4. What did you learn that you did not know before? New knowledge? New skills? New ways of looking at situations or people?

5. What knowledge, skills, or ways of looking at situations or people do you still find lacking in yourself?

6. How have you changed?

7. Do you intend to continue being involved in community service activities? If not, why not? If yes, in what way(s) do you intend to continue to be involved?

The evaluation phase of service-learning consists of determining whether the objectives developed during the planning phase were met. Although the amount of hours spent performing the service activities can be evaluated as part of a process evaluation the learning objectives are most important. What did students learn about the course content, about the population they served, about the process of health education, and about themselves and the gaps in their knowledge that need attention? Chapter 5 discusses evaluation in greater detail.

In Conclusion

In a speech at the University of Texas on April 6, 1993, Hillary Clinton stated:

> And if we ask, why is it in a country as wealthy as we are, that there is this undercurrent of discontent, we realize that somehow economic growth and prosperity, political democracy and freedom are not enough— that we lack meaning in our individual lives and meaning collectively, we lack a sense that our lives are part of some greater effort, that we are connected to one another. . . . We need a new ethos of individual responsibility and caring.

Yes, we need to care. We need to cry. We need to act. No parent should have to watch his or her child go hungry, or die in the streets, or become ill because of inadequate health care. No child should have to watch his or her parent search for food in a garbage can, or arrange cardboard boxes to provide shelter on a rainy night spent sleeping outdoors. No youth should have to fear leaving his or her home, walking around his or her neighborhood, attending school or a concert, or hanging out with friends. For health educators to bemoan this situation, to stand by and watch it with concern, to give speeches suggesting what to do about it are all not enough. We need to *do something* to make life in our village better. We need to do something collectively as individuals, as citizens; and we need to do something as professionals. Service-learning is a way to respond to societal and community health-related needs while simultaneously enhancing the learning of program participants.

CHAPTER FIVE

Conducting Health Education

This chapter discusses the various settings in which health education typically occurs, aspects of planning for health education, implementation of health education programs, and how these programs may be evaluated.

Health Education Settings

Health education can occur anywhere, and often does. For example, when parents instruct their children on the importance and the proper way of brushing their teeth, that is health education. When friends discuss sexuality on the street corner, that too is health education. However, some settings are more apt to result in accurate information. These settings are usually those specifically established for health instruction. Obviously, the street corner and even the home do not meet this criterion. The street corner too often leads to beliefs based on misconception; and the home, although more likely to present valid information, too often passes along inaccurate family and/or cultural beliefs that are inconsistent with current knowledge. This does not mean you cannot acquire accurate health information on the street corner or from friends and relatives. It is not the setting that is the problem here, so much as it is the competence and knowledge of the person conveying the information. Generally speaking, people associated with formalized health education programs possess more accurate health information than the lay public.

In addition to the accuracy of information that they convey, formalized health education programs are often more conducive to learning than are programs in other settings. For example, a classroom that is organized and relatively quiet is more conducive to learning about health than is the bathroom at home, with siblings arguing about the need to use it and Dad also needing to shave. Furthermore, when the setting is specifically designed and designated for health education, the focus is more likely to be on that topic. Everyone knows (or at least should know) why they are there, and distractions can be held to a minimum.

The formalized settings that are typically established for health education include academic, community, workplace, and medical care facilities (such as hospitals and health maintenance organizations). Each of these settings is discussed here.

The Academic Setting

There are both advantages and disadvantages to any setting in which health education is conducted, and the academic setting is no exception.

Advantages   Health educators in academic settings often have a captive audience. That is, often students have to complete a health education course to graduate. If health education credit is not a school requirement, at least students have to attend school, thereby providing the health educator with a good chance of attracting students to the program — they have to take some course, so why not an interesting one like health education?

In addition, the school health education budget is usually fairly fixed: teachers know about how much they will have from year to year (even though those amounts are often inadequate). Fixed budgets allow for better planning than budgets subject to wild yearly fluctuations.

Also, the fact that learners are in their developmental years means the impact of health education may be significant, and there is less need to work with learners to unlearn unhealthful behaviors and lifestyles. The opportunity to help mold learners' health values and affect their health behaviors is relished by many health educators and considered a most meaningful responsibility.

Other advantages of health education in academic settings relate to the body of literature in this area and the professional organizations available to help. For example, the *Journal of School Health* and the *American Journal of Health Education* contain many practical articles that can be quite useful to the academic health educator. These journals and others also publish articles describing research studies that lend guidance to the practice of health education in academic settings. Professional organizations such as the American School Health Association and the American Association for Health Education conduct meetings and publish monographs to help school health educators as well.

These and other health education organizations have published National Health Education Standards (American Cancer Society 1995) to provide a foundation for curriculum development, instruction, and assessment of student performance in school health education programs. These standards are presented in Appendix E at the conclusion of this book. Standards in health education are designed to help students achieve national health objectives.

Several widely used and effective national school health education curricula are available for either wholesale adoption or local adaptation. *Growing Healthy* (formerly the *Primary Grades Curriculum Project* and the *School Health Curriculum Project*) is an example of such a curriculum. Others have also been evaluated as quite effective (Abt Associates 1985).

Disadvantages   The disadvantages of health education in the academic setting are several. As previously noted, the budget for health education is often disgraceful; that is, it is not adequate enough for the health education program to accomplish its objectives. Unfortunately, health education is too often considered a "fringe" subject, not as important as English, mathematics, or history. Consequently, limited resources often mean that health education is served last.

Not only is the budget affected by this perception, but so is the time allocated to health instruction. The crowded curriculum often dictates that health education be given only limited instructional time, if any. Several states do not even require health education. A national survey of school health education (the School Health Education Policies and Programs Study) found that 10 percent of states do not require health education. At the elementary school level, only 10 percent of all states require a separate course devoted to health education; at the middle/junior high school level only 28 percent of all states require a separate health education course; and at the senior high school level only 55 percent require a separate course. Furthermore, only 55 percent of all school districts have a school health education director (Collins et al. 1995).

Even when health education is taught, it is often taught by unqualified instructors. Only 69 percent of states require health education certification for secondary school health education teachers, and only

6 percent of states require such certification for elementary school teachers who teach health education (Collins et al. 1995).

The population that academic health educators work with also places limitations on the program's perceived effectiveness. By and large, that population consists of healthy, young males and females. Consequently, the effects of health education are difficult to objectively determine. That is, the goal is usually to maintain good health (no change) rather than to recover from illness or disease (a change that can be measured).

Academic health educators argue that the result of their instruction is that their students form attitudes and develop skills that will serve them throughout their adult lives, and that expecting to measure these effects is either naive or unrealistic. Though this may be true, the problem is that health educators in academic settings are placed in the unenviable position of not being able to demonstrate any significant impact of their programs. That makes it difficult to argue for more time in the curriculum or more dollars from the budget. The fringe-subject status ascribed to health education means that even though mathematics and history educators, for example, do not have to demonstrate the immediate utility of their disciplines, health educators do. The difficulty of measuring long-term benefits of health education in academic settings and important short-term effects are two disadvantages of working with a young and healthy population.

Finally, health educators are too often restricted in the content with which they can deal or in the manner in which they can present this content. Several years ago, I conducted a study of the effects of a high school unit on homosexuality. One part of the unit called for representatives from the local Mattachine Society—a group consisting of homosexuals—to visit class as guest speakers. When I originally discussed the research project with the school's principal, he objected to homosexuals visiting class. Disappointed but not beaten, I suggested that we videotape an interview with representative homosexuals as opposed to bringing them to class. The principal would not agree to that either, fearing objection from the students' parents. Almost in jest, I then suggested we audiotape an interview with these homosexuals and, lo and behold, the principal agreed! It seems that this principal believed it okay to hear homosexuals but not okay to see them! Interestingly, when the unit was presented, the only objection raised by either students or parents was by one father who suggested that the next time the unit was offered it might be a good idea to bring some homosexuals to class to speak with the students. Many academic health educators have similar stories about being specifically prohibited from presenting certain topics—for example, abortion, contraception, or morality—or from presenting these or other topics in certain ways—for example, values clarification instructional activities. Such restrictions are less prevalent in other settings.

The Community and Public Health Setting

Health education is also conducted by government agencies, community health departments, voluntary health agencies (for example, the American Heart Association), and for-profit organizations. It is not surprising that even in programs conducted in the community there are both advantages and disadvantages.

Advantages Usually community and public health education programs target readily identifiable and legitimate community needs. For example, educational programs to alert the community to the dangers of lead poisoning from lead-based paint can have a significant effect on the health of children in that community. As a result, health educators can get the sense that their activities are valuable and valued.

Another advantage of community health education programs concerns the voluntary nature of the program's participants. Unlike schoolchildren, individuals enrolling in community health education programs generally do so because they want to, not solely because they are required to do so. The result is that they are usually highly motivated to learn and to incorporate what they learn into their daily lives. Working with such motivated learners is a real peak experience for health educators.

Resources are also readily available to the community and public health educator. These resources can take the form of professional organizations—such as the American Public Health Association or the Society for Public Health Education—or professional journals such as the *American Journal of Public Health* or the *Journal of Community Health.* This advantage of community health education settings is not insignificant, especially when one is at a loss as to how to organize or evaluate a program. Still another advantage develops out of the appreciation that the potential participants for any program must be recruited to that program. Consequently, community and public health educators often have a budget—small though it may be—to advertise and market their programs. Brochures, mailings, and media advertisements may be developed to attract participants and make the program cost effective.

Recently there has been renewed appreciation for the potential of community health education. For example, in 1995 the Pew Health Professions Commission published the results of a study concerning how the health professions could meet the challenges of the twenty-first century. Among the recommendations was to "restructure the mission and organization of allied health education programs to focus on local community health needs identified through partnerships with delivery systems, professional associations, educators, regulators, consumers, and the public" (Pew Health Professions Commission 1995, vii). Everyone interested in health education, regardless of the setting in which it is practiced, ought to read this report.

An organization has been formed to foster partnerships between communities and campuses around health issues. This organization, Community–Campus Partnerships for Health (CCPH), publishes reports, identifies funding sources to support these partnerships, and maintains a listserv for its members. CCPH can be reached on the Internet at http://www.futurehealth.ucsf.edu/ccph.html.

Disadvantages   One of the most serious disadvantages of health education in community and public health settings pertains to the perception of the health educator. Often the most underserved community members and the most needy are those who may also feel alienated from the community's institutions. When the health educator is seen as a representative of the "establishment" from which the potential participants feel alienated, recruiting for health education programs may be more difficult and frustrating. Even if program participants can be recruited, they may remain suspicious of the health educator, and the educational process may therefore be uncomfortable and ineffective.

In addition, community health education may suffer from a "second cousin" image, as we found was the case in the academic health education setting. The result may be insufficient funding, facilities, or equipment. Health education with suspicious and distrusting populations is difficult enough. To compound the difficulty with inadequate facilities and equipment seems especially cruel and unjust. This too often occurs because administrators of community health programs themselves may not know what health education is or what skills health educators can bring to their organizations.

Another disadvantage is that the programs usually have to go to the people. We have already seen that those most in need of the programs are probably from disadvantaged neighborhoods, so that means the health educator may have to frequent unsafe areas of the community. Placing oneself in jeopardy of physical harm is certainly a disadvantage of community and public health education settings. On the other hand, too often community health educators exaggerate such danger because they are unfamiliar with the neighborhoods. That is, health educators are, by definition, educated. Most probably grew up in neighborhoods that afforded them the opportunity to become educated. Consequently, many may not be familiar with other environments, and that fear of the unknown can be disconcerting.

Serious-minded and caring health educators may also find the problems in particular communities to be so severe that no remedy seems available. The frustration about not being able to make a meaningful (at least to the desired degree) impact on the lives of the community's members may make the job intolerable. The only action that may be evident is to become an activist in the community, and that requires a great deal of time and energy and may threaten the career development of the health educator (for example, being promoted or rehired).

The Medical Care Setting

Health education occurring in medical care settings such as hospitals, health maintenance organizations, and physicians' offices has several advantages over programs conducted in other settings and several disadvantages as well.

Advantages   When a health educator is perceived as part of the health care team, program participants may ascribe greater status and more expertise to that person. Consequently, participants may be more attentive and more likely to follow the advice conveyed by the health educator. In addition, program participants may be more motivated to learn and to work on adopting healthful behaviors because they are in a medical setting, often because of some diagnosed health problem. Health educators can then pretty much ignore the need to convince program participants of the worthiness of the actions recommended and can instead devote most of the instructional time to strategies to help the patient comply with these recommendations. Instructing motivated program participants can also be motivating and stimulating for the health educator.

Furthermore, because many program participants in medical care settings will have some identifiable health malady, the health educator often feels as though the instructional time is very meaningful. That is, actions recommended can have a significant and relatively immediate effect on the health of the participants. For most of us, meaningful, important work is rewarding in itself, and more so if that work has beneficial value for others.

In conducting health education in medical settings, health educators have at their disposal a unique set of resources. They have the backup of expert health specialists—for example, physicians, nurses, and laboratory technicians—who can enliven and embellish the instructional process. Imagine the effect of pretesting program participants and then retesting them some time after the program to demonstrate the changes their new health behaviors have brought. For example, analyzing blood samples for amounts of blood fats prior to the start of a nutrition program can validate new diets program participants adopt. Measuring the effect of an exercise program on blood pressure can reinforce a continuation of exercising.

In addition to medical resources, health educators in medical care settings often have the financial and logistical resources to advertise their programs and obtain sufficient enrollment. It is not unusual, for example, to see notices posted in hospital corridors announcing health education programs, or to be handed a flyer from a physician describing an upcoming program. Health maintenance organizations and other prepaid health insurance or health care entities also readily publish announcements of health education sessions they are offering.

Working in managed care organizations has its own particular advantages. Theoretically, these organizations make more money by keeping enrollees healthy so they do not have to access health care. Reasoning that it costs less to teach people preventive health behaviors than to care for them after they become ill, managed care organizations are willing to invest in health education and promotion activities. Consequently, health educators working in this setting may be perceived as an important cog in a machine designed to be profitable. Because profitability is consistent with helping people maintain their health, there is no ethical dilemma faced by the health educator. More profit, better health — and everyone wins.

Disadvantages   Although health educators in medical care settings can be perceived by patients and other program participants as part of the health care team, within the team itself they are often considered and treated as second-class citizens. Too often only after other resources — for example, room assignments or funds — are doled out does the health education program get its share. When budget cuts become necessary, the health education program is often the first to feel the purse strings tighten. This treatment can be disheartening and frustrating for the health educator, and many have left positions because of this situation. Too often this is due to administrators in medical care settings not understanding the potential contribution health education can bring to their programs.

Another frustration for the medical care setting health educator is the lack of compliance with recommendations. It is well known that significant numbers of patients do not follow prescribed medication regimens; they either forget to take their medication or decide they no longer need it once they begin feeling a little better. Health education programs have been demonstrated effective in motivating patients to adhere to physician recommendations. However, many patients still do not comply. One need only visit the cardiology wing of a large hospital and notice the patients and visitors who are overweight or who order fatty foods in the hospital cafeteria to find cause for the kind of frustration experienced by health educators in these settings.

To make matters even worse, program participants in medical care settings are often already ill. As we discussed, that can be an advantage because many are motivated. However, for health educators who believe the best approach is to prevent illness in the first place, the focus on disease can be irksome. When patients are ill to the point of not being able ever again to regain their health — for example, with emphysema — and can be helped only to maintain the status they presently have, health educators further confront the limitations of their capabilities.

Last, when the program is considered a fringe and not an integral part of the total operation, it becomes even more imperative to justify its existence by cost–benefit analyses. The difficulty of demonstrating the cost benefit of a program that affects many variables that are not easily quantifiable has already been discussed. The health educator, then, may find himself or herself in the unenviable position of being threatened fairly regularly with program elimination at worst or severe curtailment at best.

The Worksite Setting

Health education in the workplace does not escape having both advantages and disadvantages specific to its setting.

Advantages   One of the most significant benefits of conducting health education at places of work is the support that often accompanies such programs. If unions can be recruited to back the program, management will often join in as well; and with the support of these two groups, workers will usually value the educational program available to them. Even when union support is not obtained, if upper management can be offered the program, and the program is a good one, they often will arrange for the program to be more widely distributed in the workplace. With management's support, adequate facilities are usually made available, and necessary instructional materials can be acquired.

The availability of microcomputers and health education software has transformed some physician and clinic waiting areas into ideal settings for health education.

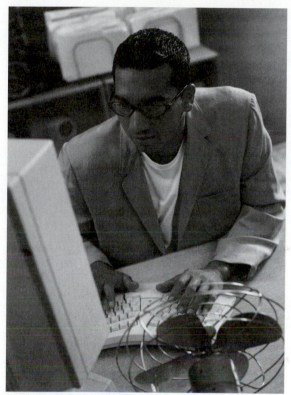

Source: Ryan McVay/Getty Images/PhotoDisc

Since businesses exist to make money, the rationale for all of their activities typically is the profit motive. Businesses that adopt occupational health education programs believe that the benefits (such as recruiting and retention; favorable publicity; the increase in worker productivity resulting from healthier workers and therefore less absenteeism; and the decrease in the use of insurable health care, resulting in a lower health insurance premium) will outweigh the cost of the program (Aldana 2001; Jee et al. 2001; Pronk et al. 1999). Consequently, there often is an initial high level of commitment to these health education programs to help them fully achieve these goals.

In addition, because participation in occupational health education programs is usually voluntary, workers who volunteer are usually motivated to adopt more healthful lifestyles. It is a pleasure for health educators to work with program participants who are so motivated. The focus of the educational sessions can then be on the health content rather than motivational strategies.

Last, businesses that commit to an occupational health education program also commit to offering that program to as wide a distribution of workers within that company as possible. If the program will save money for the organization, why not save lots of money? Consequently, a marketing budget is

Employees are often encouraged to join groups of other employees to enhance their physical fitness. Some companies have extensive physical fitness facilities on site, while others have fitness facilities nearby.

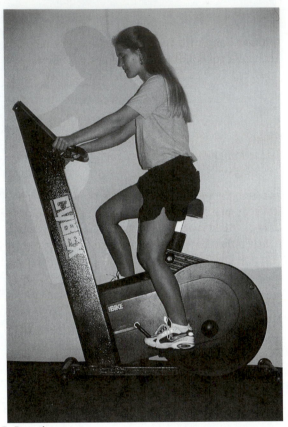

Source: Courtesy William E. Prentice

usually available to recruit program participants. Posters placed around the workplace and advertisement brochures or flyers mailed to workers are not unusual.

Disadvantages   If the health education program is perceived as a management ploy to get greater productivity from the workers rather than to respond to their needs, suspicion and distrust can develop, which can interfere with achievement of the program's objectives. It won't be much longer before the program is then discarded. This is not an unusual occurrence, especially if management and the health educator have not anticipated it and, therefore, have not attempted to involve all potentially affected groups in the planning stages.

Health education in this setting is also limited in the health content areas with which it deals. Sexuality education, for instance, is usually not one of the concerns in the business setting, and even though workers could benefit by education in this area, it is not offered. Topics most frequently associated with occupational health education are alcohol and drugs, hypertension and cardiovascular health, stress, physical fitness, cancer prevention, mental health, and safety and emergency medical care (O'Donnell 1997).

The staff of occupational health education programs is often quite small. It is not unusual to find relatively large organizations hiring just one or two health educators who are responsible for planning and implementing the program. The evaluation component, if it exists at all, is often a function of some other entity within the company. It must be remembered, though, that health educators need to evaluate programs as they are being conducted and again shortly thereafter to be able to identify adjustments that may be necessary to achieve program objectives. The workload that results from understaffing large programs in this manner is often a frustration expressed by occupational health educators.

Given these limitations, to be held accountable for cost benefits is unfair to health educators. And yet in the business setting this is often expected. Making this situation even more irksome is the realization that many benefits resulting from the program are not quantifiable — for example, employee morale or the effects of the program on the families of the workers. When health educators "sell" worksite health education on the basis of its cost benefit — that is, telling management it will save money in the long run — they must expect to be held accountable for the realization of that expectation. However, it is often difficult or impossible to achieve identifiable cost benefits given the staffing, limitations on content, and other factors (for example, are workers expected to attend the program after or before a workday?).

Last, there may not be long-term employee or employer commitment to the program. Given the difficulty of demonstrating a cost benefit, the threat of "pulling the plug" on the program at any time always exists. Since the program's objectives and activities are often not directly related to the company's production goals, its relevance is constantly being tested, and its existence threatened. To live under the ax in this way is not appealing to many health educators and may not be healthful for them!

Planning for Health Education

Once the setting in which health education is to be conducted is identified, the next step involves planning the program. This necessitates that a needs assessment be done, objectives be developed, and other program components be selected.

Needs Assessment

In every health education setting, unique features need to be identified through a *needs assessment*. Green and Anderson (1982, 87–92) outline the following necessary steps as part of the planning for health education:

1. *Social diagnosis* — Determining the social concerns of the people for whom the program will be developed. This can be accomplished through interviews or through an inspection of relevant data (for example, statistics on the pregnancy rate in a community or on its rate of unemployment).

2. *Epidemiological diagnosis* — Reviewing health statistics to determine the health problems of the people for whom the program is being developed. Subpopulations — such as different ages or races — should be studied to see if unique needs exist; if so, the program should take these into account.

3. *Behavioral diagnosis*—Identification of the behavioral problems or barriers to good health. For example, what is the rate of cigarette smoking, how early in pregnancies is prenatal care usually sought, or how well are safety rules followed?

4. *Educational diagnosis*—Determining how much knowledge potential program participants have regarding health and related issues, and which health-related skills they possess.

5. *Administrative diagnosis*—Assessment of the resources available to achieve the program's objectives—for example, the budget, resource people and organizations in the community, and the level of staffing.

A needs assessment, then, "involves the collection of data concerning a population of interest regarding (1) their health problems, needs, and concerns; (2) behaviors related to those health problems, needs, and concerns; and (3) the determinants associated with those health behaviors" (Greene and Simons-Morton 1984, 33). These data can and should be obtained in various ways: interviews, questionnaires, focus group meetings, administration of standardized tests, literature searches, and inspection of health and other statistics relative to the population for whom the program is being planned.

Just looking at needs, though is not enough. Assets or resources should also be identified for several reasons. First, a "needs-only" approach is incomplete. It ignores the existing community resources available to respond to the needs. Second, it is disparaging. In any community there are both needs and assets. To focus only on the needs connotes that the health educator is coming into this "needy" community, with outside resources, to solve *their* problem. A more acceptable approach is to consider the community's needs with community representatives who know that community best, together identify projects and objectives designed to respond to these needs, and then identify and employ community resources that can contribute to the satisfaction of these needs. This approach connotes working *with* the community rather than working *on* the community. The result will be a better relationship between the health educator and members of the community, and more effective community and public health programs. After the needs assessment and identification of community assets, program objectives can then be developed.

Developing Objectives

Program participants should be involved in the development of the program objectives. Not to do so is to chance being undemocratic and ineffective. Furthermore, the validity of these objectives—their appropriateness for the population being served—will be enhanced by involving the learners in their development, and learners' commitment to achieving the objectives will be greater.

Writing Measurable Objectives   To develop objectives that provide guidance for the conduct of the program and for its evaluation requires a special skill. Too many planners of health education programs ignore the importance of writing objectives carefully, only to find later that they are at a disadvantage because they either promised more than they intended or they wrote objectives that could not be evaluated, thereby leaving them unable to demonstrate the program's effectiveness. As one expert on objectives puts it, "If you are teaching skills that cannot be evaluated, you are in the awkward position of being unable to demonstrate that you are teaching anything at all" (Mager 1962, 47).

To write a measurable objective, Mager recommends three criteria (1962, 12):

1. Identify the terminal behavior—that is, what the learner will be expected to do at the end of the learning experience.

2. Describe the important conditions under which the behavior will be expected to occur.

3. Specify the criteria of acceptable performance — that is, how well the learner must perform to be acceptable.

An example of a health instructional objective that Mager might be expected to approve is "Given two different people — one with a diet high in saturated fats and with a sedentary lifestyle, and the other with a diet rich in fruits and vegetables and who is physically active — the program participant can identify which person is at greater risk for coronary heart disease."

If stated more generally, such an objective might be impossible to evaluate adequately. In this objective, the terminal behavior is to "identify which person is at greater risk of coronary heart disease"; the important condition is "given two different people — one with a diet high in saturated fats and with a sedentary lifestyle, and the other with a diet rich in fruits and vegetables and who is physically active"; and the criteria for acceptable performance is implied in that the program participant should identify the person at greater risk each and every time (total accuracy).

Objectives may be written for cognitive learning (knowledge), affective development (emotions, feelings), or the psychomotor domain (skills, behavior). Using HIV education as an example, here are objectives illustrative of these three areas:

1. The participant will be able to list three behaviors that are known to put one at risk of HIV infection (cognitive domain).

2. Given a scenario describing a situation in which a woman insists on a male partner's wearing a condom but the partner refuses, the program participant will state that the woman should refuse to engage in the sexual activity (affective domain).

3. The participant will be able to place a condom on a model of a penis so that there is room left at the tip of the model penis for the accumulation of semen (psychomotor domain).

The PRECEDE Model   One way to make use of educational objectives is to use the popular model for program planning developed by Green and associates (Green et al. 1980). It is called the PRECEDE model and consists of predisposing, enabling, and reinforcing factors. The model requires the program planner to identify factors that should be included in the program that can *predispose* the learners to achieving the health education objective — such as knowledge, attitudes, values, and perceptions; factors that will *enable* the learners to incorporate the objectives into their health styles — such as the availability and accessibility of resources, referrals, and skills; and the factors that will *reinforce* healthful lifestyles — such as attitudes and behavior of other health personnel, parents, and employers.

By way of example, let's consider a stress management program offered for high school students. The knowledge students would need to be able to manage their stress and the attitudes and values that would help them do that would need to be identified. These would be the predisposing factors. Next, having access to a relaxation lounge in the school and learning how to meditate (a relaxation skill) would enable students to adopt effective stress management strategies. These would be the enabling factors. Educating parents and schoolteachers regarding the need to encourage students to regularly practice their stress management skills would reinforce that behavior. These would be the reinforcing factors. The PRECEDE model, then, provides guidance for the planning of health education programs.

The PRECEDE model has since been expanded into PRECEDE–PROCEDE (Green and Kreuter 1999) to account for the broader mandate of health promotion. PROCEDE stands for "policy, regulatory, and organizational constructs in educational and environmental development." Once the PRECEDE portion had been developed, the PROCEDE portion is designed to "promote the plan or policy, regulate the environment, and organize the resources and services, as required by the plan or policy" (Green and Kreuter 1999).

Implementation

Once the program is planned, it must be implemented. Implementation involves "bringing programs into reality" (Greene and Simons-Morton 1984, 33). That requires consideration of funding, facilities, equipment, scheduling, and marketing.

Funding

Without adequate funding, achievement of program objectives is problematic. Funds are needed to hire staff, and the more funds for this purpose, the larger and more qualified the staff will be. Funds are needed to purchase instructional materials (for example, videotapes or slides), and the more funds for this purpose, the more instructional equipment will be available and the better that equipment will be. Funds are also needed to advertise and market the program. Certainly, effective programs have been conducted on shoestring budgets, but those are the exceptions rather than the rule. With inadequate funding, program objectives should be scaled back to what is realistic and feasible. If not, the program will be set up for failure, people's expectations will not be met, and support for the program may erode.

Facilities

If school health education is conducted in the gymnasium with basketballs bouncing around, it will be difficult for significant learning to take place. If patient education programs are conducted adjacent to the emergency room, with constant traveling in and out of medical personnel and other patients, learning will be impaired. And if worksite health education is offered next to a noisy factory production area, significant learning will be difficult.

Distractions aside, the location of the facility can create a problem. For example, if an alcohol education program is offered to workers who have a drinking problem in a room next to the shop foreman's office, workers may not sign up for the program because of the fear of being identified as alcoholics and of the effect that might have on their promotions, raises, or other job factors.

For health education to have a chance of success, facilities should be well ventilated, temperature controlled, and well lit. Distractions should be kept to a minimum and the classroom should be attractive.

Equipment

Health education programs that don't actively involve learners ignore one of the cardinal laws of learning: learners learn best by doing. Too often health educators will convey a great deal of information by lecturing, thinking they have taught a lot. However, there may be a large gap between the educators presenting information and students learning that information. If the educational sessions are varied, students' attention will be taxed less than if not. One way of varying the instruction is to use equipment to show slides or PowerPoint presentations, to run computer health educational games, or to play audio-

Many different types of instructional materials are available to liven up health education. For example, some excellent software has been developed to teach health-related topics to program participants in a way in which they remain interested and motivated.

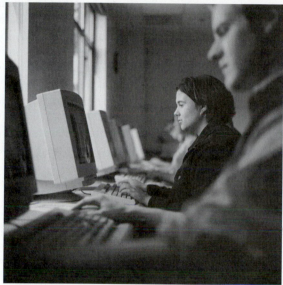

Source: Ryan McVay/Getty Images/PhotoDisc

and videocassettes. Video- and audiocassette tape recorders, synchronized slide/tape players, overhead projectors, computers, and carousel slide projectors can help enliven instruction, result in more learning because students are paying attention for longer periods, and achieve more of the program's objectives. Without the variation this equipment can provide, instructional sessions too often become boring and ineffectual. That need not be the case, however. The following chapters delineate activities that do not require equipment and that activate learners. Still, instructional equipment can add much to the program.

Scheduling

The time of day when the program is conducted can significantly influence how successful it will be. For example, a worksite health education program held during regular work hours, with workers being released from their usual work tasks to attend, will generally be more successful than a program conducted either after work hours or before. A school health education class scheduled just after lunch or physical education can mean students will be more inattentive and more difficult to get on task than a class scheduled at some other time. A patient education session conducted with patients before they are treated—for example, prior to surgery—will find different learners than one held after treatment. Although health educators do not always control when their programs are scheduled, they should at least take scheduling into account when planning the instructional sessions and the strategies they will employ during these sessions.

Marketing

In some health education settings, recruitment of program participants is not of concern. For example, when students are required to take health education in order to graduate, there is no need to advertise the program and attract students to it. However, in other settings recruitment becomes a major issue. In fact, some programs' existence and some health educators' jobs depend on the ability to attract program participants. Usually, when this is the case, a budget is provided to help recruit program participants, with funds being used for publishing brochures and flyers announcing the program, advertisements in local newspapers, and posters hung in places where prospective program participants congregate. Other useful marketing strategies include press releases to the news media (print as well as radio and television), contacts of community groups (religious organizations, fraternal orders, and cooperative service groups), and personal contact with community leaders. When developing marketing strategies, involve community leaders and have them help identify places to announce the program, people who should be notified of its existence, and the manner in which the announcement should be stated (which community needs should be appealed to and what language should be used in making that appeal).

Evaluation

In order to determine a program's effect on its participants, it must be evaluated. To modify the program to better achieve its objectives, it must be evaluated. And to justify the continued existence of the program, it must be evaluated. For all of these reasons, health educators should pay particular attention to the evaluation process and should consider it an integral component of their programs.

Evaluation can relate to the outcomes identified in the objectives or the processes employed to achieve these objectives. The former is termed *outcome evaluation,* and the latter is termed *process evaluation.*

Outcome Evaluation

If objectives are stated in a way that allows for the measurement of their achievement, the evaluation of objectives becomes relatively easy. It is when they have been globally stated in such a way that measurement is not possible that a problem develops. In that case, just what to evaluate is uncertain because the objective itself is uncertain. However, let's assume the objectives are measurable. Then the changes in learners' health knowledge, attitudes, skills, and/or behaviors, previously identified as objectives, need to be determined. This can be accomplished in several ways. For example, knowledge tests administered before and after instruction can identify increases in knowledge that have occurred. Psychological inventories or scales (for example, self-esteem scales, alienation scales, or locus of control scales) administered pre- and postinstruction can identify attitudinal changes. Tests of skills (such as CPR, brushing and flossing, behaving assertively, and resistance skills) can determine the program's effects on the ability to perform certain health-related behaviors. And self-report behavioral inventories can be used to find out if the program had any impact on the participants' actual health-related behaviors.

Process Evaluation

A dilemma arises when the evaluation determines that the outcome objectives have not been achieved. What led to that unfortunate finding? Was it the nature of the objectives? For instance, were they unachievable given the amount of available instructional time? Was it a problem with the instructional strategies employed? Were they ineffective in motivating students? Or was it the instructional materials that were used? Were they below or above the comprehension of the program's participants? In order to be able to use the evaluation to improve the health education program, the components of the program must also be evaluated. This type of evaluation is called *process evaluation* (Windsor et al. 1994; McDermott and Sarvela 1999).

Process evaluations involve techniques that are somewhat different from those used for outcome evaluations. Feedback from students regarding the components of the health education program may be sought through questionnaires or interviews. In this way, problems with the objectives, content, instructional strategies, or instructional materials can be identified. In addition, evaluation of the educational process may be obtained from parents, other school or worksite personnel (for example, other teachers or administrators), or from the health educator who conducted the program. This is not to say that more objective evaluations of the educational process cannot be obtained. It is also possible, for instance, to administer a reading comprehension measure (for example, the SMOG Index) to the written program materials to determine whether they are at an appropriate level for the learners. Or it may be possible to ask a panel of experts (perhaps health educators at the local college) to judge the program's content for accuracy or its relevance to the learners.

Formative and Summative Evaluation

When evaluation occurs in the midst of a program with the intent of using that information to revise the program as it is ongoing, that evaluation is called *formative evaluation*. When evaluation occurs at the completion of a program in order to determine its effectiveness in achieving program objectives, that evaluation is called *summative evaluation*. Both forms of evaluation are valuable and should be employed by health educators in all settings. In this way, programs can be revised immediately if necessary to be more responsive to their participants and can be revised at their completion to be more effective for the next group of participants.

Evaluation of Long-Range Objectives

A word needs to be mentioned here about the difficulty of evaluating long-range health education objectives. Health educators argue that it is unfair to ignore the effects of their programs on learners many years after being enrolled in their programs, and yet these effects cannot be measured. There are just too many intervening years and variables for this analysis. Furthermore, they argue, how can the potential for health education be determined if these programs are understaffed, the staff are inadequately trained, and the programs are underfunded and relegated to a low priority by employers, administrators, parents, and/or students? Such problems for the valid evaluation of health education programs need to be recognized, even if solutions are not readily forthcoming.

Summary

1. Health education can take place in various settings. Some of the more usual settings are academic settings, the community, the medical care setting, and the workplace.

2. Each setting in which health education occurs has both advantages and disadvantages. These usually pertain to funding and related issues (for example, facilities and equipment made available), status ascribed to the health educator and the program, the needs of the program

participants, the ability to market the program, and accountability for meeting program objectives (including, but not limited to, demonstrating a cost benefit).

3. Planning health education programs necessitates conducting a needs assessment and identification of resources, and developing valid objectives that are stated in a manner that allows for evaluation.

4. Needs assessments collect data concerning the population of interest regarding (a) their health problems, needs, and concerns and (b) behaviors related to those health problems, needs, and concerns. Needs assessments include social, epidemiological, behavioral, educational, and administrative diagnoses.

5. Objectives that are not stated in a manner to allow measurement of their achievement cannot be used to judge the program's success or to determine which parts of the program need to be adjusted. Behavioral objectives identify the terminal behavior, describe the important conditions under which the behavior is expected to occur, and specify the criteria for acceptable performance.

6. The PRECEDE model includes predisposing, enabling, and reinforcing factors and provides a framework that can be used to plan health education programs. In 1991 the PRECEDE model was expanded into PRECEDE–PROCEDE (Green and Kreuter 1991) to account for the broader mandate of health promotion. PROCEDE stands for "policy, regulatory, and organizational constructs in educational and environmental development."

7. The implementation of health education programs depends on the level of funding, the availability and nature of facilities, the ability to purchase instructional materials and equipment, factors related to scheduling, and the resources necessary to advertise and market the program.

8. Evaluation of health education programs is necessary to determine their effectiveness and to provide guidance for adjusting and improving program components. Evaluation can focus on program outcomes (outcome evaluation) or on the educational processes (process evaluation).

PART TWO

PREREQUISITE INSTRUCTIONAL STRATEGIES

GROUP PROCESS AND THE EXPLORATION OF VALUES AND HEALTH

This section describes numerous ways in which the important knowledge and skills of working in groups and of understanding one's values can be learned. Because researchers tell us people learn best by doing, each activity is designed to actively involve the program participants during the learning process.

The importance of learning how groups function, which roles group members play, and how to be a functional group member is related to the instructional activities presented later in this book. Many of these activities require the learners to participate in groups, and for those groups to be most effective, group members must contribute to their functioning. In addition, the role of the instructor in the group is also discussed. The chapter on group process is designed to accomplish this goal.

Furthermore, many of the instructional activities that follow require program participants to express their values regarding health-related issues. These values often dictate which behaviors they adopt and which they don't. The chapter on values and health helps learners identify which values are most operative for them, thereby helping them better understand their health-related decisions.

CHAPTER SIX

Instructional Strategies for Development of Group Process Skills and the Learning Environment

Requisite to learner-centered educational processes are human relations skills. To expect learners to initiate and conduct their own learning activities without prior human relations training seems unrealistic. For program participants to function effectively as a group, they must be acquainted with group dynamics and able to operate as productive group members (Goldman 2000). This chapter consists of learner-centered activities that health education programs may use to develop the following requisites to subsequent learner-centered instruction:

1. Familiarity with and trust in other program participants.
2. Friendship with at least one other participant.
3. Listening skills.
4. Knowledge of and experience with roles assumed by members and leaders of groups.
5. Knowledge of and experience with the decision-making process.
6. Cooperation and participation among all members of the program.
7. An understanding and appreciation of both one's own feelings and the feelings of others.
8. Open communication among disagreeing factions and empathy with those of opposing viewpoints.
9. Recognition of unfulfilled needs of program participants and of the means of satisfying those needs.
10. Appreciation of individual differences and of unique potentials.

We start off with the role of the health education instructor and his or her responsibility for developing a climate conducive to learning.

Various Roles of the Instructor

The health education instructor will initially be viewed as the person with all the answers. By the nature of his or her position, the instructor is usually depended on for health information, clarification of misconceptions, and the organization and conducting of program sessions. In terms of health education as freeing, this view of the instructor may be dysfunctional. When the instructor selects the content to be learned, time restraints dictate that certain content must be omitted. Some ethicists have described that process as coercive and manipulative in that it allows for the shaping of attitudes and behaviors. For example, if a tobacco education program does not consider the relaxation many people describe as a benefit of smoking, it is one-sided and inconsistent with the concept of health education as freeing.

Therefore, the learning climate established by the health educator is of vital importance. Program participants should feel free to suggest additional content, to search out other sources of health information and opinion, and to disagree with the instructor and/or other program participants. To do so, they must feel comfortable and unthreatened in the class. To get them to this point is the responsibility of the health educator. Several instructional activities are presented here that can accomplish this end.

Developing Trust among Program Participants

One of the most important roles of the health educator is to help program participants trust one another and the instructor. Several activities to develop this trust are described next.

Introduction Skits

If sessions are to be conducted in an open, informal manner, and if program participants are expected to verbally interact, then the more each person knows about every other person, the better each can evaluate what is being stated. It is often helpful to know where a person stands when he or she speaks. Another point worth mentioning is that we tend to fear that which is strange to us. We are more likely to fear—or at least be uneasy with—things or people we don't know than those we do know. Prejudice is often a result of inaccurate generalizations directed at strange people—people we don't know very well.

To build trust among program participants, then, it is recommended that they know one another. Of course, one class period is not sufficient time for learners to feel comfortable with one another. As the history of a group develops, however, trust can be developed—thereby enhancing an open, informal, verbally active class format. A beginning of this process can take several directions. It is possible for each person to stand up in class and mention a few facts or thoughts about himself or herself. It is possible for one person who knows another person to introduce that person to the group. However, a more interesting activity can be organized.

Divide program participants into groups of six members each. With 20 minutes' preparation time, each group is responsible for presenting a three-minute skit that will introduce the members of that group. During the author's experience with this technique, several interesting skits were developed. One group role-played a drug raid, with one person playing a policeman who asked the others questions about their lives as he was searching them for drugs. Another group established one student as psychiatrist and the others as patients who one by one visited the psychiatrist's office to talk about their lives.

The health educator or the learners may decide to associate a particular theme with the skits. For instance, when the author established a television-show format as the theme for introduction skits, one group set three chairs on a table, another chair on the floor separated from the table, and three other chairs by a partition. When three female students sat on the three chairs, the *Dating Game* television format was used to introduce the actors to the class. Another group used a late-night talk-show format with a host who had guests stopping by to be interviewed. Still another group adapted an interview of famous sports figures by a television sportscaster to help learn something about group members. A variation of this approach would allow time for the class to direct questions at group members to get to know them better.

Pyramiding for Introductions

Introduction skits introduce group members to one another. Though these introductions are initially useful, their superficiality is evident, and further activity directed at getting to know one another is needed. There are several approaches to this end, but the one the author has found of most worth is pyramiding. In *pyramiding,* the participants are asked to look at someone in the group that they know, then forget that person and choose someone they do not know very well to be their partner. Each pair is told that they are to discuss no other topic than themselves — their aspirations, family history, interests, and so on. After 20 minutes of this, each pair is to combine with another pair to form quartets. On combining, each person must introduce his or her original partner to the new pair. Once these introductions have been made, the members of each quartet begin a freewheeling discussion about themselves. After another 15 minutes, quartets can be combined to form octets (groups of 8); then these can become groups of 16; then 32; and so on.

A variation of this approach is to be concerned with content as well as process by suggesting a topic to discuss after introductions. The topic might be any health-related one in which the participants are interested. As an example of this type of pyramiding, the instructor requires students to form pairs and talk only about themselves for 10 minutes. At the conclusion of that time, the teacher asks the pairs to direct their discussion to the question: How can I be safer as a pedestrian (or any other health education–related topic)? After 15 minutes of discussing this issue, the original pair combines with another pair to form a quartet. The quartet members begin their discussion by talking only about themselves (*not* the health-related topic) until they feel properly introduced. When they feel comfortable with one another, they discuss the content question. Pyramiding might also be used more than once to allow all group members to meet one another in pairs or quartets.

The advantages of pyramiding over introduction skits are several. First, the one-to-one basis of the original pairing lets students get to know someone and talk confidentially with that person. No one is eavesdropping, and because the topic is limited to oneself, talking about oneself is perceived to be neither boastful nor in poor taste. Second, each learner is responsible for introducing his or her partner to another pair, so he or she is required to pay attention to what that partner says, and will more readily ask for statements to be clarified. Third, group sizes of two and four provide for and necessitate verbal interaction among all the group members. And last, program participants exit pyramiding feeling secure in that class because they have gotten to know a number of their classmates in an informal, nonpressured setting. Class discussions and learner-centered activities should then be more easily conducted and more educationally rewarding.

Developing a Trusting Learning Environment

Another important characteristic of effective health education is a trusting climate. Developing such a learning atmosphere is the responsibility of the health educator. Several ways to develop a trusting learning environment follow.

Tell Me Statements

Provide program participants with statements to which the pairs, quartets, and so on must respond. These statements can be content oriented. However, statements related to the feelings of each participant will better allow them to get to know one another. The reader can develop statements that would be appropriate to the pyramiding exercise. Statements like the following have been successfully used for this purpose:

1. Tell me something you like.
2. Tell me something you don't like.
3. Tell me something that makes you laugh.
4. Tell me something that makes you cry.
5. Tell me something that frightens you.
6. Tell me something that comforts you.
7. Tell me something you want to say to me.
8. Tell me something you don't want to say to me.

Responses to statements like these will develop discussions of interest and accomplish the objective of establishing rapport among students in the class. It should be noted that each of these statements relates to the feeling level of the participants. No right or wrong answers are possible. The usual "name, rank, and serial number" types of information are omitted, and the participants are free to show what they wish of their inner selves as well as of their already-evidenced exteriors. It should be emphasized throughout that anyone who feels threatened or uncomfortable participating in any of these activities is free to choose *not* to participate.

Trust Test

This exercise affords the health educator the opportunity to test trust in the group. With the group seated in a circle, each person thinks of a problem or secret that he or she does not usually share with others. Without relating that secret to the group, each person goes around the circle telling the group how he or she thinks each other person would respond if the secret were told. In this manner, the degree to which each person is trusted by the group is readily perceived.

Trust Walk

Another way to test trust or to develop trust initially is known as the *trust walk*. In this exercise, people are paired with someone they don't know very well. Each person is then asked to share a concern with his or her partner. After 10 minutes of conversing, each pair is asked to take a walk for 20 minutes. In the first 10 minutes of the walk, one partner must keep his or her eyes closed and is not allowed to talk to the other person, who is leading. After 10 minutes the leader and the blind walker reverse roles. On return, each pair shares their feelings about the exercise. Those who have participated in trust walks often mention that their feeling of trust increased as the walk progressed.

Developing Listening Skills

If program participants do not listen to one another and to the health educator, learning will be minimal. The following activities can help develop listening skills.

It is difficult to trust other people if you do not trust yourself. Some programs, such as Outward Bound, are designed to help participants learn to trust themselves as well as to trust others. Schools, businesses, and other organizations send employees to these programs to enhance their organizations' productivity and provide a more satisfying work environment.

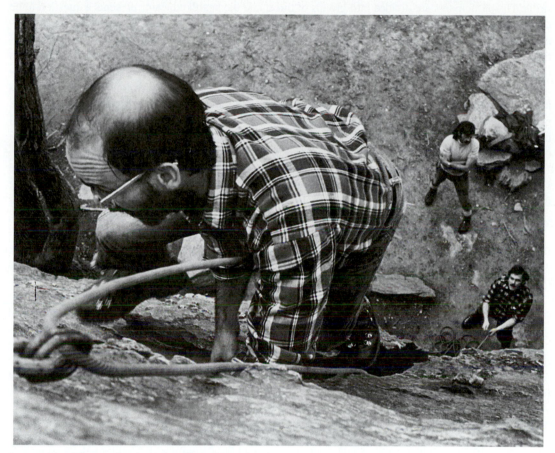

Source: The Diamondback, University of Maryland

Paraphrasing

Though apparently concerned with one another, people have difficulty in listening. To be sure, they hear. But do they listen? This exercise will clearly demonstrate the absence of listening skills typical in program participants and, for that matter, in most people.

First, though, what prevents listening? Most people are so concerned with what they want to say — and with how to word their thoughts — that they can't be bothered with listening to what is being said to them.

Other things prevent listening, too. People who are biased listen to and remember best items that can be used to support that bias. Emotions can also prevent adequate listening. Anger, fear, alarm, and numerous other emotions provoked by a speaker can prevent clear listening.

Speakers who don't define their terms or who use terms inaccurately can easily be misunderstood. The speaker who uses terms inappropriately can be understood if the listener asks for clarification of terms. However, in many instances the listener either applies his or her own definitions to the term or isn't allowed to ask for such clarification.

In any case, paraphrasing can be useful in highlighting listening difficulties and developing listening skills. The participants are divided into groups of three, and the health educator presents a question to be answered in small-group discussion. The question might be, Should marijuana be legalized? or Is abortion moral? or it might pertain to any other health content area. The small groups are to discuss this question for 20 minutes in the following manner: After each participant's comments, subsequent speakers must first paraphrase what was said by the previous speaker — to that speaker's satisfaction — before they can make their comment. If the first speaker does not feel that the paraphrase is accurate, he or she repeats his or her original comments, and the paraphraser must then attempt a new paraphrase. At the outset, group members will have a great deal of difficulty in paraphrasing accurately, due to any one or a combination of the reasons previously cited relating to poor listening skills. To aid the participants in this exercise, they should be told to begin whatever they say with the words, "In other words, you said . . ."

After the question posed by the instructor is discussed for 20 minutes, there should be a 5-minute discussion in the small groups pertaining to the purposes of the paraphrasing exercise. However, during this short discussion, each speaker must continue to paraphrase each previous speaker in offering his or her comments.

At the conclusion of this exercise, a group discussion including the whole class should result in participants understanding their difficulty in listening, and desiring to develop more effective listening skills. A repetition of this exercise periodically throughout the group's history may also be required in order to provide sufficient practice in listening.

Another means of practicing listening requires the instructor to tape-record several television or radio commercials. After they have listened to these tape recordings, program participants can be asked questions to which they can respond correctly only if they have listened carefully to the recordings.

It should be noted that since listening has become such a lost art (if you doubt this statement, conduct these exercises), several repetitions of these activities and periodic referral to them will be required to develop listening skill. However, unless time is spent to develop this skill, the health educator cannot be assured that program participants are really communicating with one another.

Written Conversations

The evident frustration that results when students engage in the paraphrasing exercise can be somewhat alleviated by use of paper–pencil conversations. When the class becomes engaged in an emotional discussion in which it appears that those advocating one position are not listening to those who advocate an opposing position, the teacher can reintroduce the paraphrasing exercise or have the class conduct their conversation in writing. This requires the teacher to pair off students (in the previous example, students advocating opposing positions) who will not be allowed to talk at all. Each pair is to discuss the issue at hand, but only in writing. That is, when one wants to say something, he or she writes it and passes it to the other to read. In this manner, students can refer back to previous statements, which, being written, are matters of record. Time is required to read and write each statement, so each participant must stop to think about both what the other has said and what he or she wants to say. Because of the time required in reading and writing statements, emotional reactions are limited, and more rational thoughts and logical ideas are presented and discussed.

A discussion of this technique by the total class can result in an underlining of those factors inhibiting listening previously referred to. As with the paraphrasing exercise, written conversations can be repeated whenever a sharpening of listening skills seems necessary.

Understanding Roles of Group Members

Each group, in order to meet its goals, must consist of group members willing to assume certain roles within the group's functioning. Group members who do not assume these roles adequately or who assume disruptive, nonproductive roles usually falter and create frustration for themselves and the rest of the members. It follows then that education about these roles and how best to perform them would be useful to any potential group member. One method of developing knowledge of group roles is titled the *fishbowl technique.*

Fishbowls

The fishbowling of roles of group members is begun by selecting seven members who are willing to participate in a group discussion. They are escorted out of the room but not allowed to talk with one another until given permission to do so by the instructor. While these seven are out of the room, the health educator discusses the roles played by group members. The discussion relates to information that appears on a handout given to the total group — a handout that contains the following:

In all groups, roles are played by the group's membership. We will be observing a group discussion and should be looking for evidence of the following roles being played:

Task Roles

1. People who ask for or give information.
2. People who ask for or give opinions.
3. People who ask for clarification or elaboration.
4. People who initiate or continue work at hand.
5. People who keep a record of the group's discussions.
6. People who define the group's position or summarize in order to orient the group.

Task roles are directed specifically at solving the group's task, problem, or question.

Maintenance Roles

1. People who make jokes.
2. People who follow others.
3. People who compromise.
4. People who help to settle arguments by two or more of the membership.
5. People who make sure all the members feel involved and are involved in the group's deliberations.

Maintenance roles keep the group cohesive, relieve frustration when necessary, and keep the members friendly toward one another. Though maintenance roles are not directly related to accomplishment of the group's task, without them task roles would not be effective.

Individual Roles

1. People who want their own way all the time.
2. People who fool around too much.
3. People who attack others in the group.
4. People who always disagree.
5. People who say they are speaking for a larger group but who are advocating a particular position.
6. People who continually interrupt others.

Individual roles block the group from effectively satisfying its goals and must therefore be minimized. As a group's history develops, successful groups have members increasingly playing task and maintenance roles, with fewer and fewer individual roles being acted out.

As you observe a particular role being played in the group you will be observing, write down exactly what was said by the person playing that role.

The class is then seated around the periphery of the room with a smaller circle of chairs inside the larger one. The seven members who were not given the handout reenter the room, sit in the chairs in the center of the room, ignore the rest of the participants, and begin a discussion about anything they want. This discussion should last from 20 to 25 minutes and should not be interrupted by either the instructor or the observers. At the conclusion of this discussion, evidence should be presented by the observers pertaining to the performance of particular group roles. Productive and nonproductive performances should be noted.

The following session might be devoted to the practice of productive group roles in small-group discussions with one or several recorders assigned to each group to provide feedback on roles being played. Another way to practice positive group membership is to have an additional circle between the outside one (observers) and inside one (group members). This additional circle would consist of coaches assigned to particular group members to help them be more productive and less disruptive. Further feedback can be provided, as before, by the outside circle of observers. In any case, practice of effective group membership is necessary if, in subsequent sessions concerned with content considerations, small groups will be formed to discuss issues and prepare reports of some kind.

Leadership Exercise

In each group at particular times, a leader either emerges or is appointed. Whether emergent or appointed (either by an authority figure such as the instructor or by the group itself), a leader can better serve the group he or she leads by being aware of types of leadership and their associated levels of satisfaction and sense of achievement. To acquaint the group with these types of leadership, divide them into small groups of six members each. Assign a leader for each group, and meet at the front of the room briefly with all of the leaders to explain to them the type of leadership they should exhibit. These leaders should be told to act *authoritatively*—that is, to require members of the group to raise their hands and to be acknowledged by the leader before speaking, to comment on the value (or lack of it) of each member's statement, and to eventually come to a decision for the group. Each leader is then given the following sheet to distribute to each of the members in his or her group:

Discussion I **Rank the following eight traits in order of their importance in being a competent health educator. Place a number 1 by the most important, a number 2 by the second most important, and so on down to number 8, which will be the least important trait.**

Rank	Trait
_____	Tact
_____	Honesty
_____	Ambition
_____	Courage
_____	Warmth
_____	Energy
_____	Intelligence
_____	Friendliness

After a 15-minute discussion, a group decision is required, which the leader will communicate to the instructor. Each member of the group will also keep a record of the group's decision.

At the conclusion of Discussion I, a different person in each group is chosen leader, and the new leaders meet with the instructor. The instructor defines their type of leadership as *laissez-faire*. That is, they are to respond "I don't know" to questions, are not to call on anyone, and are not to be involved in the group's deliberations. The new leaders are then given the following sheet to distribute to each member of their groups:

Discussion II **Rank the following eight items in order of their importance in being a competent health educator. Place a number 1 by the most important, a number 2 by the second most important, and so on down to number 8, which will be the least important item.**

Rank	Item
_____	A good understanding of the community
_____	Ability to hold temper under aggravating circumstances
_____	Ability to keep order in a group
_____	Keeping program participants informed of their progress and development
_____	Willingness to accept people whose standards and background differ radically from his or her own
_____	Ability to make decisions based on fact rather than on personal feelings
_____	Ability to use time flexibly but still to keep things moving
_____	Ability to work with others

After this 15-minute discussion, the decision arrived at and agreed to by the group is communicated to the instructor and, as before, recorded and saved by each participant.

At this point a third leader from each group is selected and told to act *democratically*—that is, to attempt to hear from all group members, to offer his or her own opinion but not to require that that opinion be accepted by the group, to be concerned with supplying task and maintenance roles when necessary, and to ensure consensual decision making by the group. Each of these leaders is supplied the following sheets to distribute among his or her membership:

Discussion III   **Rank the following eight items in order of their importance in being a competent health educator. Place a number 1 by the most important, a number 2 by the second most important, and so on down to number 8, which will be the least important item.**

Rank	**Item**
_____	Talks effectively
_____	Treats program participants as individuals with unique abilities, interests, and so on
_____	Improves self by continuing formal education, reading current journals, attending workshops, training programs, and so on
_____	Relates well to other staff members
_____	Brings in new ideas
_____	Takes an active part in community affairs
_____	Has ability to effectively handle administrative details
_____	Is willing to try new techniques and methods

As before, each group's decision is related to the instructor and recorded by the group's members.

Upon completion of these three discussions (more than one day may be required), each student is asked to respond to the following items for *each* of the discussions:

1. How much satisfaction did you derive from the discussion?

   9 Completely satisfied

   8

   7 Moderately satisfied

   6

   5 Neutral; neither satisfied nor dissatisfied

   4

   3 Moderately dissatisfied

   2

   1 Completely dissatisfied

2. How much responsibility do you feel for the ranking you made as a group?

   9 Completely responsible

   8

   7 Somewhat responsible

   6

   5 Neutral

   4

3 Very little responsibility

2

1 Not responsible

3. How much hostility did you feel toward the leader?

9 No hostility

8

7 Some hostility

6

5 Neutral

4

3 A lot of hostility

2

1 Complete hostility

4. Rate the quality of the ranking you made as a group.

9 Best possible ranking

8

7 Moderately good ranking

6

5 Average ranking

4

3 Moderately poor ranking

2

1 Worst possible ranking

The totals of the four responses are recorded and compared. The higher the score, the better the discussion. In most instances the democratic form of leadership will be preferred and the laissez-faire style of leadership liked least. A discussion of the reasons for these preferences will reinforce democratic leadership when a leader is subsequently assigned or emerges within the group.

Teaching Cooperation

Another important characteristic of effective groups is that members cooperate with one another. Here is an activity designed to enhance group cooperation.

Cooperation Puzzle

Group members sometimes need to have the importance of cooperation emphasized. For the instructor to speak to the group about the need for the members to cooperate may sometimes be helpful. However, a more dramatic and effective method is available to make this point. The health educator prepares envelopes containing parts of a large square (like a jigsaw puzzle). A heavy sheet of paper cut into variously shaped pieces can be used for this exercise. The group is asked what cooperation means. Some of the following points may be made:

1. Everyone has to understand the problem.
2. Everyone needs to believe that he or she can help.
3. Instructions have to be clear.
4. Everyone needs to think of the other person as well as of himself or herself.

The group is then divided into small groups of five each and given the following instructions:

> Each member of your group has an envelope containing parts of a square. When all of the pieces in all of your group's envelopes are placed properly together, like a jigsaw puzzle, they will form one large square with no pieces left over. Your task as a group is to form this large square. However, in accomplishing this task, no communication will be allowed, either verbal or nonverbal. You will not be allowed to *take* a piece of the puzzle from another group member, but you can *offer* another group member any one of your puzzle pieces that you wish.

Upon completion of this exercise, the instructor can ask the following questions:

1. How did you feel when someone held a piece and did not see the solution?
2. How did you feel about having to depend on others?
3. Were some people more cooperative than others?

Another means of demonstrating the need for cooperation in the group employs five squares shaped like those shown in Figure 6.1. The squares are cut along the lines within them, and the lettered pieces placed in separate envelopes as follows:

Envelope 1: a, a, c

Envelope 2: a, j, d

Envelope 3: g, i, f

Envelope 4: b, e, f, h

Envelope 5: a, c, h

The participants are then divided into groups of five, each group member receiving an envelope and a handout sheet on which appear the following directions:

> As of this moment you are not allowed to talk with one another or communicate in any nonverbal fashion (no gesturing, making facial expressions, and so on). Pass out the envelopes so that each person has one in front of him or her. Take the pieces out and place the envelopes to one side. At a signal, the task of each group is to form five squares of equal size. This is not a race, but the task is not completed until each group has before it five perfect squares of equal size.
>
> You are not allowed to take or ask for a piece of the puzzle that is in front of someone else. You *are* allowed to give someone else a piece of the puzzle that is in front of you.

This exercise results in participants realizing that cooperation often means giving of oneself, not only taking from the group. As with many exercises of this type, the group will have fun while learning this very valuable lesson.

FIGURE 6.1

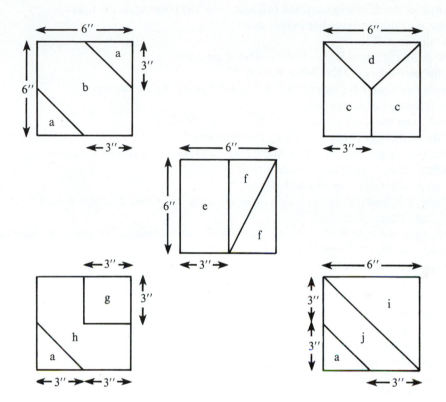

Making Sure All Participate

Often in classes, several people dominate during verbal discussion. It may be that those people are assertive, or it may be that the silent members feel that they have nothing worthwhile to contribute. In either case, the *baseball clue game* should help broaden the pattern of communication.

Baseball Clue Game

Each player gets an index card on which a clue is written. Since there are only 17 clue cards, the players will have to be divided in half, and two sets of clue cards (one for each group) will be needed. No player may let anyone else read his or her clue, but he or she may verbally relate that clue to the others in that group. The clues, of course, are needed to solve the problem, so each person rightfully feels that he or she has something of worth to contribute.

Health educators can make up their own problems and clues, but a sample relating to baseball follows:

Problem:
What are the names of the players on the baseball team, and which positions do they play?

Clues:

The shortstop, the third baseman, and Bill each won $100 betting on the fight.
Harry and the third baseman live in the same building.
Jerry is taller than Bill.
Paul and Allen each won $20 from the pitcher at pinochle.
One of the outfielders is either Mike or Andy.
Mike is shorter than Bill. Each of them is heavier than the third baseman.
Sam is involved in a divorce suit.
Paul, Andy, and the shortstop each lost $50 at the racetrack.
Ed and the outfielders play poker during their free time.
All of the battery and infield, except Allen, Harry, and Andy, are shorter than Sam.
The pitcher's wife is the third baseman's sister.
Ed's sister is engaged to the second baseman.
Paul, Harry, Bill, and the catcher took a trouncing from the second baseman at pool.
Andy dislikes the catcher.
Ed, Paul, Jerry, the right fielder, and the center fielder are bachelors. The others are married.
The catcher and the third baseman each have two children.
The center fielder is taller than the right fielder.

Solution:

Harry is the pitcher.
Allen is the catcher.
Paul is the first baseman.
Jerry is the second baseman.
Andy is the third baseman.
Ed is the shortstop.
Sam is the left fielder.
Mike is the right fielder.
Bill is the center fielder.

Once the group is accustomed to the clue-game technique, the health educator might want to vary the technique for specific purposes. For example, a group of verbally active students and another group of verbally inactive students may be in the group. The instructor could then give clues only to the quiet ones and have them sit in a circle in the center of the room working out the solution, while each of the others sits behind a quiet student and acts as a coach. In this exercise, only those in the inner circle are allowed to speak to the large group, while those in the outer circle are limited to communication with the person behind whom they are sitting.

A periodic repetition of these communication techniques is recommended. Some people need to participate in several exercises of this kind before they can feel comfortable enough in a group to speak up without hesitation when they feel they have something worthwhile to contribute.

Building-upon Exercise

One of the more serious, but correctable, examples of group dysfunction is group members failing to respond to what has been said. Rather, people are anxious to add new and often unrelated remarks. A well-functioning group builds upon each member's contribution so that the end product of that group is the collective and interrelated thoughts and ideas of its members. Such collective material is most often better than a pooling of individual ideas.

One way to help groups practice building upon one another's ideas is to structure a group discussion so that after Speaker 1 has reacted to a question posed by the instructor, Speaker 2 must cite all the ways in which he or she agrees and disagrees with what Speaker 1 has said. Speaker 3 then responds to Speaker 2 in similar fashion, and so on until everyone in the group has had a turn. A discussion of the difficulty in not being allowed to add new ideas, and in identifying points of agreement and disagreement, will prepare the group for the next phase of this exercise.

For that phase, have the participants discuss a new problem but allow them to add new ideas *after* they cite points of agreement and disagreement as they did before. This discussion should be structured as the previous one; that is, Speaker 2 responds to Speaker 1, Speaker 3 to Speaker 2, and so on.

Developing Empathy

Role-playing is often used to develop a sense of empathy for particular people. For example, a person who has evidenced a bias against African Americans may be asked by the instructor to act the part of an African American in a role-playing situation. It is hoped that putting a person in another's shoes will help that person develop an understanding of the other person's situation. Similarly, role-playing might be employed to help people empathize with parents of teenage children. In using role-playing in this manner, someone might be asked to act the part of a parent whose teenage daughter, played by another person, returns from a date two hours past her curfew. Playing the role of parents will help participants develop a greater appreciation for the parents' side of the coin and increased empathy for parents. It demonstrates the complexity of seemingly uncomplicated situations that occur between parents and children.

Likewise, role reversal can develop empathy between those advocating opposing points of view. For example, parents could be invited to a school and asked to play the role of child, while their child plays the role of parent. In this manner parent and child should better appreciate one another's point of view.

In the context of this chapter, however, role reversal is suggested as a means of developing more effective groups. It is desirable for two members of a group who are disagreeing with each other to reverse roles to develop an appreciation of the opponent's point of view. Compromise will be more easily achieved and more palatable if each group member is able to perceive some validity in the opposing viewpoint. At still other points in the group's existence, particular members might be dysfunctional in the group because of a number of reasons: boredom, need for attention, an aggressive nature, or a dislike of the group's members, for example. In these instances it is wise to provide feedback to the disruptive group member concerning his or her behavior. One effective way to provide this feedback is through role reversal. The dysfunctional person can be asked to play the role of the leader of the group, while someone else portrays the dysfunctional person. An awareness of dysfunctional behavior and its effect upon the leader of the group is often all that is needed for group members to behave productively. For fear of forgetting the nature of role reversal, it should be noted that an appreciation for the needs of individuals within the group is the responsibility of the group leader and is enhanced in the role reversal example just cited.

There are other ways to respond to dysfunctional group members. Either an audio- or videotape recording might be employed and analyzed to document disruptive behavior. However, one of the most effective manners of relating to someone who has been demonstrating antigroup behavior is to have each group member act like any other group member of his or her choosing while the others try to guess whom he or she is acting like. Often this technique causes the dysfunctional group member to realize how disruptive he or she has been. A discussion by the group about the feelings each person had when he or she was being portrayed by someone else will help to limit dysfunctional group behavior.

One other very effective manner for helping the group deal with such behavior requires first that the group stand in a circle. Each program participant then goes around the circle, standing in front of one other participant at a time, holding his or her hand, looking him or her in the eyes, and revealing feelings about that person. Only the program participant going around the circle may speak until the exercise is over. At this point, explanations about the reasons for these feelings will often reveal to dysfunctional participants what effect their behavior has on others in the group and how the others feel about them. It is suggested that no more than eight people form a circle and that, before asking the program participants to divulge their feelings, the instructor highlight the differences between feelings (see the mental health chapter) and thoughts.

Other means of responding to disruptive or dysfunctional behavior include assigning such a person a particular role to play in the group. Such roles might be recorder, summarizer, or clarifier (see the fishbowl roles of group members in this chapter) so that the person experiences and practices constructive group behavior.

Treating People as Individuals

One underlying assumption of health education as freeing is that people are different from one another. They may have different values, different goals, and different styles of living. Treating people as individuals, therefore, should be given attention in health education programs. Here are two ways to do that.

Filling Needs

This appropriately named exercise is another that can be employed to help leaders of groups fill the needs of problem members in an effective manner. A seemingly simple exercise, this activity is one of the most valuable in a group leader's repertoire. Each group member is asked to make a list in response to the question, What can we do to make you happier in this group? Upon completion of the lists, each group member may read his or her responses to the question while others react to the individual's needs. Another possibility is for the leader to collect the responses and assign group members to help fill the needs of other group members. In any case, it is important to realize that groups are most effective when the needs of their members are satisfied.

Appreciation of Individual Differences

In spite of what people list as their needs as group members, an appreciation of their individuality may be all that is needed to make them productive group members. People who join a group often neglect the individual and his or her uniqueness and exalt the group. The author has found it helpful in these instances to conduct an exercise that begins with a reading of the following excerpt (Gerhard 1972):

> In all my years of teaching, Charlie McCaffrey was the finest student I ever had. Charlie failed most of the tests I gave him; he very seldom finished his science homework; he struggled for C's and generally got D's; but Charlie McCaffrey was the finest student I ever taught. No matter how I tried to impress Charlie with the contributions of Kepler and Newton, he could just never take them seriously. But ask for a volunteer to adjust the blinds, feed the fish, or clean out the snake cage and Charlie was on his feet and moving.

I always felt like a rat giving Charlie a C (and that was really a charitable act); the kid was just too much a nice guy. He was never mad at anyone. He always smiled. And his red hair always dropped into his left eye, which gave him an excuse to be inattentive just when I was trying to make a critical point about how he hadn't even tried to grasp the contribution of Gregor Mendel. That kid! What a pain! He just didn't take science seriously.

Like the time I had a really important test. I told the class, well in advance, "This is important. It's critical to your mark." Charlie bombed it. I mean a flat F. But what can you say to a kid you like who failed your test? It was a time when "Charlie the Tuna" ads were in full swing on television. I didn't want to be too rough, so I drew a fishing line down through his paper and attached a note to the hook, which just said, "Sorry, Charlie." His mother had been a teacher and a lot of her friends were teachers. When he took the paper home they laughed and understood. I mean, she had to live with this kid who just didn't appreciate that Tycho Brahe had a gold nose.

In retrospect, I realize that Charlie was the kind of person the world needs more of. His temperament was equable. The sparkle of enthusiasm enlivened his eye. He never deviated from his way of life. He was the perfect public relations man, promoter, communicator, a potential contributor to society. And I gave him a C.

So, Charlie, you said I was your favorite teacher, the guy who treated everyone as if they were unique. But you were out of my class. I said I individualized, but in your case I didn't. What a great mayor of Boston you would have made!

I won't make the same mistake again. When, if ever, another Charlie comes along I'll be ready. I was sorry, Charlie, when you were killed in Viet Nam. I spent all that time trying to change you—and you changed me.

I'll say it again. I'm sorry, Charlie.*

Following the reading there is a discussion of the meaning of this excerpt and the lesson's transferability to each person's group. Next, the instructor reads the following two case studies and asks the participants to classify as hopeful, unpredictable, or hopeless the future of the two people described.

Case 1: This boy is a senior in high school and has obtained a certificate from a physician stating that a nervous breakdown necessitates his leaving school for six months. The teacher describes this boy as a problem. He is not a good all-around student, has no friends, and spoke late as an infant; his father is ashamed of his son's lack of athletic ability. This boy has odd mannerisms, has made up his own religion, and chants hymns to himself.

Case 2: This six-year-old boy's head was large at birth, and he was therefore thought to have brain fever. Three of his siblings died before birth, but the mother disagrees with relatives and neighbors who insist the child is abnormal. When the child is sent to school, however, he is diagnosed as mentally ill. This diagnosis infuriates the mother, who withdraws the boy from school and says she will teach him herself.

After these case studies have been presented and the two children's futures have been determined to be either hopeful, unpredictable, or hopeless, the instructor then announces that the person discussed in the first case was Thomas Edison and the one in the second case was Albert Einstein. Obviously, the point is then made that each person is unique with the potential for considerable contribution and that this uniqueness should be appreciated and rewarded in the group.

---

*Extract from "Sorry, Charlie . . ." by Victor J. Gerhard in *Phi Delta Kappan,* 53:536, 1972. Copyright © 1972 Phi Delta Kappan. Reprinted by permission of the author.

Analyzing Frustration

Often, in groups, the creative potential of group members is thwarted and frustration develops. However, frustration can develop for numerous reasons, and its manifestation can take many forms. This exercise, done with colored pieces of poster board of various shapes, illustrates reactions to the limitation of creativity and to frustration. On its completion, ways to respond to these reactions are discussed.

Participants are seated around tables—6 to 12 at each table. On each table are different-colored and different-shaped pieces of poster board, cut out prior to the session by the instructor in sufficient number so that each participant can create a design to his or her desire. After they have had 15 minutes of creating designs with the colored poster board pieces, the participants are instructed to dismantle their designs and to adhere to the following instructions:

1. Take the long, red piece in your right hand.
2. Take the round, yellow piece in your left hand.
3. Place the red piece adjacent and to the left of the yellow piece.
4. Now pick up a small, white piece.
5. And so on.

The instructions continue for 20 minutes. After approximately 10 minutes, frustration reactions begin to surface. One person may yawn (withdrawal behavior), another may protest the absurdity of the exercise (rationalization), a third may disrupt the situation (attack reaction), and still another may resort to laughter and playing (regressive behavior). After the instructions have elicited these reactions, a discussion of how people respond to frustration will help participants recognize frustrated group members. Further discussion might determine how the group should react to frustrated group members (filling needs, for example).

Managing Group Disagreement

In any group's history there are times when there is a great deal of disagreement on a particular issue. Two techniques have been demonstrated to be of great value at these times. The first technique requires the group to discuss the issue about which they are disagreeing — but before offering comments, the student speaking must first cite those aspects of the previous speaker's comments with which he or she agrees. All speakers therefore begin their comments on a positive note; for example, "I agree with you that . . . ," rather than immediately disagreeing with what has been stated. In addition, while listening to others speaking, the listener must be attuned to ideas with which he or she and the speaker are in agreement rather than only those about which they differ.

The second technique allows program participants to develop an empathetic feeling for those with whom they disagree and a better understanding of opposing points of view. This activity requires that those in disagreement switch positions so that they are, in effect, arguing for the position with which they disagree. By way of example, if A is opposed to legalization of marijuana and is arguing with B, who favors its legalization (or decriminalization), the instructor requests that for a short period A argue for legalization and B against it (just the opposite of their actual opinions). Having to think of cogent arguments for a position you disagree with results in a better understanding of that position and greater appreciation for those favoring that position.

Summary

The activities and exercises described in this chapter are recommended for use throughout a health education program but particularly at its beginning. In this way, coping skills — like listening, communicating, and cooperating; dealing with frustration, group dysfunction, and disagreement; and the development of trust, personal worth, and camaraderie — can be accomplished early and serve as prerequisites to health content considerations. These coping skills are essential in life. As will be obvious, the development of the skills, feelings, and group atmosphere referred to in this chapter will be necessary for a successful experience with the learning activities described in subsequent chapters.

It should be noted that small-group work need not command all of the instructional time. Large-group instructional activities can be vehicles for meaningful learning experiences as well. Small groups do, however, provide greater opportunity for program participants to be active in the learning process and therefore should be employed regularly.

One last word: The activities described have been employed with success by both the author and many health educators who have been enrolled in his classes and workshops. The delight experienced after people complete these exercises is so rewarding that they and the instructor alike look forward to the next health education session.

CHAPTER 7

Instructional Strategies for Exploring the Relationship between Values and Health

This chapter offers the health educator exercises to help program participants clarify their values. Knowing where one is seems important before journeying anywhere. Therefore, the activities included in this chapter are directed at establishing, for learners, the point from which they are beginning their educational journey. A reintroduction of these activities at the end of the program will determine the changes in values associated with that time period.

It should be noted that the activities included in this values clarification section are not directed at *developing* values. Rather, they seek to help the individual become aware of the values he or she already possesses. That individual may then determine that changes in values are appropriate and seek the instructor's help in changing particular values.

Because our decisions are based on the values system we share, exploration of our values seems a necessity. To make more rational decisions relative to our health and health-related behavior, we must understand ourselves and our motivations. A study of the values we possess will contribute to such an understanding. As with all of the other exercises described in this book, the health educator should be lucid on the rationale for incorporating values clarification activities in the health instructional process. Much harm can be done to the movement for humanistic health education — health education as freeing — by instructors who play "games" without an understanding of how those games contribute to the growth and development of the people participating in these activities. Although such educators usually tend to revert to more traditional health instruction, observers (employers, parents, administrators, and so on) are apt to generalize the ineffectiveness of humanistic health education to other situations. Consequently, instructors who employ humanistic education ineffectively are likely to be viewed with some suspicion.

Values are determined through three processes (Raths et al. 1966):

1. Choosing
   a. Freely
   b. From alternatives
   c. After thought given to the consequences of each alternative
2. Prizing
   a. Being satisfied with the choice
   b. Willingly announcing the choice publicly

3. Acting
    a. Consistently with the choice
    b. Repeatedly as part of a general pattern of life

Unless all 10 of the criteria for valuing (the three categories and their subcategories) are met, the item in question is not a value. It may be a belief, opinion, or attitude, but not a value. An example here might clarify this point. If one professes to value good health and has thought about the implications of and alternatives to good health (choosing criterion), is happy with that choice and talks with others about it (prizing criterion), but doesn't behave in a healthful manner by not exercising regularly (acting criterion), then good health is not a *value* for that person.

Over the years, a number of authors have advocated and described how the values clarification approach to education can be employed:

1. Dalis, Gus T., and Ben B. Strasser. *Teaching Strategies for Values Awareness and Decision Making in Health Education.* Columbus, Ohio: Charles B. Merrill, 1977.

2. Greenberg, Jerrold S. *Student-Centered Health Instruction: A Humanistic Approach.* Reading, Mass.: Addison-Wesley, 1978.

3. Howe, L. W., and M. M. Howe. *Personalizing Education: Values Clarification and Beyond.* New York: Hart, 1975.

4. Metcalf, L. E., ed. *Values Education: Rationale, Strategies, and Procedures, Forty-First Yearbook.* Washington, D.C.: National Council for the Social Studies, 1971.

5. Morrison, Eleanor, and Mila Underhill. *Values in Sexuality.* New York: Hart, 1974.

6. Osman, Jack. "Teaching Nutrition with a Focus on Values." *Nutrition News* 36(1973):5.

7. Read, Donald A. *Looking In: Exploring One's Personal Health Values.* Englewood Cliffs, NJ: Prentice-Hall, 1977.

8. Read, Donald A., and Sidney B. Simon. *Humanistic Education Sourcebook.* Englewood Cliffs, NJ: Prentice-Hall, 1976.

9. Simon, Sidney B., Leland W. Howe, and Howard Kirschenbaum. *Values Clarification: A Handbook of Practical Strategies for Teachers and Students.* New York: Hart, 1972.

It should be noted that some health educators (and educators from different disciplines) object to values clarification. Their objection pertains to the lack of rightness or wrongness about the values decisions that students might make during these activities. These opponents of values clarification argue that particular values should be inculcated in health education program participants—values such as respect for other people, sexual responsibility (which may mean different things to different people), and others. For example, former Secretary of Education William Bennett argues that schools ought to teach character. By *character* Bennett means strength of mind, honesty, thoughtfulness, kindness, fidelity, respect for the law, diligence, independence, fairness, self-discipline, and standards of right and wrong. Of course, the question of who defines these terms has not yet been answered.

In any case, health educators employing values clarification instructional strategies should assure themselves beforehand that no sanctions or prohibitions exist that discourage this approach. If they develop, it might be better not to throw the baby out with the bathwater and, instead, teach what you are able to teach. Not to do so might be to jeopardize the whole program.

Valuing Exercises

The exercises that follow are directed at identifying for program participants the nature and direction of their values. Consequently, the three valuing processes are the subject of these activities.

Values Ranking

An activity that can help people prioritize values is to have them rank circumstances according to their preference *for* those circumstances. For example, rank the following situations, indicating with a number 1 the item most preferred, a 2 the second most preferred, and a 3 the least preferred:

1. To drop a bomb on a city in a country with which the United States is at war, knowing that scores of innocent people will be killed and injured.
2. To press the button that will activate an electric chair in which a convicted killer is sitting.
3. To press down on the accelerator of your car, thereby running down and killing three men coming at you on a dark night with crowbars.

Analysis of this ranking clarifies values pertaining to life. Though professing to value life above all else, those selecting choice 3 as most preferable may actually mean their *own* lives. Those selecting choice 2, in which only one person is killed, may be those who actually do value life above all else. Students selecting choice 1 as most preferable may do so because of their distance from the results of their action. Obviously, other conclusions about values can be reached utilizing this exercise.

Below are other groupings that may be used in value ranking:

1. Disfigurement	1. Charming	1. Black African
2. Loss of intelligence	2. Reliable	2. Black Mexican
3. Poverty	3. Insightful	3. African American
1. Jew	1. Preschooler	1. Drug pusher
2. Christian	2. Teenager	2. Drug addict
3. Atheist	3. Adult	3. Drug grower

Values Grid

The values grid is similar to values ranking in that program participants have to set priorities, but the grid allows for more than three rankings at one time. Participants are asked to draw a grid consisting of four cells across and four cells down, to total 16 cells (Figure 7.1). The first column is labeled very strong, the second strong, the third mild, and the last column, no opinion. The instructor reads 16 statements, one at a time, in this way: first the statement, then identification of the key word in the statement, then a few seconds' pause. During this pause, learners are to categorize the statement just read according to how strongly they feel about the statement—regardless of whether they favor it or oppose it.

When the 16 statements have been read, each cell in the grid will contain one, and only one, key word that refers to a particular statement. It's important to remember that whether someone feels very strongly in favor of or very strongly opposed to a statement, the key word describing that statement should be placed in one of the four cells in the very strong column. When all statements have been categorized, the grid will contain four key words in each of its four columns. The participants then divide into groups

FIGURE 7.1
Values Grid

Very strong	Strong	Mild	No opinion

of four, where they discuss the grids of each of their group's members. Each member should stress their reasons for their choices and recall personal experiences relative to the statements.

Although health educators can develop their own sets of statements, the following statements, with the key words in italics, have been used successfully in school health education settings:

1. A teacher calls a student *dumb* in front of the class.
2. A senior boy tries to *seduce* as many girls in the sophomore class as he can in order to prove his manliness.
3. Someone has seen a person he or she knows rifling *lockers* but doesn't tell anyone.
4. A girl is asked to *lie* for another student.
5. A girl has become *promiscuous* trying to be popular.
6. A boy does not want to participate in *sports.*
7. A student is suspended for *smoking.*
8. A student is thrown out of class for *cheating.*
9. An unwed pregnant student is advised by a friend to have an *abortion.*

10. A student decides to leave home because he doesn't have enough *freedom.*

11. A "pot missionary" gives *marijuana* to others because he thinks it is cool.

12. A student is playing the game of applying to *college* because of parental pressure.

13. A student behaves differently with different groups in order to get *elected* student-body president.

14. A student *shoplifts* as part of a fraternity (sorority) initiation.

15. Parents *beat* their daughter if she disobeys them.

16. A student is thrown out of class because she used *profanity.*

Values Continuum

Many people will claim to value seat belts in automobiles. Surprisingly, many people, though valuing seat belts, will not wear them, in spite of state laws that may require that they be worn. The values continuum is useful in helping us see the inconsistencies between what we profess to be our values and how we behave. Relative to seat belts, the reader is asked to place himself or herself at the appropriate place on the following continuum:

How often do you wear seat belts?

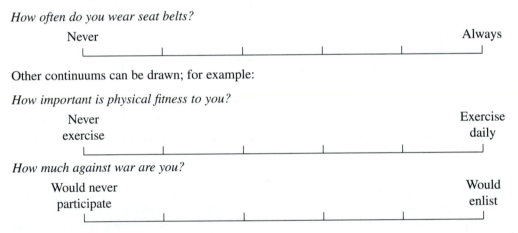

Never   Always

Other continuums can be drawn; for example:

How important is physical fitness to you?

Never   Exercise
exercise   daily

How much against war are you?

Would never   Would
participate   enlist

From these continua, participants can discuss their behaviors and develop suggestions for behavior more consistent with professed values.

Activities Enjoyed

Another useful activity to clarify the acting-out aspect of values requests people to list 20 things they enjoy doing. It is surprising how difficult a task this is in itself. After the list is complete the following instructions may be presented:

1. Place a dollar sign next to each item that cannot be done without an initial outlay of at least five dollars.

2. Place a *P* next to those items that you prefer to do with other people and an *A* next to those things you prefer to do alone.

3. Place a *5* next to any item that you would not have listed five years ago.

FIGURE 7.2
Prerequisite Instructional Stategies

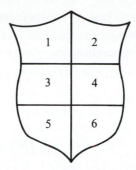

4. Place a *G,* for generation gap, next to each item that your parents would not have included on their list when they were your age.

5. Think of a person you love, and place an *L* next to each item you would want that person to include on his or her list.

6. Place an *M* next to the five items on the list that you *most* enjoy.

7. Record the date when you last did each of the items you just marked with an *M*.

An activity of this sort shows whether those things most enjoyed are the things most often done, how values may change, how materialistic one may be, and how different generations may or may not possess similar values. Of course, several other interpretations may develop during a discussion of this exercise.

An important aspect of this exercise, as well as of other values clarification activities, is that it does not force the instructor's values on the participants. All that is required is that they analyze for themselves what they think they value and how they behave relative to their perceived values. Then they will have to choose between acting more consistently with their own desired values or changing their perceptions of those values to be more in line with desirable behaviors.

Coat of Arms

By learning more about themselves and sharing a little of themselves with others, participants will be better prepared to make decisions pertaining to use of cigarettes, choice of marriage partner, choice of occupation, and so on. The assumption is that the more one knows about oneself, the more one's motivations for behavior are recognizable and accounted for in the decision-making process. To help in this respect, group members are asked to do the following:

1. On a large sheet of paper draw the shape you see in Figure 7.2—but *do not* write in the numbers. Draw the figure as large as you can, because you will be adding pictures or words to each of the six sections.

2. In section 1, draw two pictures: one showing something you are very good at, and the other showing something you're not very good at but would like to do better.

3. In section 2, draw a picture depicting one value to which you are deeply committed.

4. In section 3, draw a picture representing the material possession that is most dear to you.

5. In section 4, draw two pictures: one describing your greatest accomplishment during the past year, and the other representing your biggest failure during the past year.

6. For section 5, assume you had one year to do whatever you wanted and were guaranteed success. Draw a picture in section 5 representing the activity you would choose to do for that year.

7. Finally, in section 6, write three words that you would want others to use in describing you if you were to die today.

Emphasize that how well the person draws is unimportant. Some will be good drawers, others not so good. All should be encouraged to participate. This is not an art course. The purpose of this activity is to help program participants learn more about themselves. They all can draw well enough to accomplish this goal.

On completing the seven steps, participants will each have a coat of arms. They should be encouraged to share their coats of arms in small-group discussion at this point. In this manner, they will learn more about themselves and about other program participants.

Values Quadrant

Still another exercise that can be employed for self-analysis begins with a large square containing four quadrants. In the upper left quadrant, participants are to list 10 people with whom they would like to be friends or with whom they are friends. In the lower left section, they are asked to list 10 places that they like to go—that is, 10 places where they enjoy spending their time.

In the upper right section they should list five people with whom they do not want to be friends, people not liked. In the lower right space they should list five places at which they do not enjoy spending time.

The completed quadrants can then be examined and discussed or analyzed separately. Questions should be related to why certain people are liked and others disliked; why certain places are enjoyed and others are not; what would happen to the places enjoyed if the people that are disliked went to them; how would the people that are liked be viewed if they were associated with places that are not enjoyed; and how people and places can be transformed from the right side of the grid (disliked people and unenjoyed places) to the left, or positive side. How often people who are liked are taken to places that are liked is still another question to help analyze the values quadrants.

Who Should Survive?

When people are asked to make decisions about the relative worth of people, the value ascribed to particular skills or to personality attributes surfaces. For this exercise, participants are divided into groups of six, and each person is given a handout sheet containing the following information (the instructor should make it clear that there are no right or wrong answers):

Survival Problem

An atomic war has occurred, and the 15 people listed here—who are in a single atom-bomb shelter—are the only humans left alive on the earth. It will take two weeks for external radiation to drop to a safe survival level. Supplies in the shelter can just barely support seven people for two weeks; the rest must be turned out to die so that those seven can survive. You, and the other members of your group, must decide who the survivors will be — and the group decision must be unanimous.

1. *Dr. Dane:* 39, no religious affiliation, Ph.D. in history, college professor, good health, married (one child, Bobby), active in community, white.

2. *Mrs. Dane:* 38, Jew, A.B. and M.A. in psychology, counselor in mental health clinic, good health, married (one child, Bobby), active in community, white.

3. *Bobby Dane:* 10, Jew, special-education classes for four years, mentally retarded (IQ 70), good health, enjoys his pets, white.

4. *Mrs. Garcia:* 33, Latino American, Roman Catholic, ninth-grade education, cocktail waitress, prostitute, good health, married at 16, divorced at 18, abandoned as a child, in foster home as a youth, attacked by foster father at age 12, ran away from home, returned to reformatory, stayed till 16 (one child, three weeks old, Jean).

5. *Jean Garcia:* 3 weeks old, Latino American, good health, nursing for food.

6. *Mrs. Evans:* 30, African American, Protestant, A.B. and M.A. in elementary education, teacher, divorced (one child, Mary), in good health, cited as outstanding teacher, enjoys working with children.

7. *Mary Evans:* 8, African American, Protestant, third grade, good health, excellent student.

8. *Saheb Arat:* 13, Muslim, sixth grade, good health, excellent student.

9. *Mr. Newton:* 25, African American, claims to be an atheist, starting last year of medical school, suspended, homosexual, good health, seems bitter concerning racial problems.

10. *Sister Mary Kathleen:* 27, nun, college graduate, English major, grew up in upper-middle-class neighborhood, good health, her father was a businessman.

11. *Mr. Clark:* 28, African American, college graduate, B.S. in electronics engineering, married (no children), good health, enjoys outdoor sports and stereo equipment, grew up in a ghetto, homosexual.

12. *Mr. Blake:* 31, white, Mormon, B.S. graduate, mechanic, Mr. Fix-it, married, 4 children, good health, enjoys outdoors and working in his shop.

13. *Miss Allen:* 21, Latino American, Protestant, college senior, majored in nursing, good health, enjoys outdoor sports, likes people.

14. *Father Evans:* 37, white, Catholic priest, college plus seminary, active in civil rights, criticized for liberal views, good health, former college athlete.

15. *Dr. Gonzales:* 66, Latino American, Catholic, M.D., general practitioner, has had two heart attacks in past five years but continues to practice.

The instructor can conduct a discussion with the total group, at which time each group can report the reasoning behind its choices. During such a discussion, emphasis should be placed on why certain people were chosen over others. Groups that disagree should be encouraged to be accepting of others' values and not feel compelled to encourage others to agree with their choices.

This is an excellent activity for the study of prejudice and discrimination. It can also be used to discuss how some segments of society treat people with HIV/AIDS.

FIGURE 7.3
Exploring the Relationship Between Values and Health

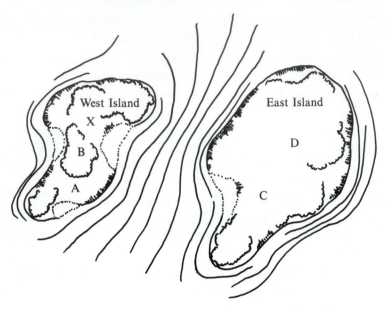

Value Judgment

Like the exercise just described, the value judgment exercise ranks people in order to investigate the worth attributed to particular behaviors. Again, participants are divided into groups of six, and a handout containing the following information — and Figure 7.3 — is distributed to each person:

> There are two islands close together in the ocean, but because of sharks in the water it is impossible to cross from one to the other without a boat. On West Island there are one woman (X), two men (A and B), and a boat. On East Island there are two men (C and D) but no boat. X is in love with C and wants to go to him, but she doesn't know how to handle the boat. She asks A to take her to East Island, but he does not want to hear about her problems or become involved in them. He wants to be left alone.
>
> B offers to take X to East Island, but only if she spends the night with him first. She agrees. Next day, after X has gotten over to East Island, C discovers the circumstances under which she got there, and wants nothing more to do with her.
>
> D, on the other hand, doesn't care what she's done or why. He'll take her under any circumstances.
>
> Your task is to rank these people in order, from the one you respect most to the one you respect least.

A discussion of each group's rankings will elicit conclusions similar to those of the "who should survive?" activity.

Proud Statement

Everyone has something of which to be proud. Often, however, people do not stop to think of how proud they should be and at what specifics their pride should be directed. The time taken to ask group participants to verbally complete the statement "I am proud that I . . ." is time well spent. The proud statement exercise is just one method in which to use the positive nature of people. When the rationale for each proud statement is discussed by the person making the statement, it often evokes very heartwarming feelings in the listeners. People usually become more thoughtful and appreciative of their own worth and of the value of their fellow participants as a result of this exercise.

Fantasy Questions

When people are confronted with open-ended questions calling for imagination, their answers often indicate their values. Some examples of such questions follow:

1. If you were a color, what color would you like to be?
2. If you were a food, what food would you like to be?
3. In which period in history would you have liked to live?
4. If you were a piece of furniture, which piece of furniture would you like to be?
5. If you were a flower, which flower would you like to be?
6. If you were an animal, which animal would you like to be?
7. If you could perform one miracle, what would that miracle be?
8. If you had a million dollars, what would be the first thing that you would buy?
9. During next weekend what would you like to do?
10. If you were a television program, what program would you like to be?
11. If you were a day of the week, what day would you like to be?
12. If you were an electrical appliance, which one would you like to be?
13. If you were a parent, what would you like to do with your children?
14. If you were a smell, what smell would you like to be?
15. If you were a part of a body, what part would you like to be?

A discussion of these responses in small groups is recommended. Because no answers are wrong or right, participants should be instructed to ask questions of one another that will help clarify why they responded as they did, rather than to persuade one another that their responses were the most creative.

Epitaph

The purpose of having program participants deal with values choices is perhaps best served by confronting them with the purpose of their very existence. This exercise requires them to imagine their own deaths and to compose their own epitaphs. In this manner they decide what they would like to be able to say about themselves at the conclusion of life. In other words, the question becomes, What do I want my life to have meant? When the epitaphs have been written, and the discussion turns to how the participants can best deserve the epitaphs they have written for themselves, the result will be that each one will devise means of being what he or she wants to become.

Similarly, participants can be asked to write their own obituaries or to develop collages that include pictures, words, and items around the theme "If I had two days to live. . . ."

Making Lists

The development of lists can help clarify values and help people behave consistently with the values they profess. For example, they can be asked to list things that would make them feel good. Next they list obstacles to achieving those things, and the resources and strategies they can employ to overcome these obstacles.

Likewise, participants can list things they have to do—then ways of feeling better about these things (perhaps by combining them with activities they enjoy).

The possible listings are limited only by the health education instructor's creativity and ingenuity.

Values Check

A grid can be handed out to periodically check one's values. Utilizing the three aspects of values clarification processing, the grid takes the form shown in the accompanying box. The numbered columns at the right coincide with the seven questions at the bottom of the grid. The task is to check those boxes representing the criteria (the seven questions) that a person has met. A subsequent task becomes an attempt to meet those criteria for which the person has not previously accounted. The development of strategies to account for the unmet criteria should then occur.

STATED ISSUE	1	2	3	4	5	6	7
I favor rational decisions.							
I am opposed to abortion.							
I care about people.							
Etc.							

1. Are you *proud* of (do you prize or cherish) your position?
2. Have you *publicly affirmed* your position?
3. Have you chosen your position from *alternatives?*
4. Have you chosen your position after *thoughtful consideration?*
5. Have you chosen your position *freely?*
6. Have you *acted* consistently with your position?
7. Have you acted with *repetition* or *consistency* on this issue?

-ly Descriptions

On a two-foot-square sheet of heavy paper, participants can be requested to list, using large letters, six descriptions of how they think they act—four positive and two negative ways. These descriptions must end in the letters *ly*—for example, cruelly, sweetly, crazily, interestingly, and so on. A piece of yarn can be placed through two holes—one at each top corner—so that the sheet with the six descriptions can be worn around the neck, like an "Eat at Joe's" sign. Then they are requested to walk around the room and nonverbally show agreement or disagreement with others' descriptions of their behavior. For instance, after stopping to read *A*'s descriptions, *B* might point to one of these descriptions and shake his head vigorously yes or no to indicate strong agreement or disagreement with it. This phase of the *-ly* descriptions exercise gives participants the opportunity to receive feedback from others about their behavior as well as to engage in some introspection.

The second phase of this exercise requires participants to trade one or more of their six descriptions to someone else for one or more of that person's descriptions. So, for example, *A* might trade a "cruelly" for *B*'s "belligerently." In this manner, participants inspect their values pertaining to these behaviors and must judge some to be more worthwhile than others. Obviously, in the example just cited, *A* values "belligerently" more than "cruelly," since he was willing to part with "cruelly" and substitute "belligerently."

The last phase of this activity is conducted in small groups where the traders present the rationale for each trade.

Role Trading

Somewhat like *-ly* descriptions, this activity calls for participants to place a role that they play on an index card. Each person writes six roles for himself or herself — one per index card — so that he or she has six index cards. Possible roles are brother, sister, student, friend, athlete, and so on. When all have written their cards, they walk around the room and, nonverbally, give to some other players the three roles that they *least value.*

A small- or large-group discussion should then relate to the following questions:

1. How would you feel about giving away these three roles if you *really* had to do that?
2. How would you feel about *really* accepting the roles others gave you?
3. How important to you are the three roles you were unwilling to give away?
4. How well do you perform the roles you valued most?
5. How could you perform better the roles you valued most?

Learning Statements

Because the health education setting is one in which learning is expected to occur, and because the purpose of values clarification is related to introspection and cognizance of one's values, program participants should periodically be asked to write a couple of sentences, paragraphs, or pages beginning with the phrase I learned that I . . . Participation in values clarification activities is very valuable for understanding one's values, but the additional task of specifying what one has learned about oneself adds considerably to the worth of these exercises.

After conducting values clarification exercises with a heterogeneous group of teachers and students in a workshop setting, learning statements were submitted to this author. It seems appropriate to end this section with some of those statements:

I learned that I am one hell of a lot better off than I thought I was.

I learned that I can communicate with older people quite easily when I want to, that we can learn to live together in society, that I can respect their views if they respect mine.

I learned that I find young people fun, interesting, and concerned.

To Follow

The following chapters are divided by health content study areas and are meant to employ the knowledge, attitudes, and skills developed through group process and values clarification activities. Because valuing is such an integral part of health behavior, activities are provided to explore values related to each of the content areas. Likewise, activities for small- and large groups are interspersed throughout. In all cases, however, the activities involve active participation in the learning process.

PART THREE

HEALTH EDUCATION

INSTRUCTIONAL STRATEGIES TO ACTIVATE LEARNERS

This section presents numerous instructional strategies that can be used to actively involve health education program participants in the learning process. The rationale for this section is based on research findings that indicate learning by doing results in greater learning. One of the reasons for this is that passive learners — perhaps those listening to a lecture time after time — do not pay as much attention to what is going on as those learners who are required to do something with the content and who therefore must be attentive. Besides, being actively involved during educational sessions is more fun. If it's more fun, learners will pay more attention and will feel better about being a part of the program.

The activities presented are organized by health science content areas: mental health, drug education, sexuality education, and so on. The instructional activities are purposely not defined for any particular learners or for any particular settings because only strategies that could be adapted to various program participants and to various health education settings were included. Specific adaptations should be made by the health educator who knows the learners and the settings best.

In addition, some of the activities may seem either too juvenile or overly sophisticated for the setting or the group of learners with whom you are most interested. In that case, these activities probably need to be adapted more than some of the others. However, there is no reason that you cannot use each and every instructional strategy presented once it is modified for your particular situation, be that a public or community setting, a worksite setting, or an academic setting.

Certain settings may limit the health educator's freedom to employ some of the instructional strategies that follow. For example, in some communities valuing activities may be proscribed, in other communities certain sexual issues (for example, abortion or masturbation) may be specifically eliminated from the health education programs, and in still other communities instructional strategies related to death and dying may be judged too sensitive for certain age groups of learners. The health educator needs to be aware of these local sensibilities and choose health education content and instructional strategies consistent with community standards.

The intention, then, is that this book will serve as a resource to help you conduct health education in various settings with various program participants, making adaptations that you judge are needed.

CHAPTER EIGHT

Instructional Strategies for Mental Health

The title of this chapter refers to a state of well-being. Some excellent mental health education programs are being conducted by health instructors. Some other programs are preoccupied with mental *illness* as opposed to mental *health*. Since educators are not prepared for the role of therapist, deep-seated psychological disturbances characteristic of some program participants cannot be adequately responded to by the health instructor. In cases of this type, the responsibility is to refer such people to those who are better able to help them. To be sure, an understanding of mental illness is worthwhile. However, the view expressed in this chapter is one of prevention and exploration. Feelings of alienation and self-deprecation will be prevented; one's feelings toward oneself and others will be explored, as will the means of bettering one's mental health status and of decreasing loneliness and isolation.

Introductory Activities

This section concerns itself with instructional strategies to increase trust in the educational setting while providing the opportunity for introspective deliberations.

Tell Me Statements

The "tell me" game can be organized to be played in pairs or in small groups of four to six. The object of this exercise is to help program participants get to know one another better and to feel more comfortable with one another. In order for these objectives to be met, statements beginning with "tell me" are developed and responded to by the participants. Though participants familiar with the exercise can develop their own tell me statements, it is recommended that initially the instructor create them. Once a number of such statements are developed, each person chooses one to ask another person. Should a person who was not asked to respond to a particular tell me desire to, he or she should be allowed that opportunity. Participants should be cautioned to react honestly and in some detail to these statements for the objectives of this exercise to be best served. Examples of tell me statements are

1. Tell me something about your family.
2. Tell me something that you like about yourself.
3. Tell me something that you dislike about yourself.
4. Tell me what you like and dislike about health education.

 5. Tell me which parts of your body you like least and which parts you like best.

 6. Tell me your most vivid elementary school memory.

 7. Tell me about the best thing that ever happened to you.

 8. Tell me a secret.

 9. Tell me how you feel about this group.

10. Tell me what you enjoy doing.

11. Tell me about a turning point in your life.

12. Tell me about your greatest success.

13. Tell me about your greatest failure.

14. Tell me what you would like to do after you retire.

15. Tell me about the person who has most influenced you in your life.

16. Tell me how you feel about dying.

17. Tell me what you like to eat.

18. Tell me what you look for in a friend.

19. Tell me what you fear.

20. Tell me what you think of yourself.

Conversation Starters

Similar in purpose to the tell me game, this exercise utilizes incomplete sentences rather than tell me statements.

 1. Other people usually . . .

 2. The best measure of personal success is . . .

 3. Anybody will work hard if . . .

 4. People will think of me as . . .

 5. When I let go . . .

 6. Marriage can be . . .

 7. Nothing is so frustrating as . . .

 8. People who run things should be . . .

 9. I miss . . .

10. The thing I like about myself is . . .

11. There are times when I . . .

12. I would like to be . . .

13. When I have something to say . . .

14. As a child I . . .

15. The teacher I liked best was a person who . . .

16. It is fun to . . .

17. My body is . . .

18. When it comes to the opposite sex . . .
19. Loving someone . . .
20. Ten years from now, I . . .

Once the group becomes more trusting of each another, more intimate sentence completions can be discussed. Some possibilities are

1. In the bathroom . . .
2. I used to daydream that . . .
3. At night I . . .
4. When I first heard a profane word I . . .
5. When I first saw a naked person I . . .
6. My religion is . . .
7. I feel most ashamed about . . .
8. I'm turned on by . . .
9. Right now I'm most reluctant to discuss . . .
10. I feel that you . . .
11. The thing I dislike most about this group is . . .
12. The opposite sex thinks I . . .
13. I need . . .
14. My body . . .
15. The first chance I get, I'll . . .

You're Like Statements

Rather than having one person reveal something about himself or herself to others, this activity requires others to reveal their perceptions of the person they are focusing upon. In small groups of five, four people give their responses to statements that refer to the fifth. Each person in turn has his or her chance to be focused upon. Examples of you're like statements are

1. Your childhood . . .
2. You get angry at . . .
3. You enjoy . . .
4. You care deeply about . . .
5. You will . . .
6. You think this place . . .
7. You would like to be . . .
8. You would like the instructor to . . .
9. You would like us as group members to . . .
10. The thing you dislike most about yourself is . . .
11. The thing you like most about yourself is . . .

12. You like people who . . .

13. People don't like you when . . .

14. You feel hurt when . . .

15. You really are . . .

16. In front of the opposite sex you feel . . .

17. When you lose a game you . . .

18. When you're alone you . . .

19. You feel like smiling when . . .

20. Right now you feel . . .

Perceptions Survey

Another means of aiding people to see themselves as others see them is through the survey technique. Having organized participants into groups of six, the instructor hands out the following perceptions survey:

Directions: Fill in the name of the person in your group, other than yourself, who you think *best* fits the descriptions here. Place that name on the line to the left of the description. Each description *must* have one, and only one, name associated with it, but the same person's name can be used to answer more than one question. Do not discuss your answers with anyone in the group until the instructor requests you to.

_____	1.	Who is the kindest?
_____	2.	Who is the cruelest?
_____	3.	Who is likely to do anonymous favors for people?
_____	4.	Who is afraid of mice?
_____	5.	Who might cheat on exams?
_____	6.	Who is careless?
_____	7.	Who is very careful?
_____	8.	Who enjoys music?
_____	9.	Who enjoys sports?
_____	10.	Who wears seat belts?
_____	11.	Who likes chocolate layer cakes?
_____	12.	Who rarely has a cavity?
_____	13.	Who dislikes school?
_____	14.	Who butters up the teacher or boss?
_____	15.	Who wakes up often with nightmares?
_____	16.	Who will make a good parent?
_____	17.	Who was a good child?
_____	18.	Who is most materialistic?
_____	19.	Who enjoys danger?

_____	20.	Who would be a good teacher?
_____	21.	Who would be a good friend?
_____	22.	Who likes pets?
_____	23.	Who might use drugs?
_____	24.	Who is afraid of being alone?
_____	25.	Who would like to be someone other than who he or she is?
_____	26.	Who cares a lot about his or her reputation?
_____	27.	Who enjoys classical music?
_____	28.	Who feels most sad?
_____	29.	Who is most happy?
_____	30.	Who has the most secrets?
_____	31.	Who doesn't sleep enough?
_____	32.	Who feels most comfortable with his or her body?
_____	33.	Who needs something?
_____	34.	Who will most likely smoke cigarettes?
_____	35.	Who will most likely be unhealthy?
_____	36.	Who would make a good judge?
_____	37.	Who would make a good scientist?
_____	38.	Who would make a good guidance counselor?
_____	39.	Who is most serious?
_____	40.	Who will be most religious?
_____	41.	Who will be most popular?
_____	42.	Who will spank his or her children?
_____	43.	Who will choose not to marry?
_____	44.	Who reads the most?
_____	45.	Who reads the least?
_____	46.	Who daydreams the most?
_____	47.	Who has enjoyed filling out this questionnaire the least?
_____	48.	Who has enjoyed filling out this questionnaire the most?
_____	49.	Who is most likely to become a television personality?
_____	50.	Who would want to change his or her name?

When all have completed the survey, they are asked to write each group member's name on a separate sheet of paper, then to place the *number* of each description under the *name* they associated with that description. The results of this procedure might look like this:

John	Harry	Beth
2,6,23,33	1,3,7,16,22	14,20,27,44,48

The next step requires the participants to discuss the results of this survey in their groups by focusing on one person at a time. In this manner, each person will have insight into how five others perceive him or her and his or her behavior. Generalizations should be drawn from each set of perceptions. For example, the results cited might lead to the following generalizations:

1. John needs help to change. If that help doesn't come, he might one day abuse drugs or turn to some other deviant behavior.

2. Harry interacts well with others. He is well liked and will therefore relate well with other people regardless of the situation.

3. Beth is very smart. She will do best at things requiring thought and logic. Her enjoyment will probably be derived not from other people but rather from things (books, classical music, questionnaires, and so on).

Some people might object to negative perceptions and generalizations such as those concerning John. These instructors could change the negative descriptions in the survey to positive statements. However, the value of this exercise might then be subverted. If the objective is to afford people the opportunity to see themselves through others' eyes, they must be allowed to receive — and should expect — honest responses. The attitude that ignorance is bliss, and that therefore a program participant perceived by others in a negative manner should not be made aware of these perceptions, is one that will not help them grow and develop in a socially functional manner. The first step to becoming a better person is to find out the kind of person we are. Exploration of the perceptions others have of us is a necessary ingredient for our improvement. Of course, the instructor and participants should understand and agree with this posture, or this activity might be dysfunctional. Some may not be ready for such honesty.

Perceptual Set

A logical follow-up to the perceptual survey is an exercise that will demonstrate the importance of how others perceive us in relation to how they treat and receive us. Probably two or three sessions will need to be devoted to this activity. The instructor arranges for a speaker to visit one day to talk about some controversial topic, such as some aspect of sexual behavior. The speaker is told to give a "neutral" speech — that is, to neither advocate nor reject the sexual behavior about which he or she is talking. Three different health education groups, preferably similar to one another in terms of intelligence, age, and so on, are prepared for the speaker in different ways. One group is offered a positive perceptual set of the speaker by being given and asked to read the following biographical data sheet at the beginning of the speech:

> Bob Jones is a young activist who has worked continually for sexual freedom for people like yourselves. He has even been arrested and locked in jail when he interfered with the police as they were hassling a young girl outside a local high school. The young girl was being bothered by the police for using profanity. Bob often talks with young people about sex and has just turned down a job paying much more than he presently makes so he can continue to meet with people as he is today. I'm sure that you'll enjoy Bob's stay with us.

The second group is offered a neutral perceptual set of the speaker and his visit:

> Robert Jones is a man who speaks to people about sexuality. Mr. Jones will talk for 15 to 20 minutes today about this topic. I now present Mr. Robert Jones.

The third group is presented a negative perceptual set for the presentation:

Robert Jones is a speaker who has the reputation of often distorting the truth. He is regarded as interested only in himself and his own sexual hangups. Mr. Jones's experiences have led many organizations to prohibit his speaking, since people have always been appalled at his lack of knowledge and disregard for others. Let me just add that I would prefer not having to introduce Mr. Jones in this way, but I want you to view his presentation very critically and not be taken in by his act. I now present, quite reluctantly, Mr. Robert Jones.

No questions are allowed after the presentation (15–20 minutes) is finished. Instead, the participants are asked to complete the following questionnaire:

Speaker-Reaction Form

Name _____   Session_____

Directions: On the basis of your impressions of this person, check one alternative in each set that you feel would most accurately describe him. Work quickly, and check the alternative that most closely matches your impression.

1. In general, how does he get along with other people?
_____   a.)   Very well, with friends, but only if he knows them well.
_____   b.)   People are impressed until they really get to know him.
_____   c.)   Is well liked, meets people easily.
_____   d.)   Is respected rather than liked.

2. What does his attitude toward others seem to be?
_____   a.)   Cold and distant.
_____   b.)   Somewhat indifferent to others.
_____   c.)   Really likes others, enjoys meeting them.
_____   d.)   Tends to take advantage of people, uses people.

3. How responsive to people is he?
_____   a.)   Often reserved and aloof, somewhat distant.
_____   b.)   Very warm and open with almost everyone.
_____   c.)   A little distrustful of people, always on guard.
_____   d.)   Attempts to be warm but really isn't.

4. How would his temperament best be described?
_____   a.)   Somewhat excitable and emotional.
_____   b.)   Serious, cautious.
_____   c.)   Cool, calculating.
_____   d.)   Tends to be a stable person, calm, easygoing.

5. How might he behave in an argument?
_____   a.)   Remains calm, reasonable, and controlled.
_____   b.)   Agrees on the surface but is quite rigid.

_____   c.)   May side with other's point of view to avoid a scene.
_____   d.)   Becomes angry, belligerent.

6. How would he react to criticism?
_____   a.)   Shows resentment.
_____   b.)   Ignores it.
_____   c.)   Outwardly accepts it but inwardly seeks revenge.
_____   d.)   Is hurt, very sensitive, but keeps it to himself.

7. How does he feel about people like you?
_____   a.)   Sincerely likes them and shows it.
_____   b.)   Admires them but resents and envies them.
_____   c.)   Is tolerant of their beliefs.
_____   d.)   Appears to like them, but really thinks he is better than they are.

8. What is his greatest strength?
_____   a.)   Loyalty, trustworthiness.
_____   b.)   Sense of humor, keen wit.
_____   c.)   Intelligence.
_____   d.)   Shrewdness.

9. What is his primary life goal?
_____   a.)   To have enough security and be comfortable.
_____   b.)   To help others (for example, the poor, the ill); to be a "good Samaritan."
_____   c.)   Success and recognition.
_____   d.)   To receive esteem from others.

10. What about himself is he most proud of?
_____   a.)   Intelligence.
_____   b.)   Ability to understand people.
_____   c.)   Sincerity, honesty.
_____   d.)   Ability to manipulate people.

11. What is his real opinion of sexuality education?
_____   a.)   Sincerely believes in it.
_____   b.)   Acts interested but is really indifferent.
_____   c.)   Actively supports it.
_____   d.)   Tolerates it but is doubts its effectiveness.

Go on to the following exercise:

Check one adjective or phrase in each pair that best describes the person you have just heard.

1. _____   a.)   Concerned with self   3. _____   a.)   Sincere
      _____   b.)   Concerned with others   _____   b.)   Phony
2. _____   a.)   Sense of humor   4. _____   a.)   Suspicious
      _____   b.)   Stern, businesslike   _____   b.)   Trusting

5. _____   a.) Vindictive   13. _____   a.) Intelligent
   _____   b.) Forgiving   _____   b.) Shrewd
6. _____   a.) Dependable   14. _____   a.) Optimistic
   _____   b.) Undependable   _____   b.) Realistic
7. _____   a.) Progressive   15. _____   a.) Honest
   _____   b.) Conservative   _____   b.) Untrustworthy
8. _____   a.) Scheming   16. _____   a.) Kind
   _____   b.) Humble   _____   b.) Inconsiderate
9. _____   a.) Honest   17. _____   a.) Opinionated, dogmatic
   _____   b.) Two-faced   _____   b.) Flexible, open
10. _____ a.) Condescending   18. _____   a.) Warm, friendly
    _____ b.) Considerate   _____   b.) Cold, indifferent
11. _____ a.) Tolerant   19. _____   a.) Selfish
    _____ b.) Prejudiced   _____   b.) Generous
12. _____ a.) Conscientious   20. Would you like to get to know him better?
    _____ b.) Self-centered   _____   a.) Yes
                                            _____   b.) No

Prior to the next meeting of these three health education groups, the instructor should tabulate the results of the questionnaire and make copies to distribute. The results should be tabulated by the group (actual perceptual set), and the responses of all three groups to the questionnaire should be distributed. Invariably there will be a difference in the results between the group that received the positive perceptual set and that which received the negative perceptual set.

The instructor then lets the participants in on the "secret" and conducts discussions pertaining to the importance of people's perceptions of others. It is worthwhile to mention that people behave in terms of their *perceptions* of reality and not necessarily in terms of what *is* reality. Through this procedure, the perceptions of themselves gleaned through the perceptual survey exercise take on added significance.

Exploring Feelings

FEELINGS ACTIVITIES

List three feelings you have about this book. Please do not read further until this is done. Was your list similar to the following?

_____ 1. I think this book is great.

_____ 2. The author is unrealistic.

_____ 3. Some of these activities are tremendous.

_____ 4. The book is too short (long).

_____ 5. I wish this book had been available much earlier.

(continued)

FEELINGS ACTIVITIES *(continued)*

Or did your list include items such as these?

_____   1. I feel frustrated that I can't conduct health education this way.

_____   2. I feel confused.

_____   3. I feel enthusiastic and want to try some of these activities.

_____   4. I feel close to the author.

_____   5. I feel a sense of worthiness, since I've been doing exercises like these before I ever read the book.

It must be obvious now that the first set of statements above are thoughts, beliefs, or opinions—but not *feelings*. The second set of statements expresses the feelings of frustration, confusion, enthusiasm, psychological closeness, and self-worth. If you found that the three feelings you listed were everything *but* feelings, do not fret. Most respondents would exhibit the same behavior because we are not used to identifying our feelings, or writing or speaking about them. In fact, we are quite talented at hiding the feelings we have. As a means of practicing feeling responses, why not mail to this author your feelings as you read this book?

This section will be devoted to instructional methodologies designed to aid learners in developing the ability to recognize the feelings of themselves and others and to respond appropriately to those feelings they identify. As the first suggestion in this section, it is recommended that the instructor conduct the same activity as employed by the author to introduce feelings. The question might be, How do you feel during health education? The following activities will be based on the assumption that this suggestion has been taken and that now the program participants know how feeling responses differ from thoughts, beliefs, and opinions.

Acting Out Feelings

Emotional health and the study of feelings make up one of the more difficult topics to investigate. One exercise that is valuable in helping people understand their feelings and emotions in an interesting manner is to act out various feelings. Participants are asked to volunteer to act out one of the feelings in the following list, or they may be assigned a feeling to role-play. Role-playing may be limited to verbal expressions only, physical movements only, or a combination of both. Discussions of the acting and the feeling are included as a part of this exercise. Feelings that may be role-played are

1. Pride	5. Love	9. Freedom
2. Happiness	6. Sadness	10. Fascination
3. Glory	7. Joy	11. Loneliness
4. Determination	8. Warmth	12. Confidence

After someone acts out a feeling, the rest of the group must attempt to guess what that feeling was. If they are unable to, the actor must role-play another feeling. An analysis of why the group could not guess the feeling being portrayed will be helpful to subsequent role-players.

It is a lot better to provide people with a socially acceptable way for them to act out their feelings (as in the acting out feelings instructional strategy) than for them to uncontrollably express these feelings in ways that get them into trouble. The feeling of anger is particularly problematic for people who have no way to express it other than destructively.

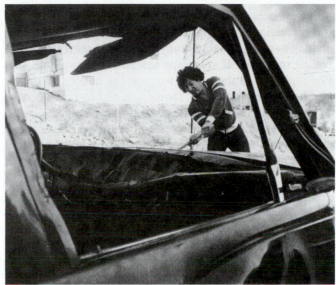

Source: The Diamondback, University of Maryland

If conducted nonverbally, this exercise highlights the relationship of body position to emotional set. For example, a happy, joyous feeling might result in a straight-backed, tall, bouncy body position, whereas a feeling of sadness might be manifested physically by a stance with shoulders rounded, head down, arms drooping. The realization that the body position often indicates feelings is one that will help participants identify what others are feeling at times when they are not communicating their feelings verbally.

Staring

The participants are divided into groups of six. One of the six volunteers to be "it" and stands, while the remaining five also stand and form a circle around "it." The instructor directs those in the circle to stare at the person in the center of the circle. They are to do nothing else; that is, they may not talk or make any attempt at nonverbal communication. The staring should continue for three minutes.

Though these three minutes will seem like an eternity, the behavior manifested by "it" will allow for a meaningful discussion of feelings at the conclusion of this exercise. Such behavior as fidgeting, nervous laughter, swaying, making funny faces at the others, looking up, or looking down will be evidence of feeling responses. If videotape equipment is available, these behaviors can be captured on tape to be replayed, as those who were on the outside of the circle guess how "it" feels from the behavior he or she shows. "It" should attempt to recall how he or she felt at that particular moment so as to verify or correct the group's guess about his or her feelings.

It is necessary for the health educator to remember that skills such as being able to detect feelings in oneself and others do not just develop. They take a lot of practice, as do other skills. The staring exercise is one method of providing this practice in a manner that is interesting and educational.

Break in the Circle

Most people have been excluded from some group at some time — whether from a country club because of background, a community because of race, a social group because of values, or a sports team for lack of ability. Not surprisingly, the feeling of rejection is intense. To demonstrate rejection from a group, have 10 people form a circle, all facing the center. These people represent a group that wants no part of another person who is on the outside of the circle; it's the in-group versus the outsider. Members of the in-group interlock hands or arms and must not allow the outsider to enter the circle. The outsider's task is to get into the circle — first by coercion and verbally requesting entry, then by physically breaking into the circle. The participants should be forewarned not to engage in any dangerous behavior such as punching, pinching, or any other means of breaking the circle that might injure a player.

There are several methods of analyzing this activity at its conclusion. The insiders and the outsiders should try to clarify for one another how they felt. If the group is effective in preventing entry, the outsider usually experiences frustration and rejection, whereas the other participants feel camaraderie, joy, and success. If the outsider does break through the circle, it should be observed whether he or she enters the center of the circle (still distinct from the rest of the players) or attempts to hold hands or interlock arms with the insiders (to be one of the group). In any case, participants should be aware of their feelings during all phases of this exercise.

A variation is for the people in the circle to face outward from the center. This indicates a conscious effort to keep out the "intruder," while facing in could connote an attitude of ignoring the outsider. It would be useful to compare these two methods, facing in and facing out, in relation to the feelings they evoke in the participants.

Shouting Names

Malamud and Machover (1965) describe a game whose function is to put people in touch with their feelings. To conduct this activity, the instructor asks for several volunteers. Then the health educator selects one volunteer at a time and instructs the remainder of the group to shout, in unison, the name of that volunteer. The name is shouted three times. When all of the volunteers have had their names shouted three times, a discussion is conducted of the feelings of both the volunteers and the shouters. Some volunteers find that they enjoy the attention, while others do not. The authors report that one volunteer winced as if being scolded, while another smiled from ear to ear, indicating the pleasure he was feeling. Relative to the shouters, some enjoy the freedom to let go a tremendous shout, while others feel self-conscious. Malamud and Machover report feelings of inadequacy and self-consciousness and needs for exhibitionism are often felt by the shouters.

Gracious Receiving

One of the more difficult tasks for people is to receive compliments in an accepting fashion. Upon being complimented, some people make strange comments and/or show strange feelings. For example:

Compliment: My, what a nice hat you're wearing.
Response: Oh, it's not new anymore.

These learners are participating in the shouting names activity. This instructional strategy can be an excellent way of introducing a discussion on feelings.

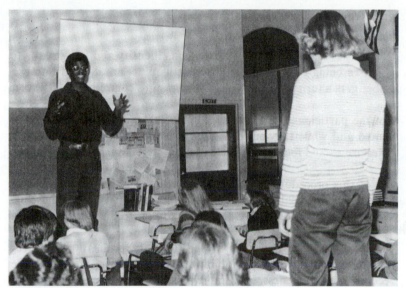

Source: Jerrold S. Greenberg

Compliment: I felt like getting you this gift.
Response: Oh, you shouldn't have.

Compliment: My, you look pretty today.
Response: You probably say that to all the girls.

Compliment: You know, you're a real nice person.
Response: Oh, go on.

The next activity is designed to have participants identify and analyze the feelings they experience when they're being complimented. The participants are divided into groups of six, and each group member gets a turn as the focus of the group's compliments. The compliments must be truthful.

The task of the participants is to attempt to understand their feelings both while they are being complimented and while they are doing the complimenting. A discussion held at the conclusion of this exercise should focus on these feelings as well as on how best to respond to compliments.

A variation of this procedure calls for "it" to tell the group a thing of which he or she is proud. The other participants continually interrupt to compliment "it" on those parts of his or her story that deserve compliments. A discussion similar to the one just described then ends this exercise.

The outcomes of the gracious receiving game are participants' realizations that receiving and expressing positive feelings can be nice, that inhibiting expression of these feelings deprives both the giver and the receiver, and that expression of positive feelings brings people closer to each other. These are indeed important lessons.

Blocking

It is often difficult for people to identify with those different from themselves. Blocking is an activity that can be employed to develop empathy for others. The health educator should supply enough two-inch-by-two-inch wooden blocks for each person in the group. The instructor distributes these blocks, requesting that each person carry the block from that moment until the same time the next day (24 hours). The block is *never* to leave the hand except when sleeping. Participants will have to hold the block while eating, showering, playing sports, and so on.

At the next meeting, the instructor should discuss participants' experiences and feelings related to carrying the block. Some will have felt self-conscious, others ridiculous, and still others burdened. The instructor then draws an analogy between the block and some burdens that people carry with them all the time. For example, fat is the obese person's "block"; pimples are the blocks for people with acne. The feelings of self-consciousness, ridiculousness, and being burdened that the participants felt for a short period are often felt by people with different blocks *all* of the time. That some people make fun of others different from themselves, thereby making their blocks even heavier to carry, should be discussed.

Friends and Enemies

To help people experience and investigate a wide range of feelings, have them think of one friend and one enemy. On one sheet of paper they should list five adjectives that they think their friend would use to support them; on another sheet of paper they should list five adjectives describing themselves that their enemy might use to tear them down. These adjectives should be words that actually are, or have been, used by others to describe these people. The group is then organized into pairs to discuss the feelings evoked when the supporting adjectives are used by the friend and the degrading adjectives are used by the enemy — *and* what would be felt if the friend used the negative adjectives and the enemy the positive ones in a description of that person. Is it the word, the person who uses the word, or a combination of the two that most affects the feeling response?

How/When Questionnaire

One device to help people identify how they feel during various occasions is the how/when questionnaire. Participants are asked to identify *how* they feel *when* something happens. The questionnaire should be completed individually and then discussed in pairs or small groups. Discussion should relate to why such feelings are experienced at those particular times. Some how/when items might be

_____	1.	How do you feel when you fail at something?
_____	2.	How do you feel when you lose a game?
_____	3.	How do you feel when you get turned down for a job or a date or a promotion?
_____	4.	How do you feel when you're called to answer a question in class?
_____	5.	How do you feel when you are reprimanded?
_____	6.	How do you feel when you are complimented?
_____	7.	How do you feel when you get a bad haircut?
_____	8.	How do you feel when you disappoint your relatives?
_____	9.	How do you feel when it rains?

_____	10.	How do you feel when it snows?
_____	11.	How do you feel when the sun shines?
_____	12.	How do you feel when you cheat at something?
_____	13.	How do you feel when you have a big problem?
_____	14.	How do you feel when you've won a prize?
_____	15.	How do you feel when you are selected?
_____	16.	How do you feel when you are with your best friend?
_____	17.	How do you feel when you get hurt?
_____	18.	How do you feel when you go to the dentist?
_____	19.	How do you feel when winter comes?
_____	20.	How do you feel when you come to school or work?

Responses should be placed on the line to the left of the item to which that response relates.

Feelings Drawings

Feelings may be expressed by colors (red for active and pale blue for passive, for instance) or through drawings. This activity requires participants to depict their feelings in a drawing. They might be asked to draw their feelings about

1. Competition
2. Winning
3. Losing
4. Surprising
5. Loving
6. Caring
7. Cooperating
8. Sharing
9. Learning
10. Parenting

The artists then display their drawings and briefly report to the group what they drew and why they drew it the way they did.

Activities to Affect Behavior

This section includes activities designed to specifically relate to the ways in which program participants act, and the means of behaving more consistently with their desires. Several of these exercises reflect the major concept of this book: as a popular song once said, _people need people._ Therefore, participants are organized to help other participants meet their goals.

Prescriptions

This exercise is intended to result in suggested behaviors that program participants could adopt to feel less frustrated. The exercise requires people to list things they feel frustrated about on one side of a sheet of paper, and the way they feel about these frustrations on the other side of that paper. After trying several methods of processing these data, the participants form quartets to discuss their frustrations and feelings about them. Each quartet is asked to choose one member's frustrations to focus on and to prescribe a specific behavior that person could follow for one week to attempt to relieve some of that frustration. The prescribed behavior has to be reasonable and of a type that could be expected to provide some measure of relief in a week's time. Each person in the quartet takes a turn to be focused on.

Two particular means of prescribing these behaviors are recommended. The first approach calls for the person whose frustrations are being considered to sit with his or her back to the other group members. The three others then discuss that person's frustrations for three minutes, not allowing any verbalizing from the "focus." After three minutes of such discussion, in which specific behaviors are recommended, the focus reacts for one minute to what has been said.

The second method of prescribing behaviors requires each member to touch each other member of the quartet, one at a time (shake hands, place hand on shoulder or arm, and so on), and tell him or her, This week I want you to. . . . The physical contact is designed to create a feeling of closeness and concern on the part of the group's members.

Regardless of the method of prescribing behavior, time should be provided the next week for the quartets to reconvene and report to one another which behaviors they tried and the result of these attempts. The quartet might then want to suggest additional actions for its members to take.

A word about suggested behaviors: These should be specific. Suggestions such as "Talk to someone" or "Have fun" are not as meaningful as "Talk to your wife about . . ." or "Go to the school basketball game this Friday."

The results of this activity are severalfold:

1. Participants come away with specific things they can do to overcome some of their frustrations.

2. A feeling that others care about them enough to want to help them relieve some frustration makes participants feel less isolated.

3. Peer group pressure is utilized positively by being directed at making the group members feel better.

Telegramming

Though suggestions to help people achieve their goals are useful, often these suggestions are not adopted nor their goals accomplished. This activity is designed to remind participants where they want to go (their goals) and how they can get there (suggested behaviors). Each person in the group is asked to send himself or herself a telegram specifying what he or she wants to accomplish in one month's time and what should be done to meet this end. The telegrams are written on sheets of paper, which are then placed in envelopes distributed by the instructor, and the envelopes are sealed. The health instructor requests the participants to address the envelopes to themselves and then collects them. In one month the instructor mails the envelopes to the learners. After the participants have received the envelopes, they can, if desired, discuss the degree to which they have been successful in achieving their short-range goals. At this point, another telegram might be written that specifies a second goal, or if the original goal has not been met, cites other behaviors that would aid in the achievement of that goal.

It is best to limit the number of goals to approximately four. Goals may relate to various parts of participants' lives: work, school, management of time, getting along better with others, or physical changes.

Permanent Grouping

Another means of aiding program participants to establish and move toward the satisfaction of short-range goals involves the establishment of small groups that meet every other week for one class period. These groups will be established for the life of the class to help their members develop rapport and caring for one another, and to allow for continuity in movement toward the goals cited by the group's members. At each meeting, once goals have been determined, the group should focus on identifying the forces present that seem to be assets in achieving the goals, and those that seem to be inhibiting their achievement. The task of the group then becomes one of developing strategies that members can employ to maximize the assets and minimize the inhibitors. Feedback on the effectiveness of these strategies should be a part of each group session. In this manner, the group serves as an ongoing advisory body concerned with the accomplishment of its members' goals. The phrase "All for one and one for all" comes to mind.

Justification of Self

For this exercise, the participants are divided into groups of five. To bring participants' past behavior into focus and to confront them with the meaning of that behavior, the following handout should be distributed to each group.

> An airplane on which you were flying to Europe from the United States has crashed in the middle of the Atlantic Ocean, and you are one of only five survivors. A life raft has been located, but it can support only three people without sinking. There is no possible way of switching people in and out, and, therefore, the *only* solution is to save three people in the raft and leave the other two behind. By describing your past deeds and explaining why they make you valuable to mankind, you must convince the other four people that you should be one of the three saved.
>
> Each of the five people in your group will make a three-minute presentation in an attempt to get into the life raft. After all of the presentations have been made, each person, in secret, will place on a sheet of paper the names of two other people in the group whom he or she wants to save. When this is done, count up the number of times each person's name appears on the sheets of paper. The three people whose names are most frequently mentioned are to be saved. If there is a tie for the third person, have the group vote between those who have tied.

This exercise requires participants to consider the worth of their past behavior in relation to the needs of all people. Some will conclude that they have been self-centered and have not functioned as contributing members of society. Others will determine that they are proud of their concern for their fellow human beings and will have their behavior reinforced.

Self-Concept Activities

The activities included in this section are meant to help the program participants determine who they really are. They are designed to answer the existential question, Who am I?

I Am Statements

People in general seldom stop to think about who or what they are, so it is not surprising that program participants don't either. This exercise asks learners to *list* as many characteristics of themselves as they can muster that will fit on one-half of a sheet of paper (which does not include their name). The instructor collects these descriptions and tapes them on the walls of the room. The participants are then told to walk around the room and write (in small letters, so as to leave room on the paper for others) the name of the person they think those characteristics describe. At the end of this phase of the exercise, the participants are asked to take their own descriptions off the wall and determine who they were judged most often to be. Themselves? Someone else? If someone else, did they realize that they were perceived to be like this person? And whom would they rather have been perceived as similar to?

People will often find that their real self perceived by others differs from the self *they* perceive. The question then becomes, Who am I really?

Self-Portraits

A variation of the "I am" game entails the drawing of one's self-portrait rather than the listing of characteristics. The portraits should be revealing, in some way, of the self the participants perceive. As in the previous exercise, the portraits are taped to the walls and students wander about the room writing the name of the person they believe is being portrayed. A discussion of how the group's perceptions differ from the individual's perceptions (or how they are similar) should include feelings elicited by and during this exercise.

Bravissimo

The purpose of this exercise is to help program participants learn more about themselves and others in their group in a positive, experiential manner. In groups consisting of four people, each person in turn states—in only one sentence—something that he or she does, has done, or soon will do about which he or she feels good. After each statement the group shouts *Bravissimo,* which means "Very well done." After 10 minutes of this activity, the groups should be allowed 5 minutes to have any of their members clarify a statement that has been made.

By allowing, and even requiring, participants to focus on their positive behavior, and by having others cheer this behavior, two main objectives are accomplished:

1. Learners begin to realize, if they haven't before, that they have much of which to be proud.

2. Learners' concepts of self are enhanced.

Fantasy Play

Many people desire to be someone other than who they are. The act of daydreaming about being someone else can be structured and used in fantasy plays. Participants are organized into groups of six and then asked to imagine being someone other than themselves. The instructor should hasten to add that the someone else they are imagining should not be a real person, but rather an *imagined* one who possesses the personality, knowledge, skills, and so on that they would like to possess. Each person then takes a turn to act out a one-minute play he or she developed that depicts this imaginary self. After each play, the other group members question the playwright to identify more clearly the traits of the imaginary self, then they suggest how the playwright might go about developing some of these characteristics. As stated elsewhere in this chapter, such suggestions should be realistic, with some chance of succeeding.

This activity gives participants a clearer concept of their real self, as well as concrete means for narrowing the gap between their ideal self and their real self.

Stress Management Activities

This section presents instructional strategies that help program participants understand the relationships among stress and illness and disease, and ways to manage that stress.

Mind Control (Greenberg 2002)

The mind and the body are interconnected. When the body is relaxed, the mind cannot be tense; and when the mind is relaxed, the body cannot be tense. That is why relaxation techniques that relax the body (such as progressive relaxation) will also relax the mind, and relaxation techniques that relax the mind (such as meditation) will also relax the body. To demonstrate the mind–body connection, first have program participants learn how to determine their pulse rate (how fast their hearts are beating). Pulse rate can be determined in several ways: (1) Place the first two fingers (pointer and middle fingers) of one hand on the underside of the wrist, on the thumb side. (2) Place the first two fingers of one hand on the lower neck, just above the collarbone; move the fingers toward the shoulder until the pulse is found. (3) Place the first two fingers of one hand in front of the ear near the sideburn, moving the fingers until the pulse is found.

While seated in a comfortable position, participants determine their resting pulse rate, or how fast their hearts are beating at rest. This number is written on a sheet of paper. Next, participants close their eyes and think of either someone they really dislike or some situation they experienced that really frightened them. This image should be seen in great detail; sights, smells, sounds, and taste should be noted. Participants are instructed to sense the dislike, to feel the fear, to place themselves with that person or in that situation. After approximately five minutes of this visualization, participants again determine their pulse rates. Invariably most of the group's pulse rates will increase when thinking of a strong emotion — that is, of someone they dislike or a situation in which they were frightened. The pulse rate will increase even though participants engaged in no physical activity. This activity demonstrates the relationship between the mind and the body, how the mind can actually change body processes.

Stress Emitters (Greenberg 2002)

Most participants will be concerned with their health and managing stress will be of interest to them for this reason. They will want to be able to decrease the amount of stress they are "given" by others: the boss, a coworker, the teacher, relatives, friends. However, they do not realize that they, too, cause stress for those with whom they interact. Further, they can decrease the amount of stress they cause others if they choose to. "Stress emitters" is an instructional strategy that can help them do that. To begin, participants identify three people in their lives with whom they have a relationship and about whom they care. One person is a relative, the second a friend, and the third someone else.

Next, for each person listed, participants identify three ways they cause that person stress. For each person listed, participants write down three things they will do to cause each of the people they listed less stress.

Now, form groups of four participants. In turn, participants will share their commitments to cause less stress for people in their lives and describe how they intend to accomplish that goal. If possible, reconvene the groups in two weeks, at which time group members will describe their attempts to cause others less stress and whether they were successful. Having to report back to the group provides added incentive for program participants to follow through on their commitments.

Time Pressure Buster

One of the most stressful factors of people's lives is their inability to manage their time well. The "time pressure buster" activity can help them free some time for activities for which no time was available previously. This time management technique requires participants to make four lists daily: an *A* list a

B list, a *C* list, and a *not-to-do* list. On the A list are things that have to get done that day. For example, you are getting married tomorrow and you have yet to choose a wedding gown. Not realistic? Well, perhaps a more common example is having a term paper due tomorrow and, therefore, needing to type it today. Typing the paper goes on the A list.

On the B list are things you would like to get done today, and need to get done soon, but they do not have to be done this day. They can get done in a couple of days and that would be okay. For example, your term paper is due in 10 days and you have yet to begin researching the topic. You need to get to the library to do that soon. However, if you don't get there today, that would be okay. As long as you get to the library in a couple of days, submitting the term paper will not be a problem. Going to the library, then, goes on the B list.

On the C list are things you would like to get done today but they can really wait almost indefinitely to get done. For example, you have a friend who lives out of town whom you have been meaning to telephone. You would like to do this today, but even if you do not get around to calling for several weeks, that really would not be a problem. If you never call your friend, you might lose a friend. But if you do not call your friend for several weeks, the friendship will probably remain intact. Telephoning your friend, then, goes on the C list.

On the not-to-do list are things that have been wasting too much of your time, and, therefore, you want to make sure not to do that day. For example, you have been watching too much television lately. Today you want to purposely not watch television. It then goes on your not-to-do list.

After being presented with this description of the four lists and their purposes, program participants are instructed to develop these lists daily for a week. Each day they are to accomplish the A list items first, moving to the B list only after all the A items have been done. Attention to the C list items occurs only after the A and B list items have been completed. In addition, participants periodically refer to their not-to-do lists as a reminder to not engage in the activities identified as time-wasters.

The Stress Interview (Geiger 2001)

Before discussing stress and illnesses associated with it, have program participants interview someone they know who has experienced a stress-related illness. This person can be a relative, friend, acquaintance, or anyone else that has had such an experience. Participants are given Figure 8.1 to guide the interview and the paper they will write based on the interview. When writing the paper, participants will not divulge the name of the person interviewed but rather describe that person more generally (age, sex, ethnicity, socioeconomic status, and the like). A group discussion conducted by the health educator will pertain to what participants learned about stress and its consequences, and about stress management.

Progressive Relaxation

One of the contributing factors in the development of disease is stress. The stress response can alter the body physiology to make it more susceptible to illnesses and diseases or to exacerbate already existing illnesses or diseases (Greenberg 2002). There are many ways to respond to stress, but perhaps one of the best requires the person to be able to relax the body to counteract the stress response. Several effective relaxation techniques can be employed for this purpose; three of them are described next.

Several methods have been suggested for the relief of muscular tension, one of which has been developed by Edmund Jacobson and is termed *progressive relaxation* (Jacobson 1938). Progressive

FIGURE 8.1

Stress-Related Interview Guide for Students

1. Specify the gender, race, age, and occupation of the adult you interviewed. Do not reveal the individual's name, address, or telephone number.

2. Please describe the stress-related illness for which you were treated.

3. What do you think caused this illness?

4. Which other members of your family have had problems with stress?

5. Before you became ill, how did you manage work, family, or other stressors?

6. Describe mental health treatments that were most helpful to you.

7. What types of health service providers offered these services?

8. Which treatments were not helpful?

9. Have you made any lifestyle changes since your illness to manage stress?

10. How can we improve the mental health knowledge of American adults?

11. When should people learn about mental health and stress management?

12. What are the roles of schools, public health agencies, and businesses to assist youths to manage their stress?

13. (Compose any other related questions to ask your subject.)

14. Finally, write about your reactions to the content of the interview. What did you learn about stress management from this activity?

---

relaxation involves the contraction of muscles to help the learner become more aware of the presence of muscle tension, and then a complete relaxation (letting go) to experience a relaxed muscle. The following is an example of instructions the health educator could provide to experience the progressive relaxation technique.

> Sitting in your seats with your eyes closed, extend your right arm, with the palm upward, to the right. Now make a fist and bend your arm at the elbow and contract your biceps. After 10 seconds just stop concentrating all at once, and the whole arm should fall to your side. Experience the muscle tension when the muscle is contracted, and the relief when it is relaxed. Learn to recognize both feelings and to be able to call upon either when desirable.

Jacobson (1973) has adapted progressive relaxation to the educational process. His book describing that adaptation is recommended to instructors interested in doing further reading in this area.

Autogenic Training

Another method of muscle relaxation, *autogenic training,* was developed by Dr. J. H. Schultz (1959). Autogenic training results in feelings of heaviness and warmth in the parts of the body focused on and a general relaxation of muscles in that area. The following is an example of instructions for one autogenic training exercise.

> Sitting with hands rested on your thighs (not touching each other), back straight against the chair, head hanging loosely forward, and both feet flat on the floor, close your eyes. Imagine you've just come from a long walk and you're very tired.
>   Your legs are most tired.
>   Feel the heaviness in your legs. They are very heavy.
>   Just let your legs weigh themselves down.
>   Now they are feeling very warm. Just relax them, but feel how heavy and warm they are. Enjoy this feeling. Retain it.

The whole group can participate in this activity, concentrating on various parts of the body. The whole body can be made to relax through autogenic training.

Meditation

Still another method of muscle relaxation and stress relief is *meditation.* Though there are many different forms of meditation, the one whose benefits have been most validated by experimental research is Transcendental Meditation. TM is a simple, natural, effortless technique that allows both mind and body to gain deep rest, releases stress, and leads to clearer, more powerful thinking and more effective, dynamic action. Although TM is simple to learn, the technique must be learned from a qualified instructor. The health educator could invite a TM teacher to give a presentation and to answer questions for the group. Those who would like to begin TM could sign up for a course taught by the TM teacher, either at the health education facility or at the local TM center.

Another method is the relaxation response described by Benson and Klipper (2000). The *relaxation response* is the name coined to describe the physiological reactions of the body to meditation. These reactions include decreased body metabolism, lowered heart rate, lowered respiratory rate, and muscle relaxation. In fact, the relaxation response is described as just the opposite of the much-publicized fight-or-flight reaction. To obtain the relaxation response, participants should be told to sit quietly with their backs against an upright chair, their feet on the floor, and their eyes closed. This position is similar to that prescribed for autogenic training. While keeping this position for 20 minutes, participants should repeat the same word (for example, *calm)* over and over again. When they realize that other thoughts have entered their minds, they should return to the word being repeated. It is recommended that to be most effective this meditative process not be attempted shortly after eating and should be repeated twice daily (once in the morning and once before dinner). A discussion with the group regarding their subjective experience of the relaxation response and a physiological explanation of what has occurred will be of interest.

If you are particularly interested in stress management, let me refer you to an excellent source of numerous instructional strategies—although I may be a little biased because I wrote the book I'm about to refer you to. That source is a book titled *Comprehensive Stress Management* and was published in 2002 by the same publisher of this book—McGraw-Hill.

Valuing Activities

Values clarification can be employed to explore aspects of mental health. The examples that follow are but a few of the ways in which valuing activities can be incorporated into mental health education. Many of the other valuing strategies described in Chapter 7 can also be adapted to this content area.

Values Grid

This technique requires participants to give priority to their values and to publicly affirm them. The 16 traits here should be placed in a grid, one trait per cell. When the values grid is completed, there will be four traits valued very highly, four highly, four mildly, and four for which there are no opinions. The following traits can be used:

1. Peaceful
2. Kind
3. Open
4. Tactful
5. Confident
6. Courteous
7. Fearful
8. Masculine
9. Feminine
10. Anxious
11. Careful
12. Materialistic
13. Happy
14. Lonely
15. Popular
16. Religious

A discussion of the completed grids should be concerned with the relationship between the placement of the traits and the learners' own lives. The following questions are suggested for discussion:

1. Which of the traits that you valued very highly do you possess?
2. Which of these traits do you hope to possess in five years?
3. Of the very highly valued traits that you do not possess, how might you plan to acquire them? Who can help?
4. How many of the very highly valued traits does your best friend possess?
5. Why did you express no opinion about the four traits in that column?

Values Continuum

In this activity each person is asked to reflect on the following 10 statements and then to identify where each statement would fit on the continuum.

Agree   Neutral   Disagree

1. A friend should not criticize you.
2. Everyone should learn how to relax.
3. People should not keep secrets about themselves.
4. First impressions are usually accurate.
5. Feelings are private and should not be expressed.

6. It is difficult to receive a compliment graciously.

7. Doing things is more important than whom you're doing them with.

8. People need privacy.

9. Stress can be a positive influence.

10. When anxiety develops, medication should be taken.

Students can then be organized to share their responses and the reasoning underlying their answers.

Proud Statement

This is an activity that, if program participants have developed trust and honest communication with one another, can help identify values related to mental health, and that can be emotionally very touching. Participants are asked to complete the statement "I am proud that I . . ." and take turns telling the rest of the students how they responded. As stated previously, people usually become more thoughtful and appreciative of their own worth and of the value of others as a result of this exercise.

Values Ranking

The process of ordering value statements by their importance is an important component of the valuing process. The following groupings relate to mental health and can be used to identify and clarify values in that area:

1. Popular	1. Open	1. Anxious
2. Honest	2. Secretive	2. Calm
3. Reliable	3. Ashamed	3. Excited
1. Success	1. Child	1. Pets
2. Happiness	2. Adult	2. People
3. Pride	3. Senior citizen	3. Things

Values Sheet

The values sheet consists of a provocative statement and a series of questions related to that statement with application to people's personal lives. Here is a values sheet for mental health education:

Directions: Read the following statement and then answer the given questions honestly and thoughtfully.

Paul is a friend of Todd's. When Todd stopped dating Nancy because, as he said, "Nancy isn't good-looking enough," Paul called Todd aside.

"You are too concerned with what other people think," said Paul. "It was a mean thing to drop Nancy because other people might not find her attractive. She has a great personality and is real fun to be with."

"Mind your own business," said Todd. "If you were a good friend you'd understand how important it is for me to have the other guys and girls think well of me. How can they think I'm cool if I date an unattractive girl?"

Questions

1. Do you know anybody like Todd? Describe him or her.

2. Have you ever felt rejected as Nancy must have felt? When?

3. How could you make someone who feels rejected feel better?
4. What have you learned because of this exercise?

Summary

You will note that this chapter does not concentrate on mental illness. Rather, the concern is for mental *health,* and the learning experiences described are consistent with that emphasis. In a preventive education program, such as health education, the focus should be on prevention of illness through the maintenance of health. The rationale for the study of illness should be related to its prevention and not its treatment. Consequently, this chapter presents activities designed to prevent feelings of alienation and self-deprecation through the exploration of feelings toward oneself and others, which will better one's mental health status and decrease feelings of loneliness and isolation.

The learning experiences are directed at the development and maintenance of each person's mental health status, rather than at an academic, generalized study of mental health. An outcome of such an approach is a much closer-knit group, better rapport between instructor and students, and a more efficient group of learners when subsequent health content areas are studied.

CHAPTER NINE

Instructional Strategies for Substance Abuse

The quest for a solution to the "drug problem" in our society has been unending. Unfortunately, simplistic solutions have been proposed for a very complex situation. As a result, no one is assured that any one method of substance abuse education is more effective than any other. There are, however, a number of research reports and supported hypotheses of experts in substance abuse education upon which to base a sound theory of substance abuse education and a methodology consistent with that theory.

The Pimple Theory

To better convey the kind of substance abuse education presented here, it will be helpful to employ an analogy that, though admittedly not physiologically sound, will crystallize some of the thoughts presented. Imagine a pimple roaming about a body seeking a place to surface. From head to toe the pimple roams until a potential place to appear is sighted. Now the person about whose body we are talking, deciding not to allow any pimples to surface, places his hand over the location the pimple seeks. The hand presses down hard and the pimple pushes up with all its might. Suddenly realizing there are only two hands to protect abundant potential "surfacing spots," the pimple gives up the fight and proceeds to an unprotected area, at which it surfaces unmolested.

Health educators seem to be pressing down in isolated areas (substance abuse, health faddism, juvenile delinquency, and sexual irresponsibility, for example) much as the hand attempts to prevent the pimple from surfacing. Unfortunately, even when the pimple spots are pressed down on, the pimple will surface at some other unsuspected location. It is therefore recommended here that the underlying cause of substance abuse be determined and responded to, rather than the drug behavior itself. If one were able to eliminate the pimple (or the *causes* of substance abuse), then one wouldn't have to protect all parts of the body (or the total of potential unhealthy and antisocial *behaviors)* because there would be nothing left to surface

What are these pimples that lead to such seemingly irrational behavior as substance abuse? Granted, there may be severe psychological problems associated with the use of particular addictive drugs. However, the causes of substance abuse have implications for a *preventive* substance abuse program—that is, education.

For several reasons, poverty can be disregarded as a cause of substance abuse. First, the economic background of program participants is a given element and nonmanipulative. Second, as will be discussed in the following pages, the *outcomes* of poverty rather than the condition itself contribute to substance abuse. And third, the incidence of substance abuse among wealthy and well-known people is evidence that substance abuse is not a result of lack of material possessions alone.

Similarly, lack of knowledge of the consequences of substance abuse can be ruled out as a prevalent cause. Witness that among physicians, substance abuse is greater than in the general population. It seems that intelligence or academic achievement is not related to abuse of drugs.

It has been suggested elsewhere that a negative concept of oneself *is* related to substance abuse. Levy (n.d.), for instance, states,

> The users of the nonnarcotic drugs seem to be doing more than just avoiding the pains and conflicts of living. They are seeking some way of overcoming their feelings of inadequacy and differentness. They have not been able to cope with existence satisfactorily. They feel unfulfilled and want meaningful experiences. They desperately want answers to the existential questions of: Who am I? What am I doing here? Where am I going? and How am I going there?

Dusek and Girdano (1987, 20–27) write of the social aspects of drug usage. Among other factors related to substance abuse, they cite social alienation, low self-esteem, peer pressure, and self-identity. Schlatt and Shannon (1990) concur with Dusek and Girdano but add that drugs may help people obtain "group entry" and are sometimes used to rebel against any number of people or situations (for example, one's life, one's parents, societal decisions, and so on).

Although some effective school drug education programs exist (Bennett 1986), substance abuse education occurs in other settings as well. Programs for workers with drug problems are not too difficult to find (employee assistance programs), and programs offered through local hospitals are also quite prevalent.

Drug education programs have been conducted in various settings with varying degrees of success. This chapter describes some instructional strategies that can be employed in programs that try to prevent and/or respond to drug problems. In particular, learning activities to respond to poor self-concept, negative peer influence, alienation, and values confusion are presented. The goal is to help health educators be more responsive to the human beings they are instructing, rather than to focus too much on the content they are teaching.

Peer Group Exercises

One of the most pervasive factors related to drug misbehavior is peer group influence. The following exercises are designed to explore the existence of peer group pressure, how influential it is, how to react to negative peer pressure, and how to employ this phenomenon for beneficial purposes.

Reversed Seats

The effect of peer pressure is so impressive that people often engage in ridiculous behavior because of this influence. To demonstrate this point, send five volunteers out of the room on a pretense of picking up pamphlets for distribution to the group. The person to whom these students are sent should know they are coming and should delay them for several minutes. In the meantime, the instructor tells the group that (1) when those participants return, the group will continue its discussion as usual; (2) some time later, upon a signal from the instructor (perhaps pulling on the ear), the group members will sit on their desks (or tables) and face the rear of the room; and (3) the conversation will continue just as if nothing had happened. Invariably several of the volunteers, who weren't "clued in," will leave their seats and sit on their desks facing the rear. Often at least one volunteer will refuse to perform what he or she believes to be such a ridiculous act.

The participants who left the room in search of pamphlets should then explain to the group

1. How they felt when everyone sat on their desks facing the rear.
2. What they thought about before deciding whether to do what the group was doing or not to go along with the group.
3. What they think they should have done when the group sat on their desks.

The participants should discuss generalizations that can be drawn from this exercise and how peer pressure influences behavior all of the time. They should cite specific instances when their behavior was influenced by peers in spite of their own desires. The beneficial aspects of peer pressure should not be overlooked in such a discussion. For instance, laws might be viewed as peer influence, but necessary and beneficial.

Blindfolding

The desire to impress our peers is so strong that we often are embarrassed to admit to a lack of experience. To explore this statement further, ask the participants several questions during a large-group discussion. These questions should be of a somewhat embarrassing, threatening, or revealing nature. For example:

1. How many use drugs?
2. How many have seen a person of the opposite sex naked?
3. How many have a problem with pimples?
4. How many argue with their spouses a lot?

For each of these questions, record the number of participants who raise their hands. Next, ask the participants to place blindfolds (provided by the participants or the instructor) over their eyes so that no one can see anyone else in the class. Then ask the same questions again, and again record the responses to each question. The count after the blindfolds are on is usually different from the earlier count, when everyone could see how everyone else responded. When the counts have been made, the participants discuss how they felt when the questions were read, both before and after the blindfolds were in place. As with other exercises in this book, generalizations for daily behavior should be elicited. Students can also be asked how they felt knowing the health educator was aware of their responses.

Commercial Collaging

Some of the most energetic and carefully organized efforts to affect behavior by using the desire to impress one's peers are made by the advertising and marketing complexes. To further analyze the extent and use of peer group influence, participants can be asked to examine advertisements appearing in local newspapers and magazines. Advertisements utilizing peer group influence can be cut out and used to create a collage for display. Participants may also find interest in creating their own posters counteracting the message of the advertisements. For example, an ad implying that smoking cigarettes will help one to become a he-man or beauty contest winner might be placed beside a participant-created collage of pictures of unattractive people smoking cigarettes in unappealing settings.

When it's realized that advertisements motivate large numbers of us to spray, squeeze, and rub smelly substances under our armpits, the power of ads becomes evident. Why not employ that power to encourage healthful behaviors and decisions? The commercial collaging, commercial recording, and commercial creating instructional strategies can be used in this manner.

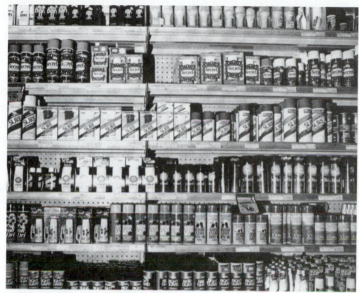

Source: The Diamondback, University of Maryland

Commercial Recording

Because advertisements are not exclusive to the written medium, television and radio appeals to status in peer groups should also be investigated. One way to accomplish this is to have participants agree to listen to a radio or television station for three hours on a Saturday morning and to record, in writing or on tape, instances of peer group pressure. Such recordings should be discussed in the group the following Monday. To acquire a more complete picture, it is recommended that different participants be assigned to listen to different television channels and radio stations. In this manner it will be possible to generalize television and radio as a whole and not be limited to data from only a few stations.

An analysis of the data brought by participants will indicate that all ages are subject to peer group influence.

Both commercial collaging and commercial recording can be used to increase awareness of how certain groups of people—certain ethnic groups, certain age groups, certain genders—are targeted with respect to drugs.

Commercial Creating

While examination and analysis are useful learning activities, a more complicated behavior is creation. Using the knowledge and insight gleaned from commercial collaging and commercial recording, participants can create commercials themselves. These commercials must

1. Use peer group influence appeals.
2. Advocate the nonabuse of drugs.
3. Be appropriate for the listeners' age group.
4. Be suitable for presentation over a public address system.

Subsequently, substance abuse education week can be established in a school or shopping mall, and five commercials can be broadcast over the public address system each morning (one each day).

Staged Argument

Rather like the reversed seats exercise, this activity demonstrates the effect of peer group pressure on decision making. The instructor selects four people who enjoy the sessions and thinks up some pretext for them to leave the room. While they are gone, the health educator instructs the group to stage an argument with him or her about how bad the course is. When those who left the room return, the others are to attempt to solicit their active support in the argument. Usually those who left the room will either verbally support the group or remain silent. In any case, they will seldom support the instructor, regardless of their beliefs.

A subsequent discussion of this activity will reveal the feelings of differentness, bewilderment, and loneliness experienced by those not in on the secret. The desire to alleviate these feelings is often the motivation for not expressing support for the instructor. If some do support the instructor, an examination of their motivations will prove interesting and informative.

Videotaping Plays

The use of videotape and filmmaking equipment offers endless possibilities for contributing to the health instructional process. In one such endeavor, program participants might videotape playlets that demonstrate how the need for peer approval may influence others to use drugs. These tapes might then be played for schoolchildren as part of their drug education offerings. Participants who create these videotapes should visit with the children as the tapes are shown to answer questions about the message being conveyed.

It would also prove valuable to videotape plays describing the results of several of the peer group exercises described in this chapter. Such tapes could be employed with teachers in an in-service educational activity. Thus, program participants would be teaching teachers. Similarly, if these tapes were shown to parents during an evening set aside for such an occasion, program participants could educate parents.

Crossword Puzzle

Although the cognitive aspects of substance abuse education have been overemphasized in some health education programs, knowledge about drugs might best be considered a necessary but not sufficient condition to affect drug behavior. The task of the health instructor is to explore such knowledge with participants in an educationally sound setting with little threat of negatively affecting the variables cited at the beginning of this chapter. One excellent means for cognitive learning is the crossword puzzle. The reader may want to develop puzzles more apropos to his or her local situation than the example provided in Figure 9.1.

FIGURE 9.1

Drug Crossword Puzzle

¹A	²L	³C	⁴O	⁵H	⁶O	⁷L		⁸S		⁹H
¹⁰M	¹¹A				¹²N			¹³T	¹⁴H	¹⁵E
¹⁶P			¹⁷P	¹⁸D		¹⁹O	²⁰P	²¹I	²²U	²³M
²⁴H	²⁵E	²⁶R	²⁷O	²⁸I	²⁹N			³⁰M	³¹M	³²P
³³E			³⁴T	³⁵L	³⁶C			³⁷U		
³⁸T	³⁹O			⁴⁰A		⁴¹O		⁴²L		
⁴³A		⁴⁴W	⁴⁵I	⁴⁶T	⁴⁷H	⁴⁸D	⁴⁹R	⁵⁰A	⁵¹W	⁵²A	L
⁵³M		⁵⁴E		⁵⁵E		⁵⁶E		⁵⁷N		
⁵⁸I				⁵⁹C			⁶⁰T	⁶¹O	⁶²O	
⁶³N	⁶⁴O		⁶⁵G		⁶⁶O		⁶⁷L	⁶⁸S	⁶⁹D	
⁷⁰E		⁷¹P	⁷²O	⁷³P	⁷⁴P	⁷⁵Y				⁷⁶A
⁷⁷S			⁷⁸A			⁷⁹T	⁸⁰R	⁸¹I	⁸²P	

ACROSS

1. _____ mixed with barbiturates can cause death
10. Nickname for mother
13. Definite article
17. Abbr. for police department
19. A drug made from poppies
24. Abusers of this drug often get hepatitis
30. Abbr. for marine military patrol
34. Abbr. for tender loving care
38. Toward
44. Reaction to the stoppage of an addictive drug
60. Also
63. Negative
67. Name for drug from a fungus on rye
71. Opium is made from the _____ plant
79. A drug-induced departure from reality

DOWN

1. A drug given for weight loss
2. Abbr. for Los Angeles
6. Covering
8. Classification of drugs that cause blood vessels to dilate
9. Common name for the marijuana plant found in India
14. To sing with your mouth closed
17. Slang for marijuana
18. To enlarge or get bigger
29. Abbr. for no charge
41. Poem of praise
44. Pl. of I
59. Abbr. for constable on patrol
61. Abbr. for overdose
65. Opposite of stop
73. Nickname for father
76. Abbr. for the Atlantic and Pacific Co.

Debates

One of the most valuable techniques for actively involving participants in the learning process is debate. A word of caution is in order, however. Often debates result in a discourse of ignorance due to insufficient planning on the part of the instructor or a lack of commitment on the part of the debaters. A debate is not a loosely conducted experience but rather a highly structured activity. Several formats for debating have been proposed, but regardless of which format is chosen, consideration should be given to

1. Length of time for initial presentation.
2. Length of time for rebuttal.
3. Sequence for presentations and rebuttals.
4. Length of time for closing statements.
5. Procedures, if any, for audience participation.
6. Means and criteria for selecting a winner if one is to be chosen.

The time allowed for initial presentations, rebuttals, and closing statements will depend on the number of debaters and the length of the session. Assuming four debaters (two pro and two con) and a 40-minute period, the following time allocations and sequence are recommended:

1. Initial presentation—four minutes per speaker (total: 16 minutes).
2. Rebuttal after all initial presentations have been made—two minutes per speaker (total: eight minutes).
3. Questions from audience—eight minutes.
4. Closing statements—one minute for each debater (total: four minutes).
5. Group vote to determine winning team—one minute.
6. Miscellaneous—three minutes.

It can't be emphasized enough that debaters need ample time to research the topic and prepare a debating strategy. The instructor's role as facilitator necessitates providing resource materials or directing debaters to them, planning for the debate well before the event to allow the debaters to prepare, and moderating the debate when it is conducted. The following is a list of substance abuse education topics appropriate for debate:

1. Should marijuana be legalized (or decriminalized)?
2. Is cocaine more dangerous than heroin?
3. Is marijuana more harmful than alcohol?
4. Should drug pushers apprehended with large quantities of drugs be jailed for life?
5. Do healthy people abuse drugs?
6. Is the stay-at-home mother drug user more dangerous than the heroin addict?
7. Should cigarettes be illegal?
8. Is caffeine injurious to one's health?
9. Should heroin addicts be allowed to legally obtain heroin from government distributors to support their addiction?

10. If a drug were developed that would induce violent physical reactions when heroin enters the body, should this drug be placed in our water (as is fluoride for the prevention of tooth decay)?

11. Is the use of drugs the best way to get high?

12. Should emergency contraceptives (the "morning-after pill") be dispensed only by a druggist upon receipt of a physician's prescription?

Brainstorming Highs

There are almost as many ways of getting "high" or "turning on" as there are people. An activity to demonstrate this concept utilizes the brainstorming approach, in which people supply instant ideas that may be associated either closely or remotely with the problem being discussed. The basic rules for brainstorming are

1. List ideas related to the problem as quickly as possible.

2. Do not criticize.

3. The more ideas, the better.

4. After all ideas are listed, combine and/or modify them.

5. From a discussion of the remaining ideas, decide on one or several solutions to the problem.

An example of the use of brainstorming to discuss ways of getting high will serve to clarify this methodology. This topic is to be discussed in one of the health education sessions via the brainstorming technique. As many ideas as possible would be elicited—for example, mountain climbing, playing basketball, singing, dancing, playing music—before an agreement or consensus is reached on the best approach. Since criticism of ideas is barred until all ideas are listed, insecure program participants will feel less threatened and therefore will tend to be more verbally active when brainstorming is used.

The many and varied means of getting high elicited through brainstorming could serve as a listing of alternatives to drug abuse. Some of the suggestions on this list will be judged inappropriate by the group when a discussion of the listing is undertaken. Some may be illegal, immoral, unethical, impractical, or impossible. But the remaining suggestions might present meaningful choices for people who have heretofore been unable to identify ways, other than drugs, to get excited about life.

Program Visitors

Whether due to budget restrictions, excessive distance to a site one wishes to visit, or the inability of the site to handle a number of people, field trips are not always possible. An alternative to visiting a site is to have someone from the site visit the group. Visitors offer a dimension to learning that instructors or fellow participants often cannot offer. With a frame of reference not possessed by participants or instructors, visitors tend to create interest by their dissimilarity to everyday program activities and by their expertise relative to the purpose for their visit. It would be naive to assume that every visitor will provide a worthwhile use of time. Some visitors may be knowledgeable but very poor speakers, some visitors may be excellent speakers but not very knowledgeable, and some speakers may be neither knowledgeable nor well-spoken. It is therefore recommended that the instructor or a representative group of participants meet with the invited guest prior to the visitation to

Many alternative "highs" can produce a "rush" and still be acceptable and relatively safe. Brainstorming highs might elicit such alternatives as white-water rafting, playing basketball, singing, mountain climbing, or hiking.

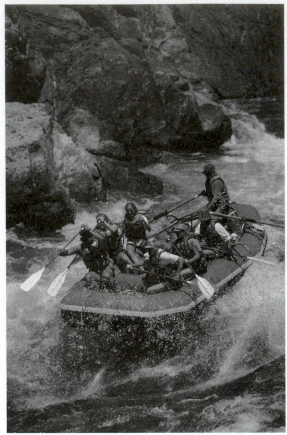

Source: Karl Weatherly/Getty Images/PhotoDisc

1. Allow the program representative to assess the potential of the visit.
2. Acquaint the speaker with the interest and knowledge level of the group about the speaker's topic.
3. Obtain from the visitor ideas for preparing the group for his or her visit.
4. Plan with the guest the format his or her visit will take (lecture, question and answer, round-table discussion, and so on).

Visitors for substance abuse education programs could be chosen from among counselors at neighborhood counseling centers, personnel of detoxification units, representatives of several organizations that offer varying modes of treatment (group therapy, methadone withdrawal or maintenance, psychoanalysis, self-help communities, and so on), and police officers from narcotics squads.

Case Study

Often learning that derives from the analysis of how others have behaved can be meaningful. Role-playing has been cited as one experience in which analysis of the actions and reactions of others can enhance empathy and understanding. Analyses of case studies also enhance learning. The cases, or stories, can be read aloud by the instructor, shown on film, or written out for the participants to read. Whatever the method, a story is presented and analyzed, and conclusions are drawn. By way of example, the instructor might read a story of a teenager whose girlfriend has deserted him, whose parents aren't responsive to his needs, to whom school is a "bummer," and who subsequently uses drugs to relieve his frustrations. Participants might then be asked how friends, parents, and teachers could have prevented the drug abuse; what other avenues of escape from one's frustrations there are; and what the implications of this story are for each of the members of the group. For the case study method to be accepted, the case must be relevant to the interests and needs of the people for whom it is intended. Stories from newspapers, books, related experiences, and vivid imaginations are several sources from which cases can be obtained. Regardless of the derivation of the case or cases to be employed, care should be taken to conclude the analysis of each case with a discussion of its implications for the participants.

Critical Incident

Whereas the case study method of instruction utilizes a story with a beginning, middle, and end, the critical incident approach does not supply an end to the story. The learner, therefore, is responsible for developing plausible endings for the story. This open-ended technique allows people to place themselves in a role that has been described and to act out the end of that story as they perceive it. The advantage of this methodology over the case study method is that people have to use their own creative abilities to end the story rather than react to a given ending. The nature of the case when employing critical incidents must be such that at the point at which the story ends a decision is necessary (thus becoming the critical incident in the story). Steps suggested for the use of the critical incident technique are

1. Reading the incident.
2. Acquiring or agreeing on assumptions about additional facts that are needed.
3. Discussing the major issues.
4. Summarizing the issues.
5. Individually recording reactions to the critical incident.
6. Forming groups to react to the critical incident.*

As can be readily determined, the critical incident technique can be used in conjunction with sociodrama as well as with other methodologies yet to be discussed.

Here are two examples of critical incidents that can be used with substance abuse education groups:

Janice's best friend (really her *only* friend) had to move out of town and, consequently, Janice had the loneliest, most miserable summer of her life. It was September when Janice started a new job, without anyone to

---

*From Cyrus Mayshark and Roy Foster, *Methods in Health Education: A Workbook Using the Critical Incident Technique*, pp. 6–7. St. Louis, MO: The C. V. Mosby Company, 1966. Reprinted by permission of Roy Foster.

whom she could confide her apprehensions. She worked next to Paula, and when Paula asked her to go with her to a party that weekend, Janice was ecstatic. When they entered the party, Janice noticed that there were a number of people smoking marijuana. Soon Paula took a marijuana cigarette from her pocketbook and asked Janice to smoke one too. Janice thought about her loneliness and then about the marijuana. Then Janice . . .

Philip was bored. He wasn't very good at sports, did poorly in his work, and did not have any really good friends. Realizing that his life was unexciting and that the future didn't look much better, Philip decided to turn within himself for excitement. He knew where all the "dopers" hung out and went there to see if he could get a drug that would help him forget about his problems. When he reached the street corner where the crowd who used drugs usually spent their time, Philip saw Jeff. Since Jeff used to go to the same high school before he decided to drop out, and Philip knew he used drugs, Jeff was the perfect person for Philip to talk with. When Philip explained his situation, Jeff said, "I've got just the thing, baby. LSD will trip you right through yourself. You'll have a religious experience, man, with all sorts of colors and shapes. Real spaced out. What do you say? Want some?" Philip said . . .

Strength Bombardment

One of the suspected correlates to drug abuse is poor concept of self. It is hypothesized that people who do not have high regard for themselves and their opinions are more apt to be influenced by others than those with a positive self-concept. Since the desire for peer status is also a suspected correlate to drug abuse, it seems reasonable to seek to improve program participants' self-concepts so that *they* can decide whether or not to use drugs with as little negative interference from others as possible. Strength bombardment is one means to improve self-esteem.

If possible, organize the group so that the participants are seated in a circle. It is important that the seating formation be circular rather than square or oblong because only a circular seating arrangement allows each participant to see every other participant. One person becomes the focus of the group's attention, and comments are directed only to that person. The others are told to tell that person as many positive statements about himself or herself as they can develop in five minutes. The statements, however, must be true; false flattery is not the intention. Though it is easier to think of positive statements for some people than others, everyone has some good traits. Therefore, every person can, at one time or another, serve as the focus.

The results of this exercise are severalfold. First, the bond between the focus and other participants becomes stronger. They tend to feel better about one another than before the exercise. Second, participants who have always felt useless, worthless, and inconsequential begin to think that they have something to contribute to the group and to others outside of the group. For perhaps the first time, these participants have focused on their positive traits and have had others do so as well. It is not unusual for some people to have positive aspects of themselves, which they never knew existed, brought to their attention for the first time during this activity. An atmosphere of camaraderie, which is conducive to subsequent health education strategies, is created as a result of strength bombardment.

It is recommended that strength bombardment be employed for short periods (perhaps two program participants in any one session) over the history of the group. An observant instructor who can perceive when participants are "down in the dumps" can employ this exercise to save the day for them. Strength bombardment is also an excellent means to end a session that has concerned itself with a topic of controversy. When participants argue a point on such topics, they often come away angry. Strength bombardment can restore the desired group atmosphere and help participants who have argued to feel better about one another.

Forced Arguing

This exercise is related to maintenance of positive self-concept once it is developed. It lets people practice feeling good about themselves and their opinions, in spite of someone else's negative remarks or feelings. This activity is organized in small groups (from four to six people per group) and requires each person to think of something about which he or she feels good. On becoming "it," each participant tells the group what he or she feels good about. The group's task is to take the opposite position from the person and argue with him or her. Name-calling *is* allowed. "It's" task is to maintain his or her good feelings in spite of the negative remarks of the other group members.

A variation of this activity is to have those who are "it" relate to the group negative feelings they have about themselves, some things they've done, defeats they have experienced, or personal weaknesses they perceive about themselves. The group's task is then to argue against "it's" self-deprecation. In this manner, each person in the group will feel better about himself or herself in spite of some negative characteristic or experience that has previously led to some self-deprecation.

Thermometer

A means of soliciting opinions and positions from participants in a more exotic fashion than just by asking for them is to take the group's temperature on certain issues. This procedure calls for the instructor, or a participant, to draw a long thermometer on a sheet of paper, which will be spread out on the floor. Chalk can also be used to draw the thermometer on the floor. Even paint can be employed if this exercise is going to be used often.

Next the instructor raises an issue (for example, arrest of alcoholics) and asks the group "how hot" they get over this issue. The "hotter" or more bothered they are about an issue, the higher they stand on the thermometer. The less concerned they feel about the issue, the cooler they are toward it, and therefore, the lower they stand on the thermometer.

A variation of this exercise is to distribute paper upon which appears a picture of a thermometer and a statement of the issue printed across the top. In this case, participants are asked to place an X at the appropriate spot on the thermometer, indicating how concerned they are about the issue. In small groups they discuss why they placed the X where they did.

Here are some issues that can be used for substance abuse education:

1. People smoking in a room where nonsmokers are present.
2. Pregnant women smoking cigarettes.
3. Methadone maintenance
4. Involuntary use of antabuse.
5. Aversive therapy (for example, electric shock administered when an alcoholic reaches for a drink).
6. Legalization or decriminalization of marijuana.

Interviews

People often come in contact with problem drinkers, users of illegal drugs, and cigarette smokers. Such is the state of affairs in our country. Rather than deny this fact, a good health educator will use it for the betterment of program participants. After studying drugs and related issues, it would be worthwhile for program participants to interview users of drugs (alcohol, illegal drugs, misused legal drugs, tobacco, properly used legal drugs) to determine

1. Their motivations for using or abusing the drug.
2. Whether they abuse or misuse other drugs and how.
3. When they first started abusing drugs and which drug that was.
4. Whether their lives have changed as a result of abusing drugs.
5. What ways the community could prevent or treat drug abuse or misuse among younger populations.
6. Whatever else is on the minds of the program participants.

Other interviews might be with parents, physicians, psychologists, school nurses, or public health officials. It should be remembered that the object of this activity is for program participants to see how what they have learned in an enclosed environment (the health education setting) applies to the community at large.

Valuing Activities

Substance abuse education provides many opportunities to use valuing exercises. Some examples of how the consideration of the relationship between values and drug behavior can be conducted are presented in this section. The health educator is encouraged, however, to adapt still other values clarification activities to substance abuse education.

Values Ranking

Asking participants to rank their preferences related to drug behavior will help them to identify and clarify values of which they may not have been previously aware. Some groupings that can be used for rank ordering are

1. Drug pusher	1. To think well of oneself
2. Drug addict	2. To be thought well of by friends
3. Drug grower	3. To be thought well of by relatives

1. Physical health	1. High	1. Drink beer
2. Social health	2. Straight	2. Smoke marijuana
3. Mental health	3. Cool	3. Pop pills

Values Statements

Another means of studying values as they relate to drug behavior is to have people complete sentences that indicate values and then discuss their responses:

1. I use drugs or medications when _____

2. My body _____

3. My friends_____

4. Marijuana _____

5. To be high is _____

6. To be straight is_____

7. To be cool means _____

8. Pills _____

9. My head _____

10. I feel alienated when_____

Value Judgment

Case studies can be combined with valuing to produce an activity that will elicit value judgments. In the following example, several values are manifested in the behavior of the story's characters. After reading the story, program participants are asked to list the characters in the order in which they like them.

> John was a drug pusher, but not the ordinary kind. When Mary came to John for some drugs, John gave them to her even though Mary had no money to pay for them. He gave her a nickel bag of marijuana (five dollars worth) and some cocaine to snort. The next day Mary felt it was unfair to hit John up for some more free drugs, so she broke into Frank's grocery store and stole $75 from the cash register. However, a policeman saw Mary leave and chased after her. When he caught her and asked Frank if he would press charges, Frank hesitated. He whispered to Mary that he would drop the charges if Mary slept with him that night. Mary was angered to hear Frank's request and slapped his face. When the policeman saw this, he charged Mary with assault as well as robbery.

> Place the names of John, Mary, Frank, and the policeman in the order in which you like them. First listed will be the one you most like, second listed will be the one you like next best, and so on until the last one listed is the one you like least.

Values Continuum

Having people place themselves somewhere between two extremes of an issue and discussing the reasons for placing themselves where they did is still another means of investigating values. This technique is called the values continuum. Here are two values continua that may be used in drug education:

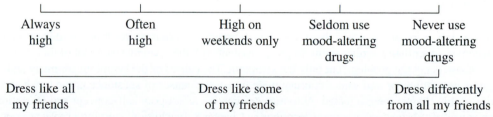

The first example presented relates specifically to drug behavior and, when discussed, may indicate inconsistency or confusion in values. For instance, if younger participants have previously indicated a value for independence quite typical of adolescence, their dependence on drugs may be cited as contrary to this professed value. The second example relates to the influence of people's peers on their behavior. As has been stated earlier in this chapter, there exists a relationship between people's behaviors and that of their peers. The extent to which this influence affects each person can be demonstrated with this values continuum. The values inherent in this influence can then be examined.

Medicine Cabinet Inspection

Many times we have values that contradict one another, and we must decide for one at the expense of the other. An exercise to demonstrate this point requires people to list everything they find in their medicine cabinets at home. Once these lists are developed, ask the following questions:

1. Did you find prescription drugs that were no longer needed? Does your family value money over safety?
2. Did you find mood-altering drugs? Does your family value highs from substances over highs from people and activity?
3. Were drugs out of the reach of children? Does your family value safety over convenience?

Learning Statements

At the conclusion of valuing activities, people can be asked to write paragraphs that begin with any of the following phrases:

1. I learned that drugs _____
2. I learned that people _____
3. I learned that isolation _____
4. I learned that getting high_____
5. I learned that drug treatment modalities_____
6. I learned that my values _____
7. I learned that I need _____
8. I learned that my health _____
9. I learned that when people are lonely_____
10. I learned that friends often _____

Summary

In conclusion, it should be noted that most of the learning experiences described in this chapter relate to objectives other than learning about drugs. Consistent with the opening statement of this chapter, substance abuse is not the problem, but only the symptom. The causes of the symptom are many and varied. Negative peer influence and values confusion are two of the causes of substance abuse to which the activities in this chapter were directed. Activities designed to affect poor self-concept and alienation, two other causes of substance abuse, were described in Chapter 8. In addition, learning experiences in which cognition about drugs could be achieved were also presented. Since many substance abuse education programs ignore the psychosocial aspects of the "drug problem," however, the focus of this chapter has been to help the health educator better respond to those needs.

CHAPTER TEN

Instructional Strategies for Sexuality and Family Living

Several factors have led to the emergence of sexuality education as an area of emphasis. There is the research base that has expanded since the work of Masters and Johnson (1966) legitimized such investigations. There are the technological developments such as in vitro fertilization (Greenberg Bruess, Haffner 2002, 307–8) and surrogate mothering (Strong et al. 2002, 393) that have led to societal and ethical concerns. There is the high rate of teenage pregnancy ("Teenage Pregnancy" 2002). There is the sexual consumerism prevalent throughout American society that is evidenced by the "home party" (similar to the Tupperware party), in which sexual paraphernalia such as French Ticklers and soft-leather ropes are displayed and sold. There are increasing sales of sexy lingerie and rentals of erotic videotapes. There is the Supreme Court's decision that, at first glance, seems to support antisodomy laws passed by the states to outlaw certain sexual behaviors even if conducted in private by consenting adults. And last but not least is the concern regarding the spread of human immunodeficiency virus HIV.

Because sexual information tends to be acquired from friends, popular literature, the Internet, and other generally unreliable sources; because polls indicate that parents of schoolchildren overwhelmingly support sexuality education in the schools; and because school administrators also favor sexuality education—these programs are being developed and offered more frequently. The former surgeon general's decree that sexuality education should be offered in the public schools to encourage "safer sex" (that is, the use of a condom during sexual intercourse and the maintenance of sexually monogomous relationships) has added the institutional support needed to get many such programs off the ground. However, sexuality health education programs are not confined to school settings. These programs are now being conducted at places of work, community health sites, and hospitals, predominantly to help prevent the spread of HIV, but sometimes to address other matters of sexuality as well.

Although prevalent concerns are about sexual disease and eroticism, or about sexual permissiveness or sexual ethical issues, health educators know that an effective sexuality education program involves more than these issues. A more comprehensive view of sexuality includes the totality of people's sexual lives: their relationships, their attitudes and feelings, their family roles, and the like. Someone once said, "Sex is what we do; sexuality is what we are." We concern ourselves here with *sexuality.*

This chapter presents instructional strategies that can be employed in sexuality education programs. The strategies are divided into content areas: the need for sexuality education, masculinity/femininity, sexual behavior, courtship and marriage, family life, violence prevention, controversy about abortion and HIV/AIDS education, and sexual valuing.

FIGURE 10.1

Even businesses use sex to attract clients. Here is an ad from a private gym that offers a variation of the "wet T-shirt contest." It offers sexually attractive couples the chance to win a prize, thereby attracting potential clients who want to watch these couples in various "poses." This is an example of how we are frequently confronted with sex in our society. Health education programs should help people understand their sexuality better and be able to manage sexual matters in their lives.

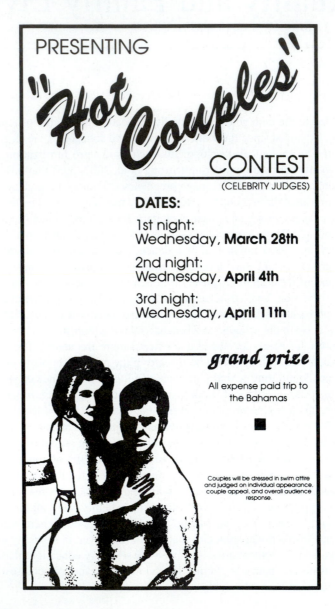

Need-For Activities

The first four activities can be used to underline the need for sexuality and family life education. It will be assumed that interest in sexuality has already begun (an assumption one can feel confident in making).

Sexy Collage

One need only glance at newspaper and magazine advertisements to notice their appeals to sexual needs and desires. Consider the "manly" man with the "sexy" woman enjoying a walk through the woods with a cigarette; the best thing (cigar) from Sweden since the blonde; the bikinied girl standing beside a car; and the candy mint that is a breath freshener and results in the user's kissing an attractive mate.

Add to these the announcements of movies about student nurses who shouldn't but do, the husband and wife who should but don't, and the rest who wish they could but can't, and the result is a society whose sexual needs are continually exploited and conditioned.

When program participants are asked to create collages on large sheets of heavy paper that reflect appeals to sex that appear in newspapers and magazines, they soon realize how such appeals influence their own behavior. The posting of these collages, and the opportunity for the group to view them,

FIGURE 10.2

This is a picture of a sexy collage created by a student. The theme of this collage is "A Man Is." Note the ruggedness of the men depicted. This collage prompted a great deal of discussion.

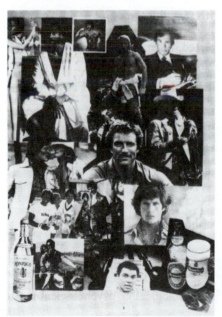

Source: Jerrold S. Greenberg

should be followed by small-group discussions of how each participant has been influenced. Here are some topics to be used in these discussions:

1. By which advertisement appealing to sexual needs were you recently influenced?
2. What did this advertisement make you do?
3. How was this advertisement presented to you? Television? Newspaper? Magazine? Would you have reacted differently if it were presented in one of the other two media?
4. What would you tell younger people to help them *not* be influenced by this advertisement the way you were?

Sex as . . . Questionnaire

Another manner in which the need for sexuality education can be demonstrated is to identify ways in which sex has been employed by the program participants, or how they feel it should be employed. The questionnaire here is designed for this purpose. It should be noted, however, that *sex* is not used synonymously with sexual intercourse or with any other particular sexual behavior. *Sex* might refer to flirting, wearing provocative clothing, or using perfume. After the questionnaire is completed, form small groups for a discussion of the manner in which sex is used as _____.

Sex As . . .*

Directions: Try to identify with this list of sex as . . . and pick those phrases that most represent your feelings. Try to identify with at least three. Place a + before the ones you choose.

_____ Sex as purely playful activity.

_____ Sex as a way to have babies.

_____ Sex as fun.

_____ Sex as an expression of hostility.

_____ Sex as punishment.

_____ Sex as a mechanical duty.

_____ Sex as an outlet from physiological or psychological tension.

_____ Sex as a protection against alienation.

_____ Sex as a way of overcoming separateness or loneliness.

_____ Sex as a way to communicate deep involvement in the welfare of another.

_____ Sex as a form of togetherness.

_____ Sex as a reward.

_____ Sex as a revenge.

_____ Sex as an act of rebellion.

_____ Sex as an experiment.

---

*From James L. Malfetti and E. M. Eidlitz. *Perspectives on Sexuality.* New York: Holt, Rinehart and Winston, 1972. Reprinted by permission of James L. Malfetti.

_____ Sex as an adventure.

_____ Sex as a deceit.

_____ Sex as a form of self-enhancement.

_____ Sex as an exploitation for personal gain.

_____ Sex as proof.

Go back over the list and place an X after those you have used but are not happy with.

Hot Line

It is now time for you, the health educator, to apply some self-appraisal. This next activity requires an instructor more comfortable with sex and sexuality than is usual for a health educator. It also requires a teacher with a great deal of knowledge about sex-related topics. This activity, "hot line," begins when the instructor announces to the health education class that a certain telephone has been designated for their calls between certain hours of the day. The telephone number and times for calls should be written on the chalkboard and each person *required* to write these in his or her notebook. Some might feel embarrassed to write down the numbers unless *all* are required to do so. The instructor then explains that any questions they want to ask that relate to sex or family life, no matter how silly, will be answered by the instructor on the telephone at the prescribed times. The health educator should emphasize that the identities of the callers will remain unknown.

As can be expected, such an activity will allow "Johnny Joker" to call and ask an embarrassing or insulting question. However, if the instructor can live through such calls, other callers will display a naiveté and lack of sophistication and knowledge that will evidence the need for sexuality and family life education. At the same time, program participants too embarrassed to ask questions in group sessions will be able to ask these questions anonymously.

Question Box

The "question box" has a purpose similar to that of the hot line — namely, to provide an anonymous means for program participants to ask, and have answered, questions related to sexuality and family life. Such a box should be placed in a convenient location to allow participants to place inside the box pieces of paper on which are written questions. The instructor should periodically remove the questions from the box and provide class time for answering them. The following is a sample of questions asked by college students enrolled in this author's sexuality class:

It has been reported that when women reach climax their nipples become erect. Is this a myth?

I think I'm a DES daughter. What should I do?

Is it possible that the fluid which comes out of a man's penis before semen causes a woman to become pregnant?

Do the same things that arouse men also arouse women?

Is masturbation harmful?

Is there a male menopause?

When is it safe to have intercourse without using any safeguards and not have to worry about getting pregnant?

How is abortion done and what laws govern it?

Sometimes, when my partner is obviously interested in sex, I'm not. It's pretty awkward. Is there something wrong with me?

Does living together before marriage increase the chance for a successful marriage?

Can older people have satisfying sex lives?

Masculine/Feminine Roles

One of the topics still being debated is the role of women and, consequently, the role of men in our society. To simplify the debate, *behaviorists* believe that much of sexual role determination is learned behavior. An example: boys learn to be aggressive and girls learn to be passive because of the games they play. *Naturalists* believe that the sexual role is inherited or related to hormonal secretions. That is, males are more aggressive than females because they have a greater amount of androgen. The following activities will help the instructor involve program participants in the study of sexual and/or gender roles.

Sex Riddle

To highlight the prevalence of stereotypic thinking relative to sex roles, the instructor should distribute the following handout.

> A father and his son were involved in a car accident in which the father was killed and the son was seriously injured. The father was pronounced dead at the scene of the accident and his body taken to a local mortuary. The son was taken by ambulance to a local hospital and was immediately wheeled into an operating room. A surgeon was called. Upon seeing the patient, the attending surgeon exclaimed, "Oh, my God, it's my son!" Can you explain this? (Keep in mind that the father who was killed in the accident is not a stepfather, nor is the attending physician the boy's stepfather.) Think about the "riddle" for a few minutes. If you think you have the answer, write it on a sheet of paper.

The answer is then read: The surgeon was the boy's mother.

The inability of most (if not all) of the class to conceive of the surgeon as a woman can then be discussed. Such questions as the following should be posed:

1. What other jobs are usually thought of as masculine? Feminine?
2. Can women (men) perform these jobs well?
3. Why do you think these jobs have been assigned to women (men)?
4. What is your thinking regarding sex role stereotyping?

Imaginary Mirror

With the purpose of further exploring stereotypes associated with sex roles, program participants can be asked to give their conceptions of masculine and feminine in a unique manner. The instructor asks the students to close their eyes and imagine that they are looking in a magic mirror. In that mirror they see someone of the opposite sex (do not mention the age of the image they see). The group is told that they can see everything about that person: what he or she looks like, how he or she functions socially, the IQ of the image, and the emotional responses the image exhibits. The group is then given 20 minutes to describe, in writing, the image they saw relative to the following four categories:

1. Physical
2. Emotional
3. Intellectual
4. Social

After the descriptions have been written, volunteers should be allowed to read their descriptions to the total group. When six descriptions have been read for each sex, the health educator then asks the class to pick out the points they have in common. It will be noted that the females imagined by the males were young, beautiful, sweet, cute, bright, cried easily, and so on, whereas the females will have imagined their male image to be brave, strong, handsome, athletic, shy, a show-off, and so on. A discussion of sexual stereotyping will then be meaningful and relate to the participants' own stereotypes as opposed to discussing, with academic disguise, stereotypes in general.

Sex Role Dislikes/Likes

To begin a discussion of what males dislike about females and what females dislike about males, divide participants into two groups—one all male and the other all female. Have each group brainstorm what they dislike about the opposite sex. After 20 minutes, one male and one female are selected to read the list their group developed. An argument should then be developed between the two groups to allow the presenting of stereotypes related to sex role that are often believed and felt, but not often stated publicly.

The next group meeting, or the end of this group session if time permits, should be devoted to a similar activity, except that the focus should be on what is *liked* about the opposite sex. Any ill feelings associated with the first phase of this activity should be eliminated as a result of phase two.

Sex Tasking

This is another activity that will illuminate sex role expectations and develop an appreciation of the sexual pigeonhole in which people are placed. It requires that females list tasks associated with femaleness that they desire to give up and tasks associated with maleness that they would like to adopt. Similarly, males should develop lists of "male tasks" they desire to drop and "female tasks" they desire to adopt. The two sets of lists should be compared in small groups for similarities. It will soon become evident that there are some tasks neither group wants to be responsible for and some tasks each group wants to adopt. The proposal of a reasonable and *just* solution to this dilemma should be the responsibility of the small groups.

Participation in "sex tasking" usually results in some of the following questions:

1. Why do women usually wash dishes?
2. Why do men usually take out the garbage?
3. Why do men usually pay for the date?
4. Why are women usually picked up on a date?
5. Why do women usually prepare the meals?
6. Why don't more women ask men out on a date?

7. Why do women usually take care of the children while men work outside of the home in families with only one salaried worker?

8. Why aren't women's athletic teams as important as men's athletic teams?

9. Why are some of these roles changing?

10. What, if anything, are the problems associated with these defined sex roles?

Head Tapes

Often an instructor will want to have program participants express their biases in a nonthreatening atmosphere. "Head taping" allows them to attribute their biases and stereotypes to the role they're playing. The instructor divides the class into small groups of six members each. Strips of adhesive tape, upon which roles are written, are placed on the foreheads of each person without the person's learning what role he or she is to play. Group members can see the roles assigned to others (since the roles are written on the tapes stuck to their foreheads) but cannot see their own role (since they cannot see their own foreheads). The group then engages in a conversation about society, and each group member is to treat the other group members as though they were the types of people identified on their head tapes. By way of example, if Johnny is to play a he-man, *he-man* would appear on the tape on his forehead. During the group conversation, the group is to react to whatever Johnny says or does as though he really were a he-man. The roles assigned should be as follows:

1. Sexy Susie

2. Athletic Abe

3. Intellectual Izzy

4. Masculine Madeline

5. Sissy Stanley

6. Ugly Augustine

As the conversation goes on, the participants are to write down their own roles when they think they know them. When all group members have guessed the role they have been assigned, the tapes are removed, and the participants determine whether their guesses were accurate. A discussion in small groups regarding why Sexy Susie, for example, was greeted with smiles but Ugly Augustine with disdain will do much to help stereotypes surface. The instructor should conclude by stating that how one is treated often becomes a self-fulfilling prophecy. That is to say, if one is treated as though one is worthless, one will behave worthlessly. If one is treated as a person of importance, one tends to behave importantly. Similarly, if females are treated as sex objects, they may tend to behave as sex objects, and if males are treated as aggressive and competitive, they will behave aggressively and competitively. The health educator should stress that escaping from our pigeonholes requires that males and females perceive each other differently from the traditional stereotypes. Consequently, more women will become partners, and more men will be able to cry.

Sexual Behavior

The following activities are offered as examples of learning experiences pertaining to sexual behavior. The limits of propriety, parental concern, administrative fiat, and participant interest are so varied that presentation of numerous activities related to many sexual behaviors does not seem warranted.

FIGURE 10.3

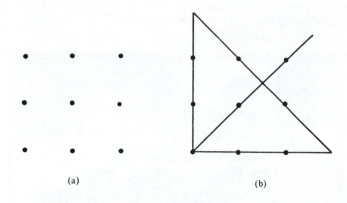

(a)   (b)

However, the activities described, and others in this book, can be adapted to the sexual behaviors chosen by the individual health educator.

Boundary Expanding

The purpose of this introductory activity in the study of sexual behavior is to develop an appreciation for varying mores, religious and home values, and personal beliefs that result in different sexual lifestyles.

A handout is distributed on which appear nine dots, as shown in Figure 10.3(a). Students are told to draw four straight lines connecting all dots without lifting their pencils or retracing a line. The solution looks like Figure 10.3(b). The teacher should ask whether students thought of going out of the boundaries (the outside dots). The relationship between unusual sexual behaviors in other cultures and within our own society — to "going out of boundaries" — should then be made. The health educator might then ask whether our society's boundaries of sexual behavior should be expanded outward (and if so, in what directions) or drawn in closer (more restrictive and prescriptive).

Sexual Orientation Grid

To investigate values relative to a specific sexual behavior, a value grid might be employed. The example here pertains to homosexuality, but the health educator might substitute another sexual behavior and revise the questions appropriately. The program participants are told to divide a sheet of paper into 16 sections and to label the columns as in Figure 10.4.

Sixteen questions are read to the group. Each person must place key words from one question (and *only* one) in one square of the grid to show how he or she feels about that question. For example, if this author were asked, "How do you feel about learner-centered health instruction?" he would place *learner-centered instruction* within any of the four boxes under "very strongly," since this author very much favors such instruction. It should be noted that one who is very strongly opposed to learner-centered health instruction would also place that item in one of the four "very strongly" boxes, since the object is to identify the *degree* of feeling — not whether the feeling is positive or negative. Participants may, and in fact will, change their responses from one column to another as more and more questions are read.

After the grid has been completed, have the participants form groups of four and discuss why they responded as they did. This exercise lets people see firsthand that values differ relative to homosexuality

Depending on who's counting, between 4 and 10 percent of the American population reports having a homosexual orientation. Some health educators argue that to ignore such a large group in health education programs is educationally unsound and socially unethical.

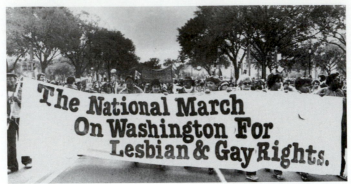

Source: The Diamondback, University of Maryland

FIGURE 10.4

Very strongly	Strongly	Mildly	No opinion

(or any other sexual behavior) and to explore why these differences occur. Questions for the homosexual orientation grid could be

1. How would you feel if your *close friend* told you he or she was gay or lesbian?
2. How do you feel about *two females* who greet each other with a kiss after being separated for a summer?
3. How do you feel about *two males* greeting each other with a kiss after a summer vacation?
4. How do you feel about a person who would *beat up* a homosexual for fun?
5. How do you feel about two *women holding hands* on the way to class?
6. How do you feel about *girls wearing boys' clothes?*
7. How do you feel about *boys wearing girls' clothes?*
8. How do you feel about two *men holding hands* on the way to class?
9. How do you feel about *males who do not like sports?*
10. How do you feel about *females who do like sports?*
11. How do you feel about taking *group showers?*
12. How do you feel about a man's taking over the *household chores?*
13. How do you feel about a *male hairdresser?*
14. How do you feel about a female who becomes a *construction worker?*
15. How do you feel about going out *only* with a person of the *opposite sex?*
16. How do you feel about going out *only with persons of the same sex?*

Premarital Sexual Intercourse Scale

Another sexual behavior that might be studied in a sexuality and family living education group is premarital sexual intercourse. Although small-group discussions could be used for such a study, the premarital sexual intercourse scale tends to be more motivating because people hold differing values relative to the topic. Program participants are instructed that they are to "weigh" their feelings about premarital sexual intercourse (PMI). The scale ranges from zero to 100 pounds. Those weighing a lot are indicating that they favor PMI, while those weighing very few pounds are stating that they are opposed to PMI. Obviously, there are weights somewhat in the middle of the scale as well. On a sheet of paper, in huge numbers, the participants write their weight. At the signal, the participants are asked to wander about the room, with the sheets on which their weights are written held up high, and to pair off with someone whose feelings regarding PMI are different from their own. The pairs are then to discuss their thoughts and feelings about premarital sexual intercourse. Pairs can later be formed into quartets for further discussion.

Processing a Contraception Decision (Dunn 2001)

Systematic decision making requires program participants to look at a problem and its potential solutions, identifying the pros and cons of each potential decision, and then select the best solution available. This activity relates this method of making decisions to deciding whether to use a method of contraception for sexually active program participants, or whether to abstain from sexual intercourse altogether. Participants should either research various means of contraception or be given a lecture regarding this content. Before engaging in this activity, they should know how contraceptives work, and understand their advantages and disadvantages, side effects, contraindications, and guidelines for selecting a contraceptive method. Once they know this information, Figure 10.5 is distributed to participants who complete the "important considerations" and the "contraceptive choice(s)" sections individually. These sections are completed in Figure 10.5 only as an example of how participants might respond. Figure 10.6 is also distributed to participants. Next program participants are divided into seven groups, with each group assigned one of the scenarios to discuss and to reach consensus on the "important considerations" and "contraceptive choice(s)" sections. The groups then report their results and their rationale to the total group. The total group then critiques the individual groups' thinking.

Dating and Intimate Relationships

Someone once said that when he spends time with someone else he has given that person his most valuable possession—an irretrievable part of his or her life. Obviously then, dating, going steady, being engaged, living together, and getting married represent important decisions relative to the finite time we have on this earth. These next few activities are designed to help program participants investigate with whom they spend time and with whom they would like to interact. In short, this section presents activities related to dating and the establishment of intimate relationships; and these activities need not be limited to heterosexual relationships.

Computer Dating

Most people have heard of computer dating services. These services seek to match people on relevant variables: age, race, religion, interests, profession, and so on. This activity, "computer dating," requires participants to create an application form that they would employ to match people for dates. All relevant options must be provided, so that rather than a question such as What are your hobbies? the application item might appear as follows:

Your hobbies are (check as many as are applicable)

_____   1. Sports

_____   2. Television

_____   3. Arts and crafts

_____   4. Painting

_____   5. Reading

_____   6. Stamp collecting

_____   7. Bicycling

The following list suggests variables for participants to consider:

1. Race
2. Religion
3. Color of hair
4. Body measurements
5. Personality
6. Hobbies
7. Age
8. Intelligence
9. Talents
10. Driver's license or not

FIGURE 10.5

Apply Guidelines in Figure 10.6 and Choose the Most Appropriate Method(s) of Contraception in the Following Case Studies.

BILL is not particularly choosy with whom he has intercourse, but it is important to him that he has it. In the last six months, he has had intercourse with three different women, two of whom he didn't know very well. Bill has a vague idea that some day, in the very distant future, he would like to settle down and have a family.

Important considerations for Bill?   Prophylactic benefit, efficacy, future fertility

Contraceptive choice(s)?   Condom and spermicide

JULIE is a healthy 22-year-old. She and John have a monogamous relationship and have been tested and are not HIV positive. Two years ago, Julie had an abortion. She does not want to have to do that again. Although they think they might like to start a family one day, Julie definitely doesn't want to get pregnant anytime soon. Julie doesn't like the nuisance and planning that some contraceptive practices require.

Important considerations for Julie?   Efficacy, future fertility, personal considerations

Contraceptive choice(s)?   Oral contraceptives, Depo-Provera

MARTIN is 37 and has been married to Mary for 15 years. They have three children. They have decided that they cannot afford to have any more children. Two of their three children were conceived by accident while Martin and Mary were trying to practice contraception. They have tried several methods but have confidence in none.

Important considerations for Martin?   Efficacy

Contraceptive choice(s)?   Sterilization

HUGH and JANE will be married soon. Both are free from HIV. They don't want any children for a few years but feel that they will want children eventually. Jane has a history of irregular and painful menstrual periods. Hugh doesn't want to be responsible for prevention of pregnancy.

Important considerations for Hugh and Jane?   Future fertility, efficacy, health benefits, personal consideration.

Contraceptive choice(s)?   Oral contraceptives, Depo-Provera

SALLY is a sexually active 37-year-old. Although she can hear her "biological clock ticking," she hasn't given up on her hope of one day marrying the right man and having a family. Until then she just keeps looking. And because her "looking" has led to sex with many different men, she does worry about contracting sexually transmitted illnesses. She is a two-pack-a-day smoker.

Important considerations for Sally?   Prophylactic benefit, future fertility, efficacy, safety

Contraceptive choice(s)?   Condom and spermicide

DEVON, an 18-year-old high school senior and has been in a relationship with Mary for about a year. He is a very good student and plans to go on to college after graduation. He and Mary enjoy a strong, committed relationship and are convinced they will have a future together. Devon is very committed to the teachings of his own religious faith, which requires strict adherence to intercourse within the context of marriage only. Although Mary sometimes attends church with Devon, her beliefs about intercourse being restricted to marriage are not as strong.

Important considerations for Devon?   Personal considerations

Contraceptive choice(s)?   Abstinence

KIM, a 25-year-old graduate student, has been exclusively dating Jack for several months, and is very attracted to him. Jack is also strongly attracted to Kim, and they both would like to have intercourse with each other but want to put off having children for at least five years. Jack recently confided in Kim that three years ago he was sexually involved with a man for a short period of time. He also has a history of intravenous drug use, but has been drug-free for over three years.

Important considerations for Kim?   Prophylactic benefit

Contraceptive choice(s)?   Male or female condom

FIGURE 10.6
Important Considerations/Guidelines for Making a Choice about Contraception

Efficacy: How well will it work?

Future fertility: Will future fertility be compromised?

Side effects: What health risks will result?

Prophylactic benefit: Will it protect against sexually transmitted illnesses?

Safety: Will it negatively affect health?

Personal considerations: Is it acceptable to both partners? Will it negatively affect lovemaking? Does it conflict with one's values? It it appropriate for the sexual lifestyle of the partner(s)?

As a follow-up to the development of the application form, participants should administer the form to friends or relatives who have an intimate relationship with one another. A discussion of how couples matched (or did not match) on the variables participants decided were important should result in several conclusions:

1. Some variables are more important than others.
2. Some couples exhibit complementary traits rather than similar. For example, one partner might exhibit a need to be domineering, whereas the other partner might need nurturance and desire to be dominated.
3. Some relationships seem to be inappropriate on the basis of the data collected.
4. There are other variables that weren't included but should be added to the application form.

Mate Recipe

Like "computer dating," this experience requires participants to list traits that are important for human relationships. However, in this activity, the relationship considered is the participant's own, rather than an analysis of someone else's. The group is told to pretend that they are each a master chef (aprons might be brought from home) and that their task is to create a recipe for *their* marriage or long-term partner. The recipe should be so exact that another chef could pick it up and be able to cook the same meal (or in this case come up with the same partner who meets the description in the recipe). Here are some items to consider:

1. What does this partner do with leisure time?
2. What does this partner look like?
3. What does this partner think about?
4. On what does this partner enjoy spending money?
5. How old is this partner?
6. What kind of clothes does this partner wear?
7. What kind of friends does this partner have?
8. How intelligent is this partner?
9. Why does this partner want to have this committed relationship with you?
10. What kind of personality does this partner have?

The recipe might develop to be

Ingredients: blond hair

nice smile

parents who are wealthy

neat dresser (no jeans)

tennis buff

measurements: 35–23–34

likes people

Mix with: 130 IQ

skimpy bikini

love for me

friends who do favors

Time: keep on ice until I'm 35 years old

Genetic Counseling Center

This activity employs a role-playing situation in which one person is a genetic counselor working for a genetic counseling center who counsels several prospective parents (other participants) on the selection of traits for their future children. The counselor should ask the parents such questions as the following:

1. How intelligent do you want your child to be?
2. What sex?
3. What color hair?
4. What handicap? (Each child *must* have one.)
5. What talents?
6. How should your child look? Father's or mother's nose? Chin? And so on.
7. What kind of personality?

At the completion of this activity the health educator should ask for a show of hands from those participants who would have been born if such a center were in existence when they were conceived. A discussion of the morality and ethical implications of genetic manipulation will then prove of value.

Pregnancy Sympathizer

How do you get someone who has never been pregnant to experience and develop sympathy for the pregnant state? To truly appreciate the effect of a bulging belly? The shortness of breath? And the backaches? Well, Linda Ware, executive director of the Birthways Childbirth Resource Center in the state of Washington, has figured out a way to do it. For the modern man eager to share his mate's pregnancy, she developed the Empathy Belly — a compartmentalized vest into whose sections approximately 30 pounds of water and weights are added. The vest costs $895 and is being used in schools, hospitals, and clinics.

The vest can be used with males who will never experience pregnancy firsthand or with females to prepare them for the reality of at least one aspect of pregnancy — its discomfort. If one of the goals of your program is to discuss pregnancy in all of its detail — positive and negative aspects — perhaps the

The Ready-or-Not Tot is a product from NASCO (www.NASCO.com) that allows health educators to program various "tending" activities, such as changing diapers, feeding, and responding to fussy periods. It also notes baby abuse such as shaking and hitting. Program participants are assigned to care for the "baby" for several days.

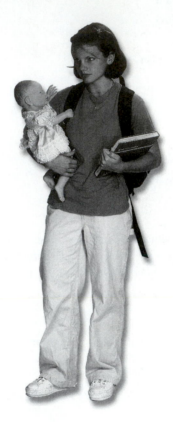

Source: Courtesy of NASCO

Empathy Belly is for you. If so, it is available from Birthways, Inc., 9225 SW Summerhurst Road, Vashon, WA 98070, by phone at (800) 882-3559, or via the Internet at www.empathybelly.org.

Family Life

Family life and role expectations of family members can be satisfying and yet bothersome. The home may be permeated with love, yet curfews, chores, and parental expectations can be viewed as troublesome by many.

The activities to follow can be employed to engage people in an analysis both of their own family life and of the family life they would prefer.

The Empathy Belly is designed to allow those who have never been or are incapable of getting pregnant to experience some of the discomfort associated with pregnancy.

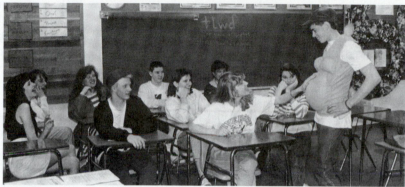

Source: Birthways, Inc.

Generation Gap

One may argue the existence or nonexistence of a generation gap. There are, however, differences in experiences and the ages at which those experiences first occurred. That can easily be documented. This activity serves as a means for such documentation.

Students are asked to compare their experiences with their parents' experiences via the following handout:

Place the age at which you and your parents *first* engaged in the following activities.

Activity	You	Father	Mother
Traveled on an airplane			
Rode a train			
A parent died			
You quit school			
Went to the dentist			
Watched television			
Got a job			
Left home			
Owned a car			
Began dating			

Implications drawn from this chart should relate to different ages at which similar responsibilities were assumed, differences in health care between the present and when their parents were children, the mobility brought about by transportation-related technology and its effects on family life, and other such items.

Family Values Continuum

Utilizing the values clarification approach to study values related to family life can be an educationally rewarding experience. Although many of the activities described in Chapter 7 can be adapted to apply to values related to family living, the values continuum is described here by way of example. Participants should be given the handout shown in Figure 10.7.

Upon the completion of the values continuum, small groups, coeducational in nature, should be formed to discuss the answers of the respondents. The rationale behind the responses should be explored through use of clarifying questions such as Why do you feel that way? It is suggested that the health educator once again remind participants that there are no right or wrong answers to this exercise and that each person should be careful not to attempt to change another's values but rather try to better understand them. The health educator should be sensitive to the many different types of family structures — blended families, gay and lesbian families, single-parent families. Adapting the statements in Figure 10.7 to meet these special needs may be required.

Build a House

Though it is useful to develop discourse in classes relative to family living, a more exotic and motivating procedure for accomplishing the same objective is the "build-a-house" exercise. The class is divided into groups consisting of five members each, with a large sheet of heavy paper and one color marker per group. The following directions are read:

> The group's task is to draw a house. Each person in the group may draw only one line at a time. You have 20 minutes to complete your task. There is to be no verbal communication from this point on.

At the conclusion of 20 minutes of house drawing, the group members write their names on the drawing and tape it on the wall. The participants are allowed several minutes to wander about looking at the other drawings and then are asked to stand by their own. The instructor then suggests that the drawings might be representative of the people in the group; for example, if one group has a good basketball player in it, that group's drawing might contain a garage with a basket attached (the directions did not state that lines drawn had to be straight lines).

Next the participants are asked to stand in front of the house in which they would most like to live. A discussion as to why they chose the house that they did will usually reveal the following:

1. Some houses were just too wild looking to be comfortable.
2. Some drawings contained people and made the house look livable.
3. Some drawings contained trees, bushes, swings, and so on that made the house seem alive.
4. Some houses had no character.
5. Some drawings reminded some people of their own house (or a friend's or relative's house).

A concluding discussion concerned with the differences between a house and a home is recommended.

Family Photos

This activity, like the previous one, seeks to develop increased awareness of the family life of each of the participants. These exercises are not concerned with a general, academic, safe investigation of family living, but rather are a study by the participant of his or her *own* family life.

FIGURE 10.7

These nine statements represent some attitudes and beliefs about the family. Place a check mark in the appropriate space, depending on whether you strongly agree with, have some agreement with, are neutral (have no opinion about), somewhat disagree with, or strongly disagree with the statement in question. If you are a health educator teaching adults, or children from single-family homes, or youth without parents, change *parents* to *parent or guardian, spouse,* or *significant other.*

	Strongly Agree	Some Agreement	Neutral	Some Disagreement	Strongly Disagree
1. My family has been the most important influence in my life.					
2. My mother should work outside our home if she wants to.					
3. My father should help my mom with the housework.					
4. The children are the most important part of the family.					
5. I have a responsibility to try to make my parents happy.					
6. I am proud of my parents as people.					
7. It is important that my parents be proud of me.					
8. Married people who do not have children are happier than those who do.					
9. What my friends think of me is more important than what my parents think of me.					

Participants are told to bring in several photographs of their family. Each photograph should include the person with at least one other family member, so that every family member is included when all of the photographs are reviewed. Each person's photographs should be pasted, clipped, or stapled on one sheet of paper. Students then exchange papers and comment on the back of the paper about the family as a whole or about individual members. Pictures are returned after numerous comments have been written on the reverse side of the sheet on which they are attached, and time is provided for participants to read the comments and draw conclusions and generalities.

Caution: Some program participants might come from dysfunctional families and this activity may cause them emotional distress. Such participants should not be required to participate in this activity.

Family Drawings

Often people's insights into family lives are such that the roles of the family members are not clear to them. Perceptions of family life are often repressed and hidden. An activity designed to bring to the surface people's feelings about their families is one in which they draw pictures of their families in group activities or some other context. At the conclusion of this activity, drawings are exchanged among the group members until each person has had the opportunity to review each drawing. On the back of each drawing they review, participants write a one-sentence comment that expresses their reaction. For example, while this author was conducting this activity with a group of graduate students, one drawing consisted of a husband, wife, and two children. However, further inspection revealed the husband, wife, and one child in one grouping, with the second child off to the side. The comments of the other students reflected the possibility that in this family one child tended to be excluded from family activity and decision making. The drawer later admitted that this was, in fact, the case, and that in the future he would make an effort to include the whole family in activities and the formulation of decisions. Comments on the back of the drawings should relate to the family as a whole (for example, was a pet drawn as part of the family?) or to the individuals depicted. Next, drawings are returned to the artists with time provided to read the comments of their classmates.

As with "family photos," students from dysfunctional families should not be required to participate in this activity.

This drawing was made by a participant in the build-a-house activity. Note that smoke comes from the chimney (indicating warmth and security) and that life is depicted (pet, tree, flower, and plant in window).

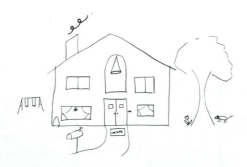

The three pictures are the result of participation in the family drawings activity. One family is attending church, another is skating, and the third going for a walk in a big city.

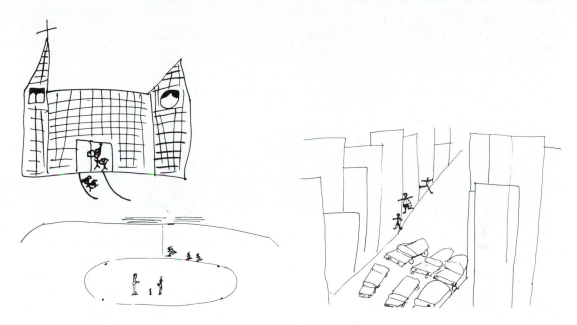

Sibling Sequencing

Often overlooked in family living classes, but very much in the minds of psychologists, is an investigation of the relationship of birth order to behavior. To begin such a study, divide the class into three groups:

1. One group of first-borns.
2. One group of youngest in family.
3. One group of middle-borns.

The task of each group is to list what their birth order has meant to them. Provide 20 minutes for this phase of the activity, after which the class discusses the conclusions reached by each group. A vote is taken regarding the number of people who would prefer to have been born to their family in a different birth order, and the group discusses why they voted as they did. This activity demonstrates quite well the principle that the grass is always greener on the other side of the fence.

Violence Prevention

Trauma physicians, frustrated with having to treat victims of family and domestic violence, have organized to advocate that violence prevention programs be included in school curricula. Given the increasing threat of violence in our society, it would be wise for all health education programs—whether located in hospitals, worksites, community health departments, colleges and universities, or schools—to include violence prevention. Space dictates that only a few violence prevention instructional strategies be presented here. However, if you are interested in expanding your library of violence prevention instructional activities, you should consult your local school district, health department, police department, or social services office. Here are a few other resources:

Preventing Family Violence
Resource Center for the Prevention of Family Violence and Sexual Assault
Massachusetts Department of Public Health
150 Tremont Street
Boston, MA 02111

Violence Prevention: Resource Bibliography
Massachusetts Department of Public Health
Massachusetts Adolescent Violence Prevention Program
Injury Prevention and Control Resource Library
150 Tremont Street
Boston, MA 02111

We Can Do It! Organizing Senior Citizens to Prevent Crime and Violence:
A Curriculum for Trainers
Massachusetts Department of Public Health
Neighborhood Justice Network
Bureau of Family and Community Health
150 Tremont Street
Boston, MA 02111

Educational Resources for Violence Prevention
CSN Adolescent Violence Prevention Resource Center
Education Development Center, Inc.
55 Chapel Street
Newton, MA 02160

Violence Prevention: Video and Curricula Catalogue
Massachusetts Adolescent Violence Prevention Program
Injury Prevention and Control Resource Library
150 Tremont Street
Boston, MA 02111

Violence Prevention: Curriculum for Adolescents
Teenage Teaching Modules
Education Development Center, Inc.
55 Chapel Street
Newton, MA 02160

Human Graph*

Different people define violence and abuse differently. In some cases, two people observing an activity may perceive it differently: one as abuse, the other as normal and acceptable behavior. To help program

---

*From Resource Center for the Prevention of Family Violence and Sexual Assault. *Preventing Family Violence.* Boston, MA: Massachusetts Department of Public Health, 1984, pp. 20–23. Reprinted by permission.

participants discuss these differing views of abuse, have them read these cases and indicate how abusive they think the person's response is. Program participants can be asked to structure their ratings according to one of the following methods:

Method 1: Have the participants clear away the furniture from the center of the room and mount a sign that says "ABUSIVE" on the wall of the room; on the opposite side of the room mount a sign that says "NOT ABUSIVE." For each case study response, each participant indicates how abusive he or she thinks the action is by standing at a representative distance from one of the labeled walls. The health educator then reads each case study and asks participants to respond.

Method 2: Have participants arrange their seats in a circle. Explain that they are to rate each response in the case studies as either not abusive, somewhat abusive, or very abusive. If they think the response is not abusive, they remain seated, just as they are. If they think the response is somewhat abusive, they raise both hands. If they think the response is very abusive, they stand up. The health educator then reads each case study and asks participants to respond.

Case Studies

1. Dinner has just ended at the Millers' house. Steve's mother is washing the dishes and his father is watching TV. The doorbell rings. It's Mr. Chambers, who owns the corner store, and he sure sounds angry! He demands to talk with Steve's father. His father calls Steve and his mother into the living room where he is talking with Mr. Chambers. Mr. Chambers stares Steve down. He tells Steve's parents that he saw Steve shoplift some cigarettes from his store.

   How abusive is each of these responses?

   Steve's father beats him with a hanger.

   Steve's parents sell his guitar.

   They slap him in the face in front of Mr. Chambers.

   They tell him he's a good-for-nothing slime.

   They don't do anything.

   They discuss it for an hour.

   They yell at him for a solid 20 minutes.

   Helen has just spent a long afternoon shopping with her three-year-old brother, Kevin. She's getting a headache. The ice cream cone she gave Kevin to quiet him is dripping down his arm. It's beginning to stain his shirt. They get onto the bus to go home. Kevin starts to sing "Row, row, row your boat." Helen looks up to see who's noticing. A lot of people on the bus are watching, and she sees a classmate of hers at the other end of the bus. Kevin continues to sing over and over again. Helen asks him, begs him, to stop, but he won't!

   How abusive is each of Helen's responses?

   She dumps the ice cream cone on Kevin's head.

   She tosses the ice cream cone out of the bus window.

   She hits him on the head.

   She pinches him on the thigh.

   She puts her hand tightly over his mouth.

She says to Kevin, "When we get home, I'm going to pull the eyes off of your teddy bear if you don't shut up."

3. Tom has been seeing Linda for a long time, only now he's developed a strong interest in another girlfriend. He decides to take Linda to her favorite restaurant to break the news to her. She gets real upset and starts crying aloud in public and calling Tom "dirty names."

How abusive is each of Tom's responses?

He slaps her in the restaurant to get her to her senses.

He walks her out and leaves her there.

He tells her she's an ugly, unattractive pig and he doesn't know why he went out with her to begin with.

4. James and Donna have been dating steadily for several months. Donna begins to feel that more and more of their time together is being spent by themselves and has gradually become quite intimate. When James picks her up tonight, she tells him that she wants to spend more time having fun together the way they did when they first started dating, and that she does not want to spend as much time making out.

How abusive are James's responses?

He grabs her arm and twists it, saying, "You can't just lead me on and tease me and then just stop all of a sudden."

He laughs and tells her he knows she likes making out with him and then he drives down a deserted road.

He listens to Donna and then drives to a deserted spot in the woods. He tells her that she's beautiful and he'd go crazy if they didn't make out when they were together. He then starts kissing her.

He gets angry and makes her get out of the car, even though it's after dark and they are several miles from Donna's house.

5. Mr. Jacobs has a terrible day at work. He gets home to his family feeling angry.

How abusive is each of Mr. Jacobs's responses?

He yells at his wife because dinner is not on the table.

He yells at her if he feels annoyed by her.

He hits her if he feels annoyed by her.

He insists that she listen to what a bad day he's had.

How Could You Handle It?

This activity is designed to help program participants differentiate between discipline and abuse. Each participant writes down a nonabusive solution for the parenting problems presented in the case studies appearing here. Then participants form pairs in which they discuss their solutions. Pairs are instructed that when they regroup, each person is responsible for presenting his or her partner's solution rather than his or her own. This will encourage partners to listen to each other when in pairs rather than merely argue their point of view.

After the solutions are presented to the large group, the health educator summarizes by differentiating discipline from abuse by making the following points:

1. Discipline is directed at changing the child's behavior. Forms of discipline include withdrawing privileges or scolding.

2. Abuse comes from the hostility or conflict the parent is feeling, more than from something the child is doing. It is very severe and it is ongoing.

3. Examples of *physical abuse:* beating, kicking, burning, shaking, throwing the child.

4. Examples of *emotional abuse:* consistently telling the child that he or she is rotten, stupid, worthless, or unloved.

5. Examples of *physical neglect:* consistently failing to provide food, clothing, or shelter, or medical care or supervision for a child.

6. Example of *emotional neglect:* giving the child no love, attention, affection, or support.

Case Studies

1. You've been home alone all day with your daughter, Lisa, who is six, has a fever, and is cranky, and with your son, Sean, who is three. You're tired of getting things for Lisa and picking up after Sean. You've already picked his toys up off the living room floor three times and now, a half hour later, you can barely get into the room. You feel yourself getting a headache, so you decide to lie down and take a nap. Lisa is finally napping herself, and you put Sean in front of the TV, turn it on, and tell him not to bother you, that you're going to sleep for a while.

   The phone wakes you up 15 minutes later. You're groggy and annoyed because it was the wrong number. You decide you'd better start supper. When you go into the kitchen you see the refrigerator door wide open, there is a milk carton on the floor and milk is slowly oozing out all over the place, and there are Cheerios spilled everywhere. You are furious. You know Sean must be responsible for the mess. You yell for him to come, but there's no answer. When you go looking for him, you find him in Lisa's room, curled up on the bed, asleep beside a pile of Cheerios.

2. Your 13-year-old daughter Julie is not supposed to have friends over after school while you are at work. One day you come home early, at 5:30 instead of your usual 6:00. It's quiet when you come in, but then your hear laughing coming from upstairs. You smell cigarette smoke. You realize that Julie isn't alone and start getting mad. You go up to her room and go in. Julie's there with her friend Mona, and two boys you don't know. You notice two empty beer bottles on the floor.

Controversy: Abortion and HIV/AIDS Education

Sexuality education is fraught with controversial content and topics. Two of these controversial topics are abortion and HIV/AIDS education. The following instructional strategies actively involve learners in these issues.

Abortion Debate

Relative to controversial topics such as abortion, program participants should be reminded to consult their clergy and others before deciding on the appropriateness of such action. However, an objective investigation can be conducted in class to analyze the arguments for and against abortion. One of the best ways to conduct such an investigation employs the debate technique. Three participants should argue for legalization of abortion and three against it. The instructor should make sure that at least the following points are made during such a debate.

1. A hospital abortion is safer than a routine tonsillectomy (Association for the Study of Abortion n.d.).

2. "Since 1869 some members of the Roman Catholic hierarchy have argued that the fetus is, from conception, a human being in the full sense of the term and that abortion is murder.

   Substantial non-Catholic theological opinion disagrees and, in fact, increasing numbers of Roman Catholics do not feel that abortion is murder. They regard the fetus as a *potential* human being, whose interests are secondary to those of its mother." (Association for the Study of Abortion n.d.)

3. "Some people believe that abortion-on-demand gives to one person (the mother) the legal right to kill another (the baby) in order to solve the first person's social problem." (Hiltz Publishing Co. n.d.)

4. An evaluation of New York State's abortion law allowing abortion on demand has shown the following (Joyce and Mocan 1990):

   a. The level of births to black adolescents fell 18.7 percent. The level of births to white adolescents fell 14.1 percent. That means that 4,091 black births and 3,128 white births were averted by the legalization of abortion over just a two-year period after the law was implemented.

   b. If abortion were banned in New York City in January 1988, there would have been 2,618 additional black births and 1,223 white births to New York City adolescents in 1988 and 1989 above what would be expected if abortion remained legal.

   c. A teenager who aborted a pregnancy was less likely to become pregnant again than was a comparable teenager who carried her first pregnancy to term.

   d. Adolescents who become parents complete less schooling, have lower wages, experience greater marital instability, and are more dependent on welfare programs than are other adolescents.

5. Although more white women have abortions, the abortion *ratio* for black women (100 per 1,000 women) is three times that of white women (29 per 1,000 women) (U.S. Census Bureau 2001).

6. One-fifth of abortions are to women under 20 years of age. Another third of abortions are to women between 20 and 24 years of age (U.S. Census Bureau 2001).

7. Eighty-one percent of abortions are to unmarried women. Married women who have abortions are older than unmarried women who have abortions (U.S. Census Bureau 2001).

8. The majority of Americans support access to safe, legal abortion.

9. People who disapprove of abortions are more likely than others to have strongly committed Catholic or fundamentalist Protestant affiliations.

10. People who disapprove of abortion are more likely than others to disapprove of premarital sexual intercourse and homosexuality, to be politically conservative, and to hold more traditional views of the female role in society.

Some sexuality education programs prohibit any education regarding abortion in an attempt to avoid offending parents and other members of the community. However, it may be argued that ignoring education about abortion is doing a disservice to the program participants and to the country, since they will be asked to make a decision when they vote for candidates who are either pro-choice or pro-life. Given the demonstrations — and, yes, even the bombings of abortion clinics — is it educationally sound to prohibit instruction about abortion?

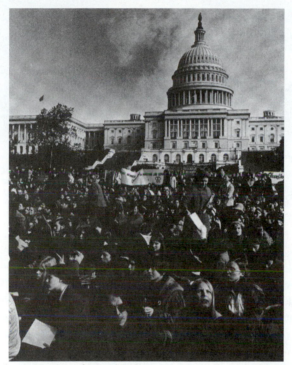

Source: The Diamondback, University of Maryland

Safer-Sex Communicating

Several strategies have been suggested to limit the spread of human immunodeficiency virus (HIV). Some advocate the teaching of sexual abstinence, others opt for valuing monogamy, and still others argue for encouraging condom use during intercourse. Since HIV is transmitted predominantly through contact with bodily fluids (such as semen and blood), the most effective means of preventing the spread of HIV is to not participate in sexual activity or intravenous drug use. Many experts believe sexual abstinence to be an unrealistic expectation to place upon the American citizenry. It just won't work, say these experts. The alternative is to teach people who do engage in sexual activity to refrain from those activities that are considered a high risk for the transmission of HIV. These include sexual intercourse without the use of a condom, anal intercourse, and coitus with numerous sexual partners.

One of the more difficult tasks for sexually active people concerned about HIV is to ask, and if necessary to insist, that their partners wear a condom. Another difficult task is to inquire about partners' previous sexual history and to insist upon a monogamous sexual relationship. These tasks are so

It's perplexing that people feel comfortable buying and sharing cookies like these but do not know how to *really* communicate about sexual issues. Unfortunately, this inability to communicate about sex can make them more susceptible to a variety of sexually transmitted diseases, of which HIV/AIDS is but one.

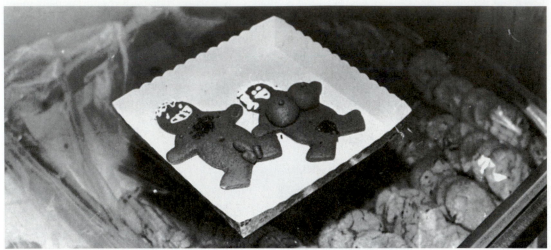

Source: The Diamondback, University of Maryland

difficult because of the sensitive nature of sex and sexuality, which, in turn, is exacerbated by a lack of assertiveness skills.

People who can be *assertive* can better assure that their needs (in this case those related to sexual intercourse) are met, while still maintaining the relationship with the person with whom they are being assertive. This is in contrast to people who meet their needs by being *aggressive* and thereby ruining their relationships. The instructional strategy presented here can be employed to help program participants learn to act assertively, both verbally and nonverbally.

Distribute the following handout to program participants.

BEING ASSERTIVE

An assertive response has several characteristics:

1. It specifies the behavior or situation being referred to.
2. It states your feelings about that behavior or situation.
3. It presents a suggested remedy for the problem.
4. It details what will happen if a change is made and what will happen if a change is not made.

Think of a situation you can anticipate in which you would like to be assertive—maybe asking for a pay raise or asking an instructor to change a grade. Wouldn't it be nice to be

BEING ASSERTIVE *(continued)*

able to assert your position in that situation? Through this activity you will learn how to be more assertive when you want to be.

To begin, imagine you have a new sexual partner. Concerned about HIV, you want to assure yourself that your new partner won't be "sleeping around," since you know that the more sexual partners, the more likely your partner is to become a carrier of HIV. Consequently, you want a monogamous sexual relationship. However, you want to make an assertive statement about your concern rather than one that will be interpreted as aggressive, since you care for this relationship and don't want to mess it up.

Make an assertive response by completing the statements below.

1. The situation you are concerned about is _____

   _____

   _____

   _____

2. Your feelings about this situation are _____

   _____

   _____

   _____

3. The change you would like to see made is _____

   _____

   _____

   _____

4. If this change is made to your satisfaction, the result will be _____

   _____

   _____

   _____

5. If this change is not made to your satisfaction, the result will be _____

   _____

   _____

   _____

After participants complete the handout, ask them to share their responses verbally with the rest of the group. This will serve as either a reinforcer for those who now know how to say something assertively or as a review for those who are still unsure. Next the instructor chooses one participant's assertive response and recites it in a verbally nonassertive manner (see the next handout). The point is then made that an assertive response that is said with accompanying nonassertive or aggressive behavior is no longer assertive. The following handout is then distributed.

NONVERBAL BEHAVIOR AND ASSERTIVENESS

Assertive, nonassertive, and aggressive behaviors differ. If you are trying to make an assertive response, you need to make sure that your nonverbal behavior is consistent with assertiveness. The behaviors associated with assertiveness, nonassertiveness, and aggressiveness are outlined here.

Assertiveness

1. Standing straight and steady and directly facing the people to whom you are speaking while maintaining eye contact.
2. Speaking in a clear, steady voice, loud enough for the people to whom you are speaking to hear you.
3. Speaking fluently, without hesitation, and with assurance and confidence.

Nonassertiveness

1. Lacking eye contact: looking down or away.
2. Swaying and shifting your weight from one foot to another.
3. Whining and hesitancy when speaking.

Aggressiveness

1. Leaning forward with glaring eyes.
2. Pointing a finger at the person to whom you are speaking.
3. Shouting.
4. Clenching your fist.
5. Putting your hands on your hips and wagging your head.

At this point, invite participants to a "party"—right then and there—at which they will roam about meeting people, while all the time *behaving* consistently with assertiveness. The health educator mingles among the "party guests" and corrects behavior to make it more consistent with assertiveness.

I have even asked a participant to interrupt two other party guests to see how they react: assertively, aggressively, or, as is usually the case, nonassertively. When they act nonassertively, they allow the interrupter to pursue a conversation with them, thereby violating their right to converse among themselves. When they act aggressively, they argue with the interrupter about how rude he or she is to violate their right to converse. And when they act assertively, they tell the interrupter they would love to converse with him or her but are presently engaged in their own conversation. They will converse with the interrupter, they tell him or her, as soon as they're through.

Draw implications for the expression of other rights and the satisfaction of other needs that relate to HIV/AIDS and in which assertiveness would serve well.

The HIV/AIDS Millionaire Game (Burnett 2002)

After program participants learn about HIV/AIDS, the "HIV/AIDS facts millionaire game" can be used as a summary or concluding activity. Program participants are divided into two teams, with the health educator being the "host." Each team, in turn, selects a player to answer the next question before it is stated. Questions are to be rotated among all team members until every team member has had an opportunity to answer a question. There are three "lifelines" per team that can be used when a team member needs help answering a question. Once a lifeline is used, it cannot be used again. Lifelines are (1) a friend from either team, (2) the entire team, and (3) 50/50 (the host will delete two possible answers). "Money" will be accumulated for correct answers and will be added to the team's jackpot; incorrect answers are ignored. The team that accumulates the most money wins the game. Questions and the "money" assigned to each appear in the accompanying box with the correct answers in bold-face. These questions can be projected on an overhead transparency or in a PowerPoint presentation.

HIV/AIDS FACTS MILLIONAIRE GAME QUESTIONS

$100
What do the letters in the acronym *AIDS* stand for?

(a) Accessed immune deficit signs.

(b) Acquired immune deficiency syndrome.

(c) Acquired illnesses and diseases syndrome.

(d) Accessed immune deficiency syndrome.

$100
What do the letters in the acronym *HIV* stand for?

(a) Human immunodeficiency virus.

(b) Human illness varieties.

(c) Hetero immunodeficiency virus.

(d) Hetero illness varieties.

$200
Why are United States high school age (ages 15–19) teens at risk for HIV/AIDS?

(a) 48% of teens have had sexual intercourse.

(b) 43% of sexually active teens did not use a latex condom during their last sexual intercourse.

(c) 16% of sexually active teens had sex with four or more partners.

(d) All of the above facts are reasons why U.S. teens are at risk for HIV/AIDS.

$200
In the human immune system, lymphocytes that kill pathogens are called

(a) A cells.

(b) B cells.

(c) T cells.

(d) Z cells.

$300
How many T cells (per drop of blood) does a healthy person have?

(a) 10–100.

(b) 100–400.

(c) 400–800.

(d) 800–1,200.   *(continued)*

$300
What is the difference between being HIV+ (positive) and having AIDS?

(a) "HIV+" means a person has the virus and "AIDS" means it shows on the test for HIV antibodies.

(b) "HIV+" means a person has the virus and "AIDS" means the person's T cell count is below 200 and/or the person has or has had an opportunistic infection.

(c) "HIV+" means the person has AIDS and "AIDS" means the person will die young.

(d) "HIV+" means a person can't give it to someone and "AIDS" means it can be given to someone.

$500
What is an "opportunistic infection"?

(a) It is an infection that has opportunity to infect once a person's immune system is "down."

(b) It is an ordinary infection that can infect anyone given the opportunity.

(c) It is an infection that is not dangerous to a person's health.

(d) It is an infection that has no effect on a person with a compromised immune system.

$500
What are two opportunistic infections common to people with AIDS?

(a) PCP (*Pneumocystis carinii* pneumonia) and KS (Kaposi's sarcoma).

(b) CMV (cytomegalovirus) and toxoplasmosis.

(c) Common cold and influenza.

(d) Both a and b; all are opportunistic infections.

$1,000
How long is the "window period" (the time between HIV infection and the presence of HIV antibodies that are detectable on an HIV test)?

(a) 1 week to 2 weeks.

(b) 2 weeks to 6 months.

(c) 6 weeks to 1 year.

(d) 6 months to 1 year.

$1,000
How long is the "incubation period" (time between HIV infection and actual AIDS symptoms or illness)?

(a) Overnight to 2 weeks.

(b) 2 months to 1–2 years.

(c) 6 months to 10–15 years.

(d) 1 to 10 years.

$2,000
What are four possible symptoms of HIV infection?

(a) Flulike symptoms, uncontrollable hiccuping, whooping cough, herpes blisters.

(b) Night sweats, no symptoms at all, weight gain, having a sore that does not heal.

(c) Swollen glands, flulike symptoms, night sweats, extreme fatigue.

(d) Extreme fatigue, weight gain, whooping cough, having a sore that does not heal.

HIV/AIDS FACTS MILLIONAIRE GAME QUESTIONS *(continued)*

$2,000
What symptom of HIV infection is unique to females?

(a) Not having a menstrual period.

(b) Constant vaginal yeast infection.

(c) Tender breasts.

(d) PMS (premenstrual syndrome).

$4,000
What are the five ways that HIV is transmitted?

(a) 1. Blood transfusion before 1985; 2. mother to baby; 3. accidents with body fluids; 4. unprotected sexual intercourse; 5. sharing drug, tattoo, or body piercing needles/syringes.

(b) 1. Donating blood; 2. blood transfusion after 1985; 3. living in the 21st century; 4. being heterosexual; 5. being homosexual.

(c) 1. Getting bitten by a mosquito; 2. traveling in a foreign country; 3. drinking water in a foreign country; 4. getting immunized; 5. doing a regular self-breast or self-testicle exam for cancer.

(d) 1. Being in a bus; 2. being in a car; 3. being on a plane; 4. riding a horse; 5. riding a bike.

$4,000
What are four ways that HIV is not transmitted?

(a) Hugging, kissing, coughing, using the same toilet.

(b) Swimming in the same pool, being in the same room with an HIV+ person, being homosexual, being heterosexual.

(c) Honestly talking with your partner about your sexual limits, sexual abstinence, listening to a friend, talking to a friend.

(d) All of the above are ways that HIV is not transmitted.

$8,000
HIV is transmitted through the exchange of which four body fluids?

(a) Blood, saliva, mucus, semen.

(b) Blood, semen, vaginal secretions, breast milk.

(c) Blood, sweat, tears, mucus.

(d) Blood, sweat, earwax, vaginal secretions.

$8,000
What do the four body fluids that transmit HIV have in common?

(a) They're full of carbohydrates.

(b) They're full of fat.

(c) They're rich in protein.

(d) They're rich in vitamins and minerals.

$16,000
What percentage of babies born to HIV+ moms will be HIV+ if their moms take the medication AZT starting early in the mom's pregnancy and continue to take AZT until the baby is born?

(a) 25%.

(b) 5%.

(c) 50%.

(d) 100%.

(continued)

HIV/AIDS FACTS MILLIONAIRE GAME QUESTIONS   *(continued)*

$16,000

What are the three types of unprotected sex that can transmit HIV?

  (a) Vaginal, oral, anal sex.

  (b) Hugging, kissing, touching.

  (c) Masturbation, mutual masturbation, watching a sexy video.

  (d) Phone sex, Internet sex, masturbation.

$32,000

What behaviors are 100% effective in preventing HIV infection?

  (a) Correctly using a latex condom every time a person has oral or vaginal sex.

  (b) Using a latex barrier (dental dams or cut condoms) when a person has oral or anal sex.

  (c) Abstinence from sex, alcohol, and drugs.

  (d) Drinking or using drugs only on the weekend.

$32,000

What behaviors are less than 100% effective in preventing HIV infection?

  (a) Correctly using a latex condom every time a person has oral or vaginal sex.

  (b) Using a latex barrier (dental dams or cut condoms) when a person has oral or anal sex.

  (c) Not sharing dirty needles or syringes.

  (d) All of the above behaviors are less than 100% effective.

$64,000

What statements are true in relation to "confidential testing" for HIV/AIDS?

  (a) The person's name is used with the test results and a record exists of the results, which are kept secret from everyone except medical personnel.

  (b) The person's counselor can contact him or her to see how he or she is doing.

  (d) The person's counselor can contact him or her about medical or support services.

  (d) All of the above statements are true for "confidential testing."

$64,000

What does it mean if a person gets a negative result from his/her first test for HIV antibodies after engaging in risky behavior?

  (a) The person definitely does not have HIV.

  (b) The person may have been infected with HIV within the last 6 months but antibodies have not yet developed.

  (c) The person definitely has HIV.

  (d) The person can now forget about "safer sex" and just have fun!

$125,000

Universal precautions include using a barrier between the blood and body fluids of people, never picking up needles, wearing gloves when cleaning up any body fluid spills, and thoroughly washing hands after any accident with

HIV/AIDS FACTS MILLIONAIRE GAME QUESTIONS *(continued)*

body fluid spills. The purpose of using universal precautions with everyone is to

(a) Make everyone afraid of germs.

(b) Make everyone afraid of helping in an emergency.

(c) Keep someone's body fluids preserved for scientific research.

(d) Prevent any contact of the body fluids of one person with the body fluids of another.

$125,000
What is the most generally accepted theory about the origin of HIV/AIDS? It first appeared in

(a) African mosquitoes that infected gay men in the 1970s.

(b) Experimental polio vaccines made from chimpanzee tissue that was tested in the Belgian Congo (Zaire) in the 1950s.

(c) Infected animals who passed it on to humans in the 1930s.

(d) Haitian homosexual men who had sex with U.S. men in the 70s.

$250,000
As of July 1, 2000, approximately how many people in the United States were estimated to be living with HIV/AIDS? As of July 1, 2000, how many people in the United States have died from AIDS (since 1980)?

(a) About 100,000 living with HIV/AIDS; 250,000 have died.

(b) About 250,000 living with HIV/AIDS; 375,000 have died.

(c) About 422,000 living with HIV/AIDS; 439,000 have died.

(d) About 1 million living with HIV/AIDS; 1 million have died.

$250,000
As of the end of 2000, approximately how many people worldwide were estimated to be living with HIV/AIDS? As of the end of 2000, how many people worldwide have died from AIDS (since 1980)?

(a) 36 million living with HIV/AIDS; 22 million have died.

(b) 25 million living with HIV/AIDS; 10 million have died.

(c) 58 million living with HIV/AIDS; 20 million have died.

(d) 47 million living with HIV/AIDS; 32 million have died.

$500,000
What is the name of the test for HIV antibodies that requires no needles or skin puncturing? (This test was first approved for use by the Food and Drug Administration in December 1994.)

(a) AIDS No More.

(b) Ora Sure.

(c) HIV Be Gone.

(d) Safe 'n Sure.

$500,000
What is the name of the first class of antiretroviral drugs (used as one drug in the drug "cocktail" or combination) to treat people with HIV?

(a) Protease analogues.

(b) Nucleoside analogues.

(c) Transcriptase inhibitors.

(d) Reverse inhibitors.

(continued)

HIV/AIDS FACTS MILLIONAIRE GAME QUESTIONS *(continued)*	
$1,000,000 What is the name of the second class of antiretroviral drugs (used as one drug in the drug "cocktail" or combination) to treat people with HIV? (a) Super antibiotics. **(b) Protease inhibitors.** (c) Nonnucleoside reverse transcriptase inhibitors. (d) Protease analogues.	**$1,000,000** What is the name of the newest class of antiretroviral drugs (used as one drug in the drug "cocktail" or combination) to treat people with HIV? (a) Antibiotic inhibitors. (b) Reverse analogues. **(c) Nonnucleoside reverse transcriptase inhibitors.** (d) Nonnucleoside analogues.

Valuing Activities

Because values contribute to our choices of sexual behavior, sexuality, and family life, the use of values clarification in a sexuality and family living unit seems appropriate. The activities to follow are but several examples of how some of the valuing instructional strategies described in Chapter 7 can be applied to the study of sexuality and family living.

Values Ranking

Asking people to rank order their preferences about sex and family life will help them to identify and clarify values of which they may not have been aware. Some possible values groupings that can be rank ordered are

1. A married man should be a lover.
2. A married man should be a father.
3. A married man should be a breadwinner.

1. A married woman should be a lover.
2. A married woman should be a mother.
3. A married woman should be a homemaker.

1. Don Juan
2. Romeo
3. James Bond

1. Homosexuals
2. Heterosexuals
3. Ambisexuals

Epitaph

What we value is often evident in how we prefer to be remembered. People can be asked to write their epitaphs relative to particular sexual roles. For example, they can be asked, If you were to die today, what would you want people to remember about you as a man or woman, brother or sister, boyfriend or girlfriend? A discussion of why each person wrote what they did would then be useful to demonstrate that different people often possess different values and that no one set of values is "right."

Epitaphs need not relate to the death of the person. We all go through various stages of life and might view these *stages* we've been through as dead. Consequently, it is possible to write epitaphs for these stages of life. One way to do this is to ask the following:

1. How do you think your sexuality will change when you are

   30 years old? _____

   45 years old? _____

   70 years old? _____

2. How does a girlfriend/boyfriend differ from a wife/husband?
3. How does a mother/father differ from a grandmother/grandfather?
4. How does an infant differ sexually from a teenager?
5. How does a 75-year-old heterosexual differ from a 75-year-old homosexual?

Role Trading

An excellent means of exploring values relative to sexuality is to ask program participants to place six sexual roles that they play on six index cards (one role per card). Some possible roles are

Boyfriend/girlfriend	Brother/sister
Mother/father	Lover
Son/daughter	Heterosexual
Feminist	Male chauvinist
Exploiter	Virgin
Teaser	Male
Female	Aggressor
Womanizer	

Each person is next told to pin on his or her chest the six cards and to wander about the room trying to trade one or more of the cards for a role that another person has and that he or she would like to have. However, in the 15 minutes allotted to the trading phase, each person *must* trade at least two of his or her index cards. At the completion of the trading phase, the following questions should be considered:

1. How would you feel about giving up these roles if you really had to?
2. How would you feel about really accepting the roles others traded to you?
3. How important to you are the roles you were unwilling to trade away?
4. How well do you perform the roles you kept? How about the ones you traded away?
5. How could you better perform the roles you kept?

6. How could you better perform the roles you traded away?

7. How could you better perform the roles you received in trade?

Values Statements

Still another means of incorporating values clarification within sexuality and family living education is to use incomplete sentences that, when completed, will indicate values. Here are some possible beginnings of sentences that pertain to sexual behavior:

1. Promiscuity _____

2. Homosexuals _____

3. Premarital intercourse _____

4. Petting _____

5. Masturbation _____

6. Virginity _____

7. Oral–genital sex _____

8. The double standard is_____

9. If I became pregnant I _____

10. Transvestites_____

Summary

Sexuality and family living are subjects worthy of study, both academically and personally. The activities presented here demonstrate the manner in which such study can be made meaningful to program participants. As previously suggested, health educators should choose activities appropriate to their local situation, change others to make them more appropriate, and decide against the use of the rest. However, the fact that a segment of a sexuality and family living unit cannot be offered is no justification for discarding the whole unit.

CHAPTER ELEVEN

Instructional Strategies for Environmental Health

Environmental problems necessitate solutions based on knowledge and reason. Many of these solutions result in a compromise between what is practical and what is idealistic. For instance, when states experience a budgetary crisis, one concern is to keep as much industry in the state as possible to keep unemployment down. A means to keep industries and to attract other companies is to make environmental legislation less stringent. Such a solution would mean less expense for manufacturing firms operating in the state because they would have to spend less money to clean up waste products, and so on. Less expense to operate in a state would mean that more businesses would move there, which would mean more jobs, which would mean more taxes collected and fewer unemployment benefits paid out, and so on. Environmental health is sacrificed for economic well-being. Just how the environmental legislation should be changed, if at all, and the relative importance of the environment versus the pocketbook are decisions that involve values. The activities presented in this chapter are designed to demonstrate to the health educator that such issues can be explored in an interesting and meaningful manner. Compromises between what is healthy for the economy and what is healthy for the environment may present themselves more and more, so health education program participants should be prepared to analyze the stimuli for such compromises and the consequences of the proposed solutions.

Sensory Awareness

One aspect of ecological study, often overlooked in crisis-oriented health education programs, is the sensory pleasure that can be derived from the environment. However, to fully appreciate the joy that can be derived from one's surroundings, one needs keen sensory awareness. This section describes learning activities that can heighten sensory awareness as it relates to the environment.

Blindfolded Activities

Though eyesight is a luxury most of us would refuse to relinquish, some experiences are more meaningful without the sense of sight interfering. In particular, where sensory awareness development is concerned, seeing distracts from an awareness of the input obtained from other senses. Consequently, this activity requires participants to choose a partner and to have one of the pair blindfolded.

Once the blindfold is in place, the sighted person leads the blindfolded one on a walk. No verbal communication between the partners should be allowed, although they are always to remain in physical

Without effective instruction in environmental health issues, we may lose settings of splendor that can evoke feelings of spiritual health. Instead, the effects of acid rain, pollutants in the air and in the waterways, and soil erosion along the banks of rivers and lakes might become all that is available to our senses.

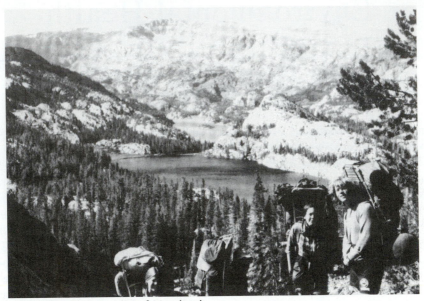

Source: The Diamondback/University of Maryland

contact (hand holding, elbow leading, and so on). For the first 10 minutes of the walk, the blindfolded person should concentrate on the sounds he or she hears, the next 10 minutes on the smells, and the last 10 minutes on feeling objects. The next group meeting should be devoted to the partner's turn to experience the blind walk. It will surprise the participants that they usually miss so much of what they hear, smell, and touch.

An additional blindfolded sensory awareness developmental activity relates to the sense of taste. Participants are blindfolded and seated at desks. From edible items brought in by each person, the health educator chooses some food for several people to taste and to guess what they've just eaten. Additional foods chosen should result in the participants having had the opportunity to concentrate on and develop their sense of taste. A similar activity—touching objects or foods and then guessing what they are—can be conducted and related to the sense of touch.

Mixing Senses

Helping program participants to look at their environment anew can be interestingly accomplished by having them mix senses. In doing so, they will develop a greater appreciation for the uniqueness of each sense and its contribution to the whole. For example, have students write compositions about

1. The *taste* or *sound* of green.
2. The *sound* or *smell* of a caring touch.
3. The *smell* or *taste* of thunder.
4. The *feel* or *look* of a murmur.
5. The *sight* or *sound* of fear.

Zoo Tripping

One interesting place to experience stimulation of one's senses is the zoo. Because the sounds, smells, and feelings present at the zoo are not those experienced usually, one's senses tend to be used more. As with the blindfolded exercises, if participants were to close their eyes for part of the visit and concentrate on one of the other senses, they would develop a greater sensory awareness. This does not mean that sight should not be utilized at the zoo; in fact, the practice of seeing and observing in a new setting is recommended. To derive even greater benefit from a zoo trip, it is suggested that, if one is available, a petting zoo be visited to provide practice in increasing sensory awareness related to touching and feeling. If a zoo is not available for visit, a farm could serve the same purpose.

Snow Romping

There are many opportunities to utilize natural settings for increasing sensory awareness. An imaginative health educator will respond to the challenge of developing increased sensory awareness through use of the environment in many diverse and varied ways. One means by which the instructor might use the environment for this purpose is called "snow romping." On a day after snow has fallen—or as it is actually coming down—the health educator has the participants bundle up and takes them outdoors. Several activities in the snow are possible, only some of which are suggested here:

1. Catch a snowflake in your mouth. How does it taste? Feel? What does it do?
2. Catch a snowflake in your hand. What does it look like? Describe it. How does it feel?
3. Look toward the sky and let the snow fall on your face. How does it feel?
4. Pick up a handful of snow. Smell it. What does it smell like?
5. Pick up a handful of snow, being careful not to squeeze the flakes together. Place the snow between the palms of both hands, bring the hands to one ear, squeeze the snow, and listen. What did the snow sound like?
6. Fall into a snow pile. What happened to you? What happened to the snow? How did it feel when you fell into the snow?
7. Listen to the snow fall. Did you hear anything?
8. Listen to the cars *swish* through the snow. What do they sound like?
9. Listen to people *slosh* through the snow. What does that sound like?
10. Act as though you are a snowflake. How does the snowflake (you) feel? Where does the snowflake want to go? From where did the snowflake come? Where will the snowflake go when the sun shines?

Other natural phenomena, such as drizzle, wind, or sun, can be similarly employed to develop increased appreciation and development of the senses.

Environmental Study

The following activities relate to the study of varied environmental factors. Once sensory awareness has been expanded, disillusionment with the state of the environment will lead to an interest in the learning experiences described in this section.

Litter Police

A police force within the health education group could be formed to meander about the building or community or worksite and observe instances of disregard for the environment. Mock violation tickets, accompanied by a handout defining ecological concerns and solutions to environmental problems, could be handed to all those observed to behave in an environmentally unhealthful manner. If it can be enforced, the violation ticket might require people cited to attend, after school or work, a short lecture or display further describing problems of an ecological nature. The "litter police force" might, in addition, decide to conduct a communitywide educational program related to environmental health education. To add to enthusiasm, unique hats could be worn by all "litter police."

Planned City

With the notoriety associated with the development and conduct of such cities as Reston, Virginia, and Columbia, Maryland, communities are increasingly setting out to develop new suburban areas rationally, rather than letting them develop haphazardly. Planned cities connote conscious efforts to make sense out of a soon-to-be community. Usually a minimum amount of recreational area per resident is planned, provision is made for an industrial complex, and both purchased and rented facilities are available.

Utilizing the planned cities concept, have the program participants plan a city that makes sense to *them*. By way of preparation for this activity, it is recommended that students read about existing or contemplated planned cities (New York State Urban Development Corporation n.d.).

Trash Treasures

To demonstrate the nature of waste and the use to which waste might be put, give program participants the time to wander about a school or place of work and its environs, gathering objects that have been discarded. From these objects they must create a work of art: sculpture, mosaic, or collage, for example. Those deemed by the group to be exceptionally interesting should be displayed prominently in an appropriate place within, or just outside, the school or worksite. A poster describing the art and its ingredients, as well as a short paragraph on the recycling of solid waste, should be placed alongside.

Trash-Container Spying

One generality about American culture is that there tends to be a great deal of waste in everyday functioning. To evidence the truth in this criticism, and to seek means for somewhat lessening this problem, send several people to bring back a waste container that tends to receive a great deal of use. After spreading a protective cover on the floor in the room (cut-open trash container liners can be used for this

These students are enjoying the trash-container spying activity.

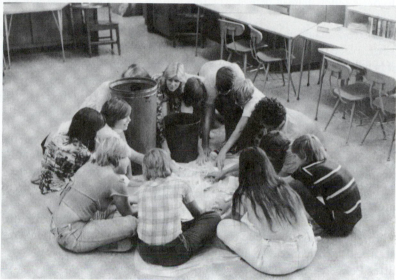

Source: Jerrold S. Greenberg

purpose), empty the contents of the trash container on the floor. Wearing old gloves, participants should rummage through the garbage and discuss

1. How some of the trash could be reused.

2. How to decrease the amount of trash deposited (for example, write on both sides of paper).

3. How industry might help decrease the amount of trash that cannot be used again.

The health educator might suggest that participants conduct a similar exercise with the trash collected from the containers in their homes.

Population Growth Experiment (CRM Books 1972)

Augment a group discussion on the population explosion by periodically halving the size of the room, which simulates doubling the population. The easiest way to do it is by using a long rope to delineate the limit of the "earth." The size can be halved at the same rate that the world population has increased and would cause the last few minutes of the session to be very hectic, leaving no time to discuss the phenomena that took place. Otherwise, the class could be roped off periodically according to convenience. The group must adapt to the changes in a variety of ways that duplicate the effects of doubling the population. For example, the decrease in amount of space per person forces many to stand, simulating moving upward as with high-rise apartment living. Occasionally some people refuse to stay within the confines of the rope, illustrating that as the pressures of more people and less space build, some of us want to drop out or push others out. This might be a reason for increased suicide and homicide. A short film that shows how population doubling time is decreasing would fit in perfectly with this demonstration.

Tug-of-War

Environmental problems and solutions relate to that thin line between *freedom* to do what one wants and *responsibility* to one's fellow human beings. The relationship between freedom and responsibility can be demonstrated by conducting a tug-of-war. Divide the group into teams of five members, each based on size; that is, each team should have comparable strength for the tug-of-war exercise. Select two teams to oppose each other; then have each team hold on to one end of a rope and tug until one team is moved five feet toward the other team's side. If the teams have been composed with concern for equal strength, the tug-of-war will be a grueling activity for the team members. Muscles will hurt, palms will feel uncomfortable, and frustration will be evidenced. What the participants *do* with these feelings is the part of this activity that should be examined and analyzed. After the tug-of-war has ended, the group should discuss such questions as the following:

1. Why did, or didn't, you stop tugging on the rope when you started to be uncomfortable?
2. Were you afraid of the reaction of your team members if you let them down?
3. When you observed someone let go of the rope, did you empathize with that person or did you deride him or her?
4. When you were close to winning or losing, did you feel that you lost your freedom to let go of the rope? Why or why not?
5. Can this exercise be generalized to any real-life situations that you recall? That you've experienced?
6. Concerning environmental problems and solutions, how do freedom and responsibility relate?

Grounds Exploring

Many opportunities for environmental study can occur on school or work-site grounds. The following activities have been suggested by one school system (Halnen et al. 1971):

1. Emphasize the *senses.*
   a. Have the participants lie on their backs in the grass quietly for five minutes. What do they hear, smell, see?
   b. Have them lie on their stomachs and do the same.
   c. Use hand lenses to discover small objects.
   d. Collect various *shades* of colors growing naturally, various colors, shapes, textures.
2. Use the *lawns.*
   a. Mark off a square foot of lawn. Count the number of plants in it. How many different kinds? Compare with an equal area of sandier, poorer soil. Discuss the differences.
   b. Dig up clover roots and look for bacterial nodules.
   c. Watch an active anthill. How do they dig a hole?

Pages ●●●-●●● and Figures 11.1, 11.2, and 11.3 are from the *Environmental Awareness Sampler* developed by the Wellesley Public Schools, 1971. Reprinted by permission of the Wellesley, Massachusetts, Public School District.

    d. Search for worm castings. How many do you find in a square yard? Discuss the important role of worms in soil formation.

    e. Are there grass, flowers, seeds?

    f. Record temperatures on various places in and on the lawn. Compare with temperatures on blacktop. Are there differences?

3. Use the *shrubbery and trees.*

    a. How many different kinds of evergreens can you find?

    b. Can you find berries? What are they good for?

    c. Has anything been nibbling on or using the leaves?

    d. How do leaves grow on a branch? Are they arranged the same?

    e. How do new leaves feel compared with old leaves?

    f. Does all bark look and feel the same? Make bark rubbings.

    g. Can you hear tree branches rubbing in the wind?

    h. Look for leaf "skeletons." What do they mean?

4. Use the *buildings, walks, and driveways.*

    a. Look for algae and lichens growing on the bare surfaces. Why do they grow there and how?

    b. Study some ivy (a safe kind). How does it cling to the wall?

    c. Look for signs of weathering and erosion (rust, corrosion).

    d. Look at stones in a wall. Compare textures, color, shine.

    e. After a rain, find miniature deltas, rivers, valleys. See how they form.

Solid-Waste Instrument Making

Since recycling has been suggested as one means of responding to the increasing production of waste products, involving program participants in a recycling activity seems to make sense. The following list of instruments that can be made from solid waste, some of which are illustrated in Figure 11.1, was developed by the Wellesley, Massachusetts, public school system.

Water whistle — A straw partly cut in two and bent at the cut with one end immersed in a bottle with water in it makes a musical note by gently blowing through the horizontal straw and raising and lowering the other part in the water.

Straw oboe — A straw with one end flattened (which acts as the double reed as in an oboe) and blown into makes a crude musical instrument. To get various notes, cut straws to different lengths.

Tuned bottles — Arrange bottles and jugs filled with water at different levels. Tune the bottles to a scale by varying the amount of water. Mark levels so they may be tuned again easily. Play a tune by tapping or by blowing across the top.

Rubber band-jo — Use various sizes of rubber bands (length and thickness) stretched over a cigar box or milk carton (with a rectangle cut from one side leaving ¼" margin for rigidity along either side and a wooden stick tacked across the opening to brace the sides). Put eight rubber bands around the carton equally spaced. The pitch of each band may be raised or lowered by tightening or loosening the band across the opening. Tune the eight strings to a scale. Make two instruments to play duets.

FIGURE 11.1

Simple Instruments Made of Solid Waste

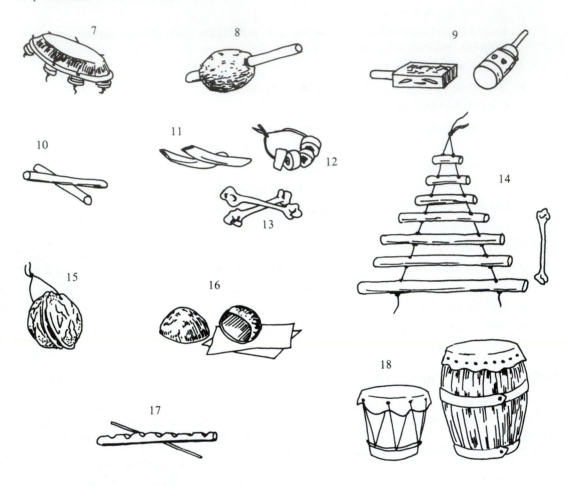

Wishbone harp—Save the wishbone from your chicken or turkey dinner for a tiny wishbone harp. String a small, thin rubber band across the opening. Wind the band over several times if necessary. Rest the open end of the wishbone on a piece of wood or empty can and pluck it gently.

Bass or contralto bucket—All you need is a large metal washtub, bucket, or large juice can; a broomstick; a length of heavy cord or venetian blind cord; and an assortment of hardware—an eye screw, two washers, and a nut. Turn the tub upside down. Drill a hole through the center large enough to fit a large screw eye. Cushion the screw with a washer, and thread it through. On the inside of the bucket put on another washer, and tighten it with a nut. Bore a hole in the end of the broomstick or a three-foot piece of doweling, and attach it with wire to the rim of the bucket through which a hole has been bored. At a convenient height near the top of the stick, drill a hole large enough so that the cord can pass through. Tie one end of the cord to the screw eye. Thread the other end through the hole in the stick. To play your bass, stand with one foot on the bucket, hold the stick with your left hand, and pluck the string with your right. This will be the lowest note.

To vary the sounds, hold the stick and string, and move your hand up and down. For the contralto bucket, hold it between your knees, tilt the stick, and pluck the string.

Panbourine—With a sharp nail, punch six to eight holes about the rim of a tin pie pan or foil plate. Cut an equal number of three-inch pieces of thin wire. For each hole you will need two metal disks—bottle tops. Remove cork or cardboard linings and punch a hole through each cap. Thread them with the wires, and attach them in pairs through the holes in the pie pan. Knot the wires at each end. (Illustration 7)

Coconut-shell shaker—Drill a hole (at least one inch in diameter) so the coconut meat can be taken out. Fill with seeds, plug hole with tape, and shake. (Illustration 8)

Coconut-shell clappers—Saw a coconut in two equal halves. These are good to imitate the sound of hooved animals. (Illustration 16)

Coconut-shell scrapers—Place paper over the two coconut shells and rub together (sounds a little like walking through the snow). (Illustration 16)

Walnut castanets—Made from perfect halves of walnuts. Drill two holes about one-half inch from the edge of each half of the shell. (Illustration 15)

Box shakers—Use a wooden codfish box, shoe polish box, baking powder box, or oatmeal cylinder. Put a number of seeds (rice or cherry pits, for example) inside and shake. (Illustration 9)

Rhythm sticks or claves—Use a six-inch-long piece of one-inch-diameter maple or old broom handle. To play, cup one in your hand, and hit it across the top with the other. (Illustration 10)

Bones—Turkey leg bones for rhythm sticks or claves. Beef ribs (minstrel bones) to click, soup bones to string and click together. (Illustrations 11, 12, and 13)

Xylophone—Maple sticks of various lengths and diameters can be strung on a string or set on two tubes of rolled-up newspaper. For best resonance, drill holes at one-fifth the distance from the end of each stick. (Illustration 14)

Guiros or notched stick—Choose a branch or a piece of scrap wood about one inch in diameter and 12 to 24 inches long. Whittle open notches half an inch wide, spacing them every half-inch or so. A metal tapper or chopstick produces the sound by being scraped across the notches or grooves. (Illustration 17)

Drums—Drums can be made from a variety of simple materials—nail kegs, wastebaskets, flowerpots, wooden chopping bowls. For the head, use a calfskin, rubber inner tube, or cloth that has been stretched and shellacked. Calfskin (from a drum shop) must be soaked in water 20 minutes, stretched over the container, and held down with upholstery tacks. Put in the first tack, then the second on opposite side. Alternate until tacks are one inch apart. For flowerpots or other nonwood forms, use cord or leather thongs to tie the head in place. (Illustration 18)

List of Questions for Environmental Study *(Halnen et al. 1971)*

Different techniques and methods may be employed in environmental studies. Given the broad behavioral objectives and the desired outcomes, a list of specific questions and samples will help the health educator direct the activities of program participants for more effective learning. The following list presents questions that may be completed by using the samples given on any appropriate choice that fits the particular unit with which the participants are involved:

What words or ideas come to mind when I
say _____?   (ecology, predator, recycle)

What do you think of when you hear the
word _____?   (conservation, SST, road)

Compare two or more _____.   (animals, bones, rocks)

Contrast _____ with _____.   (topsoil–sand, frog–toad)

What are the significant similarities between
_____ and _____?   (birch tree–beach tree, pen–pencil)

What are the significant differences between
_____ and _____?   (trains–boats, camping–backpacking)

Differentiate between _____
and _____.   (salt water–fresh water, predator–prey)

What different ways are there to solve problem X?   (air pollution, gypsy moth)

How many kinds of problems could have arisen from
situation X?   (earthquake, parking)

Questions   **Samples**

How many different ways can object Z be used?   (paper, glass)

How many different ways can you group these
objects, words, ideas, and so on?   (rocks, bottle tops)

How many different patterns do you observe in this
picture, song, and so on?   (geometric, growth)

How many different views can we anticipate in terms
of this issue?   (paying the price of pollution)

How many different predictions can we make relative
to X occurrence?   (algal bloom, drought)

How many different conclusions can we draw from
these data?   (population statistics, rising costs)

How many different errors can we make in the
process of _____?   (measuring the schoolyard, cost of a
                                                          meal)

Given the following purpose and data, develop a
plan to achieve this purpose.   (clean up litter)

Organize the following information into a meaningful   (data from written source or from direct
report.   experience)

Given the following items, construct a mobile, a
collage, a picture, a diorama, and so on.   (junk, nature specimens)

Combine the following simple machines into a
complex one.   (pulley and lever)

Given the following arithmetic operations, construct   (multiplication and division, buying and
a problem using all of them.   selling)

Combine the following data and state the interrelationships that you perceive.

(births–deaths)

Describe the pattern you discovered in a design.

(leaves, fruit, flowers)

Analyze the given data and identify the facts and fallacies.

(toads–warts, ground hog's effect on the length of winter)

Participants view a film without sound and analyze film by providing their own dialogue. Participants then replay film with sound to confirm analysis.

Tape a lesson. Participants listen and analyze their contributions and evaluate them to arrive at suggestions for improvement.

(take a tape along on nature walk)

Participants observe and analyze artifacts.

(anything goes)

Participants view a film and analyze it to arrive at the sequence of events shown in the film.

Participants view a silent demonstration and analyze to determine what they have observed.

Questions	Samples
What are the parts of a _____?	(flower, brain)
Describe the steps or procedures needed to _____.	(make a terrarium)
List the parts of X and describe how they are related.	(automobile, flower)
In solving X problem, list the steps you would take.	(snow removal)
Given the following specific situations, objects, data, and so on, what big statement can you make that applies to all?	(food chain)
Into what kinds of groups can you place these items, objects, ideas, and so on?	(oranges, toad)
Given two or more alternatives, which one would you choose and why?	(bicycle, auto)
Given X problem and solutions 1, 2, and 3, which would you select and why?	(alternatives)
Given issue and views 1, 2, and 3, select the view you would accept. Substantiate your selection.	(pollution issues, trash)
Given the following courses of action in X situation, which one would you choose to follow? Justify your choice.	
Given the following articles reporting Z event, select the one that best describes the actual occurrence. State the reasons for your selection.	(Using *Time, Life, Newsweek,* and so on, pick issue, such as SST, ABM)

Which of the following scientific inventions (X, Y, Z) was most beneficial to humanity? Why?   (airplane, DDT, polio vaccine)

How could we measure the size of this room? Which is the best method? Why?   (Use ruler, string, tape, and so on.)

Make up a story solving a problem.

Create or design a perfect world.

If you were a _____, what would you do?   (rabbit, teacher, parent)

Change the story.   (Johnny Appleseed, Pilgrims)

Invent _____.   (depolluter, a new machine)

Imagine that _____; what would happen?   (world had no grass, moon is cheese)

What would happen if _____?   (your dreams came true, you had a million dollars)

How would you feel if _____?   (your class went on a trip, but you had no permission to go; you had green hair)

What would you do if _____?   (the sun stopped shining, you were the last person on earth)

Give an imaginative account of _____.   (life of kangaroo, drop of water)

Devise a system or procedure for _____.   (taking tests, losing weight)

Correlated Activities (Halnen et al. 1971)

Following are listed a variety of sample activities in different disciplines taken from many sources. They are specific, challenging, and fun.

Language

Compose lyrics from the sounds you can hear in the natural environment. Describe what *nature* means to you.

Write poems or descriptions about something you found on a walk.

Stop in the woods and have the group, using all senses, describe the moment verbally.

Tell stories of what was seen, and listen to nature stories.

Describe the view from a given location.

As you go along, keep stopping to close your eyes and touch things — up high, on the ground, all around. Do you like how a thing feels, or dislike it? When you get back, write (or tell) about how some things felt to you. Did they feel pleasant or unpleasant? Could you tell what something was just by touch?

Write or tell a story on being an apple tree for one calendar year.

Read, write, or tell about a summary of the life of one of the following: skunk, woodchuck, mole, wild rabbit, field mouse, or any other animal.

Study a tree or flower closely and then write a haiku (17-syllable Japanese verse), simple verse, short description, prose, or drama.

Describe colors, textures, tastes, smells.

Describe an object while blindfolded.

Art

Take a "rainbow" trip—look for red, orange, yellow, and so on. Come back, and draw what you saw.

Take a discovery hike in a nearby forest. Sketch animal tracks located on the hike, and identify them. Take along paper and magic marker or crayons. As you go along, notice as many colors as you can find and mark a sample of that color (or as close as you can match it) on your paper. How does texture affect the color? How many different shades of one color do you find? When you get back, make a picture, using the colors you recorded. It doesn't have to be a picture of the woods. It could be how woods make you feel.

Collect and identify seeds, and with them make a design of different textures, colors, sizes, and shapes.

Draw different clouds; identify them and explain.

Make a study of a plot of land. Record changes with seasons through sketches.

Study changes in color, light, and shadow due to different times of day and seasons. Sketch differences.

Make rubbings of a leaf, bark, and so on.

Make leaf prints in plaster of paris. Make sand castings of cones, feathers, leaves.

Make a colored-sand painting.

Make a collection of leaves, soil, sand, moss to demonstrate textures, colors, sizes.

Make a sketch before and after going for a nature walk. (First sketch made after talking about what might be seen. Second sketch made after walk. Compare.)

Social Studies

Find out what year your house, school, or worksite was built. With other program participants, make a chart of how the acreage was used one year ago, four years ago, 50, and 100 years ago. Why was the area used for its stated purpose?

Find out where your family's water comes from, where your sewage, trash, burnable wastes, and garbage go.

What materials are used in your area for building? Why?

Look for signs of animals and birds that will tell you what inhabits the area. Where do these animals live at different times of the year? Why? Do their habits influence the balance of nature? Do other species depend on them? Do they influence humans—or humans them? Do they influence the human environment, or do humans influence theirs?

Evidence of human effect on the environment.

Nature resources found in the area. History of the area: Has it always been a forest, field, or lake?

Find causes of pollution in your neighborhood, and find ways to eliminate them.

Search for humanmade changes, roads, fire breaks, and so on, and discuss whether they may be helpful in some ways and harmful in others.

After rain, notice gullying, deltas, deposits of silt, pebbles, stones, and "minigeology."

Make a study of gravestones for plotting epidemics.

Determine the age of a tree, and associate it with a period of history past or future. Tell a story that the tree might have seen in history.

Mathematics

Pace out a given distance. Compare results with others and with a standardized unit of measure.

Measure (approximately) the surface of one average-sized leaf from a tree. Count the leaves on one branch of the same tree, and estimate how many leaves are on the whole tree. Then find the approximate total leaf surface on that one tree.

Select a tree, and determine its age by counting branches or tree rings.

Keep weather records of temperature, precipitation, length of day for a stated length of time.

Estimate how tall a tree is and how much it has grown each year.

Estimate how many times taller than a member of the class a tree is.

Estimate the age of a live tree by counting between nodes (this works well for maples, oaks, pines).

Count tree rings and explain differences in size (due to weather conditions).

Mark out an acre, quarter acre.

Calculate the percentage of a stated area that does not absorb water due to roads, buildings, and so on.

Music

Sing songs about the seasons — make up new words.

Listen to sounds of nature on a walk. Sing songs about nature. Make up songs about what you hear. (Bird songs. Sounds of forest. Wind in pines, wind in hardwoods. Bug sounds: carpenter ants, bees, and so on.)

Listen carefully for a sound or series of sounds as you walk along. Put them together, forming a melody or part of a melody. Maybe some of these could be transcribed and combined to make a "woods song."

Listen for insect, bird, mammal sounds; record on tape.

Use imagination to reproduce sounds, rhythms by simple instruments. Make instruments like sticks, shakers.

Make up a song using a nature theme.

Correlate bird songs with pictures; also frog or insect sounds.

Science

Study pond water and identify living things.

Take and study temperature deviations in an area.

Identify animal tracks.

Plant orange, apple, grapefruit seeds and so on. Grow new plants from parts such as a leaf, stem, bud.

Study weather's effect on the environment.

Find evidence of erosion. Discuss ways of curtailing it.

Choose one animal, and tell the kind of habitat it needs—food, shelter. Why must it live where it does?

Watch plant roots growing, test soils for chemical percentages, study different types of rocks.

Test soils for composition, acidity, and so on.

Town of Barnard Simulation

The following simulated game was developed by the Wellesley, Massachusetts, public school district. This activity presents realistic environmental concerns in microcosm format, requiring participants to place themselves in decision-making roles.

Directions for the Participants

1. Read fact sheets about Barnard and the gift lot.

2. Decide on a role you would like to play as a citizen of Barnard. Give yourself a name, a family, a career.

   You may wish to be

   - The moderator who will conduct the town meeting.
   - A professor who teaches biology at Lafayette State College.
   - A contractor who wants to build low-income housing and housing for the elderly.
   - A game warden who is concerned about the growing pollution problem.
   - Mrs. Nobudua, who would like to build a nature trail for nature study.
   - Mr. Dugood, a young lawyer who is politically minded.
   - Mr. Hexacre, who is concerned about housing for the growing number of retired people.
   - Mr. Goalsworthy, the high school hockey coach, who desperately desires an ice rink closer than the one in Central City.
   - Mr. Jones, president of Barnard Trust Company.
   - A member of the Barnard Rod and Gun Club.

FIGURE 11.2

The Town of Barnard

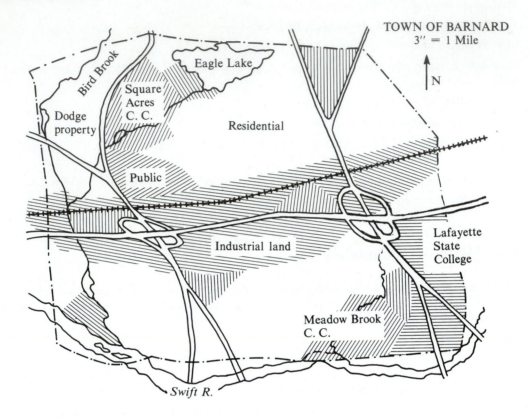

TOWN OF BARNARD
3″ = 1 Mile

- A member of the Barnard Historical Society.
- A member of the Garden Club.
- A member of the Square Acre Country Club.
- A member of the League of Women Voters.
- Any of the people listed on the fact sheet.

3. On the basis of the information given and your interest, how would you like to see this land used? Plan to come to the town meeting to put forth your own ideas and to justify your position on this issue.

Description (See Figure 11.2)

1. The town of Barnard, located 20 miles from Central City in the county of Lafayette in the state of Madison, has a population of 25,000 people.
2. Barnard encompasses 7,000 acres of land, of which 500 acres are warm-water ponds and brooks.

3. A superhighway cuts directly through the center of the town in an east−west direction and over-passes two county highways that run in north−south directions.

4. Two main bus lines and six taxicab companies service the town.

5. Running parallel to and just to the north of the superhighway is the W and B Railroad (W&BRR).

6. Many of the people in this residential community use these transportation facilities to commute to and from their places of employment in Central City and surrounding areas.

7. Barnard has an excellent centrally located shopping center, some light industry, and a growing complex of service-oriented branch offices whose main offices are in Central City.

8. There are two theaters, two bowling alleys, 10 tennis courts, two private golf courses, and many clubs, as well as two public beaches and a small boat-launching ramp on Eagle Lake.

9. Barnard has a representative town government headed by five selectmen elected by the voters.

10. The selectmen appoint the comptroller, town counsel, treasurer, tax collector, town forest commissioner, art commissioner, conservation commissioner, historical commissioner, retirement board, and constable.

11. Elected officials include a town clerk, a seven-member school committee, a board of assessors, a board of health, a recreation commissioner, a parks and trees commissioner, a board of public works, and a town moderator.

12. The moderator appoints people to help him: the advisory committee, improvement coordinating committee, and industrial development committee, and other various ad hoc committees as needed. For the town organization, see Figure 11.3.

13. There are six elementary schools of about 500 students each, two middle schools, and one comprehensive high school.

14. Lafayette State College is located in the southeast area of town.

15. A gift of a 100-acre lot of land has been willed to Barnard by a longtime resident, Jeremiah Dodge.

16. The acreage is situated in the northwest corner of town.

17. Approximately half the lot is made up of underdeveloped woodland, and the remainder is meadow and marshland.

18. A brook flows from the high area in the northeast corner of the lot to an 11-acre pond in the southwest corner.

19. Broken stone walls on the property and the remains of a stone-cellar foundation give evidence of a former farmhouse and barns.

20. The moderator has called a special open town meeting to which all interested citizens have been invited to help decide on proposals put forth for use of this gift lot of land.

Barnard's Town Government (see Figure 11.3)

The administrative officials of Barnard are led by the board of selectmen. The selectmen act as agents of the town and meet every Monday. They represent the town before officials of the federal, state and county governments, and the state legislature. They may, in the case of need, declare a state of emergency, at which time they are empowered to marshal all the resources of the community and take charge of all town departments to coordinate efforts in restoring conditions to normal. The five selectmen are the chief administrative

FIGURE 11.3

The Barnard Town Government

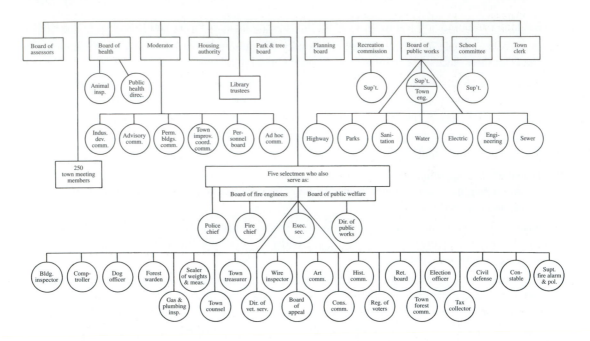

officers of Barnard. They are charged in the bylaws to "supervise all matters affecting the interests or welfare of the town," so they exercise considerable influence over town policy. The selectmen also appoint the town counsel, the comptroller, the treasurer, tax collector, town forest committee, art commission, conservation commission, historical commission, retirement board, and two constables.

This would appear, to the casual onlooker, to constitute the power structure of Barnard. However, one must look at other officials in the town who are elected and have the power to appoint various committees. Because of the rapid growth of this town, true democracy has given way to 250 elected town meeting members. The school committee (seven members) makes only one appointment, and that is the office of superintendent of schools. Three people are elected to the board of assessors, but make no appointments. The planning board has five elected members and makes no appointments. Three people are elected to the board of health and appoint a public health director and an animal inspector. (This animal inspector should not be confused with the dog officer, who is appointed by the selectmen.) A five-member recreation commission is elected and appoints a recreation superintendent. The board of public works has three elected officials, who appoint one superintendent of public works and a town engineer; these people in turn supervise the highway division, parks division, sanitation division, water division, electric division, and sewer division.

The Barnard voters also elect for a one-year term a moderator (an unpaid position). The moderator, by state statute, presides at town meetings and regulates the proceedings. The moderator conducts the meeting so that the rights of individuals and minorities to be heard are protected and at the same time the majority is able to get action.

The moderator's ruling on matters of parliamentary procedures is final. However, if seven or more voters immediately question a declaration of a vote, the law requires the moderator to verify it by polling the voters or by dividing the meeting.

The moderator is given extensive power to preserve order, including the power to order the removal and confinement of any person who persists in disorderly behavior.

The moderator exercises great influence in town affairs because it is his or her duty to make appointments to standing and special committees. The efficient operation of the town and the direction of its development depend to a great extent on the moderator's success in selecting competent and qualified citizens to serve on these committees. He or she is an ex officio member of the town meeting and may vote.

The moderator has the power to appoint a 15-member advisory committee. Each member serves a three-year, unpaid term. The terms are arranged so that one-third of the membership is appointed annually. They select their own chairperson.

The services of the advisory committee to the town are invaluable. It is required by law to consider every matter that is to be brought before a regular or special town meeting under the articles in the warrant. It consults with each town department, scrutinizing its budget and sometimes modifying proposals as the individual budgets are considered in relation to the entire financial picture of the town. It holds public meetings and sends its printed report and recommendations to all households at least seven days before a town meeting. Reasons for the recommendations are given, and a minority report is sometimes included.

At each town meeting the chairperson of the advisory committee stands ready to give its recommendations for action on each motion that is presented.

The advisory committee is empowered by statute to make transfers from the reserve fund to provide for extraordinary and unforeseen expenditures that may become necessary during the year. Thus, emergencies not contemplated at the time of the budget appropriations may be met in many cases without calling a special town meeting.

The improvements coordinating committee is appointed by the moderator also. This committee was established in 1946 "to consider the planning, coordination, financing, and timing of public word or improvement by the town" and to make annually a written report to the town before February 28. It is a long-range planning committee for the financing of major capital improvements wanted by the town. It does not pass on the desirability of suggested new town capital improvements or their priority. The report of this committee is customarily filed with the report of the advisory committee and contemplates capital improvements in light of the town's tax base, revenue surplus, and debt structure and recommends to town meeting members methods of timing and financing construction. The committee has also general concern for the long-range financial stability of the town, particularly with the level and terms of town debt.

The moderator also appoints five members to the permanent buildings committee, five members to the personnel board, and five members to the industrial development committee, who guide and plan for the expansion of small industries and encourage other businesses and companies to open branches in the town. This will help alleviate the tax burden. The moderator also may appoint special committees.

New England town government could not possibly function effectively or as democratically as it does if it were not for the work of many hard-working committees of citizens. The town creates special committees for a variety of purposes, such as the selection of school sites, the planning and building of schools or other public buildings, and the study of special problems of concern to the town. These committees are appointed by the moderator.

Robert's Rules of Order

The town meeting or hearing should be conducted in an orderly fashion by the moderator. Robert's Rules of Order should be followed, particularly during the discussion and in any voting that takes place.

All members of the group have the right to express their opinion, provided that they are recognized one at a time by the moderator and rise to address the group.

Should a member wish to make a proposal, he should place it in the form of a motion: I move that . . . The motion should be seconded by any other member. The moderator should then ask if there is any discussion, restating the motion so that it will be clear to everyone present.

A motion can be changed or amended with the permission of the person who first made the motion. This person can also withdraw a motion.

A motion can be tabled or postponed for discussion.

The chairman or moderator can appoint a committee to study the motion and report back to the group at a future meeting.

No other business can be taken up until some action is taken on the motion on the floor.

When voting, the majority of votes carries the motion. The moderator usually does not vote unless there is a tie. The moderator's job is to maintain order, recognize the speakers, and see that everyone who wants to say something is given an opportunity.

Current Environmental Threats

Global warming and terrorism are two of the current threats to the environment. The instructional strategies described next respond to these issues in a manner that involves program participants actively.

Warming to Global Warming

Carbon monoxide emissions from automobiles, chlorofluorocarbon released from air conditioners and refrigerators, and other by-products of our modern society have resulted in a greenhouse effect threatening the health and well-being of all of us. These greenhouse gases become part of a gaseous layer encircling the earth, allowing solar heat to pass through, and then entrapping that heat close to the earth's surface. The result is a climatic change manifested in drought in the Midwestern United States, flooding in India and Bangladesh, huge hurricanes, deforestation in the earth's rain forests, polar ice cap melting, forest fires, and extended heat waves in various parts of the world.

To help program participants appreciate the extent of this problem and the drastic consequences suggested by some experts, divide the group into "expert panels." Each "panel" has four to six participants and is assigned one of the proposed effects of global warming. The panel is to research changes in the parameters in question such that one group charts the change in temperature in the United States during the past century, another group researches the forestation change in the world's rain forests, another group investigates the number and severity of hurricanes, and so on. One panel also researches the recommended changes that need to be made to stop these effects. Once the panels' research is completed, they present their results to the total group.

When the presentations are done and the extent of the problem is therefore documented, advocacy groups are formed. Each advocacy group is assigned one target population to propose changes to decrease the global warming problem. For example, one advocacy group might target policy makers (politicians), another might target the public, another manufacturers of automobiles and other greenhouse gas–producing products, and so on. Advocacy groups might decide to write letters to these targets, arrange meetings to lobby for changes, submit letters to local newspapers, appear on local cable TV programs, or conduct education campaigns for the general public. Even if these activities are ineffective in bringing about the desired changes, participating in this activity will result in program participants contemplating their own behaviors that contribute to global warming and becoming more responsible citizens in this regard.

The Bioterrorism Assay

Since September 11, 2001, the United States has lived with the threat of terrorist activities. Program participants and others will naturally be concerned about the preparedness of their communities to prevent and respond to terrorist acts. The bioterrorism assay is one way of alleviating some of this concern. Divide participants into four groups to research what has been done to prevent and/or respond to terrorism. One group researches the federal government's responses, another the state government responses, a third local government responses, and the fourth community agency responses. When the research is completed, the groups write a "terrorism preparedness manual" that collates the results of their research. The existence of this manual is then advertised in the community through local newspapers and TV programs, and a copy is made available at local libraries. Although terrorism cannot be completely eliminated, the community's stress may be somewhat alleviated knowing how much has been done to attempt to respond to this abhorrent threat.

Valuing Activities

An excellent means of helping people to relate health content to their own behavior is values clarification. Environmental health seems to lend itself easily to such study. The activities here require participants to question their personal values and their own behaviors as they relate to the environment.

Baker's Dozen *(Simon et al. 1972)*

A means of aiding people to confront their own behavior and values relative to environmental concerns consists of asking them to list 13 things they use that require electricity. They then are asked to cross out the three things on the list that they could most easily live without and to circle the three things they would miss most if a power failure occurred. They might then decide to experiment for several days with not using the three items they crossed off their list. If successful in eliminating these three items relatively painlessly, the participants might select 3 items of the remaining 12 that would be least missed and try not using them. In any case, this exercise can demonstrate the existence of a gap between what people might profess to be environmental concerns of theirs (the wasting of our natural resources) and their own related behavior. An actual change in behavior often results from participation in this activity. For example, participants might decide to open cans manually rather than to use an electric can opener.

Activities Enjoyed

As described in Chapter 7, this activity asks people to list 20 things they like to do. After this list is developed, the health educator can give the following instructions:

1. Place the letter *E* next to any activity requiring energy from outside sources.
2. Place the letter *A* next to those activities you prefer to do alone and the letter O next to those you prefer to do with others.
3. Place the letter *W* next to any activity that produces waste products (for example, paper to be thrown away).
4. Place the letter *R* next to any activity that employs a reusable item.
5. Finally, place the letter *M* next to the five activities you do most often.

The following questions should then be posed by the health educator and discussed by the group:

1. Do the activities you enjoy use up our natural resources?
2. Can you use energy more efficiently by doing things with others that you presently do alone?

3. Could your activities be reorganized so as to use more materials that can be recycled and fewer materials that cannot?

4. Do the activities you do most often use up more or less energy than the activities you do less often?

5. How will you change your behavior, if at all, as a result of this activity?

Values Grid

Asking people to make values choices will help them to clarify their own values position. The values grid is one means to accomplish this end. Participants are asked to draw a 16-square grid with columns labeled very strong, strong, mild, and no opinion. Sixteen statements are then read, and they are to write the key word describing each statement in a place in the grid that represents their feelings regarding the statement. Here are 16 statements that relate to environmental health (key words underlined):

1. A man drives to work in his <u>car</u> by himself.
2. A woman takes her own <u>shopping bags</u> to the market.
3. A man takes his own clothes <u>hangers</u> to the dry cleaner.
4. A woman uses a new can of <u>tennis balls</u> each set.
5. A boy uses an electric <u>can opener</u> to open a can of soup.
6. A woman throws a cigarette <u>butt</u> out of her car window.
7. An <u>industrial</u> company pollutes the town's river.
8. A neighbor burns his <u>trash</u> in his backyard.
9. A <u>schoolteacher</u> writes on one side of the paper only.
10. A man keeps writing nasty letters to the <u>newspaper</u> about too many pages devoted to advertising.
11. A car manufacturer makes cars that can use <u>electricity</u> or gasoline.
12. A mayor proposes raising <u>taxes</u> to install a better sewage disposal system.
13. A teenager drinks a <u>soft drink</u> from a nonreturnable container.
14. A man washes his clothes with <u>detergents</u> that include phosphates.
15. A child throws a <u>gum</u> wrapper in the street.
16. A <u>mother</u> scolds her child for spitting on the sidewalk.

A discussion of the grids should focus on the reason that certain statements elicit stronger feelings than others.

Values Quadrant

One manner of organizing environmentally related data and determining what people can do to improve the environment is to develop values quadrants. Participants are asked to draw a large square and divide it into four equal parts (quadrants). In one quadrant they are to list three places they frequently attend that add pollutants to the environment; in another quadrant, three people they personally know who could be classified as polluters; in a third quadrant, three places they attend that do not add pollutants to the environment; and in the last quadrant, three people who are not polluters. The following questions should then be posed and discussed:

1. What could you do to get the polluting places to be less polluting?
2. What could you do to get the polluting people to be less polluting?
3. What could you do to prevent the nonpolluting places and people from becoming polluters?
4. Who could help you accomplish 1 and 2?
5. Who would try to prevent you from accomplishing 1 and 2?
6. In which quadrant would you place yourself?
7. What have you learned as a result of this activity?

Values Voting

As with other content areas, values voting can be used effectively to help people explore their values related to the environment. The following questions are suggested:

1. How many of you would form a car pool to get to school or work?
2. How many of you walk or ride a bicycle when going short distances?
3. How many of you have ever picked up trash lying on the street?
4. How many of you would stop someone who has thrown a gum wrapper on the street and explain the harm this does?
5. How many of your family cars have been tuned up in accordance with manufacturer's recommendations?
6. How many of you would buy soft drinks in nonreturnable containers?
7. How many of you turn lights out when you are the last person to leave a room?
8. How many of you are willing to separate your weekly trash into two piles — material that can be recycled and material that can't?

Fantasy Questions

Often questions can be used to place people in a position requiring a values-related decision. Some of these questions, as they relate to environmental health, could be

1. If you were the mayor, what would you do to improve our environment?
2. If you were a clean town, how would you have gotten that way?
3. If you were a polluted river, how would you sound?
4. If you were a landfill area, how would you smell?
5. If you were a polluter, what could stop you?
6. If you were garbage, what would you want done with you?
7. If you lived in the year 2050, what would your environment be like?

Coat of Arms

Still another means of helping people to identify and publicly affirm their values relative to the environment employs the "coat of arms" activity described in Figure 7.2. The participants should be instructed as follows:

In area 1 of the coat of arms, draw a picture that represents something with which you are very wasteful.

In area 2, draw a picture of an electric appliance you use but could probably do without.

In area 3, draw a picture of an electric appliance you use but would have great difficulty doing without.

In area 4, draw a picture of what you think to be the most important thing to do to improve the environment.

In area 5, draw a picture of what one of your most wasteful friends does that makes you judge him or her wasteful.

In area 6, write what you would like people to say about you, relative to your relationship to the environment, if you were to die today.

Introspective Questions

Not all valuing activities need involve other people. Occasionally introspective questions can help people analyze their individual behavior relative to their professed values. The following are but a few examples of introspective questions that may be used. An imaginative health educator will be able to develop many more.

1. How often do you use an electric can opener?
2. How often do you use an electric toothbrush?
3. Do you ask people to drive you places that you could walk or bike to?
4. Do you turn lights off when leaving a room?
5. Do you write on both sides of a sheet of paper?
6. Do you occasionally eat leftovers for dinner?
7. Do you buy soft drinks in nonreturnable containers?

Summary

One current societal concern is environmental health. With an increasing population, more and more waste to process, dirty air to breathe, and polluted waters in which to swim, environmental health is threatened. Several levels of our society are responding to these concerns in their unique contributory fashion: new legislation continues to be proposed, industrial firms are seeking means for recycling waste, consumers are asked to respond appropriately (for example, to keep their cars well tuned), and schools and community agencies are offering environmental health education experiences. The purpose of this chapter was to present learning experiences that make environmental health education offerings more meaningful and interesting to the participants involved. As with other chapters in this book, a prime concern was to actively involve program participants in their own learning through participation in activities requiring action on their parts.

CHAPTER TWELVE

Instructional Strategies for Nutrition

Though often an uninteresting and tedious unit of study, nutrition education can be offered in an exciting manner. That this is possible should not be surprising. Witness the interest in weight control evidenced by the development and growth of the Weight Watchers organization, and by the quantity of sales of diet books. That people in our society are concerned with weight seems obvious. That people are concerned with foods in relation to their health can also be documented. Health food consumers, health food shops, interest in books about health foods, and the purchase and ingestion of vitamins in large doses lend credence to the claim that Americans are aware of the relationship of foods they eat to their health status.

Unfortunately, some health instructors have an uncanny knack of transposing intrinsically motivating subject matter into first-rate "yawn" material. This chapter presents instructional strategies that health educators can employ to make the study of nutrition pertinent to program participants' interest.

So the study of nutrition-related educational activities begins with a concern for involving the learner in ways that relate the content to his or her life in a meaningful manner.

Sociological Aspects of Foods

Though foods can, and later in this chapter will, be related to health and aesthetics, there is a sociological aspect to foods and nutrition worthy of investigation in health education. The United States has been described as a melting pot because people of many ethnic, racial, and religious backgrounds make up its population. The use of this awareness in the study of the foods will enhance such study. In addition, the diversity in economic status of the American people means that even people from similar ethnic or religious backgrounds use different foods. This range in the ability to purchase foods should not be overlooked. Following are four activities recommended for use in the study of the sociological aspects of foods and nutrition.

Food History

Many health-related topics can be coordinated with other subject areas. One of these topics is nutrition. During earlier times in our country's history, foods other than those presently ingested were available and eaten regularly. For example, western Indians ate buffalo meat, and the pioneers ate fresh fish more often than does today's typical urbanite. The study of history can be coordinated with the study of food preparation and eating, and food history might be a means of manifesting such coordination.

The health educator should divide the class into study groups, with each group assigned to a specific period of history. Suggested divisions in American history are

1. Pre-Plymouth Rock.
2. Puritans to Revolutionary War.
3. Revolutionary War to Lincoln.
4. Lincoln to World War I.
5. World War I to the Food and Drug Administration (FDA) era.
6. FDA to present.

In addition, the instructor might want to further divide the class into geographical groups: South, Northeast, West, and so on.

Each group should be responsible for developing a skit, which they will present before the class. This skit should depict the food and the nutritional habits of the people within the group's period of history. Skits can then be combined and presented and might be titled *A Food History: Then and Now.*

Follow-up activities might require participants to develop a photocopied booklet related to food history to be distributed to other groups, or several short films of the skits with accompanying cassette tape recordings describing them.

The study of past nutritional habits and their relationship to present-day food-related behavior will provide a basis for predicting future trends related to foods and nutrition. If, as has been suggested, the purpose of the study of history is to make sense of the future through an understanding of the past, it seems worthwhile for people to examine their nutritional history as well as other aspects of their past.

Food Culturing

The melting pot concept can be employed in another manner. If people were asked to investigate their family histories, they would probably be able to identify a country or countries from which their ancestors came to the United States. Then they can be responsible for investigating the foods most common to those countries and preparing these foods for their classmates to sample. For example, program participants of Italian ancestry might prepare spaghetti, those of Portuguese background might prepare a shellfish of some kind, and those from Germany might serve apple streusel. Obviously, with such an international food feast, each person need prepare only enough food for a sampling by the others.

In addition to preparing and serving foods representative of their ancestry, participants should also *briefly* describe to the group any unique aspect of the eating habits of their forebears (for instance, eating with chopsticks) and why certain foods become characteristic of these people. For example, Asian Indians do not eat the sacred cow, and the weather of India is good for the inexpensive and nutritious rice crop; therefore, rice has long been a staple of that culture.

An analysis of the diets of various cultures should develop the attitude that the *form* in which nutrients are ingested varies throughout the world. However, the awareness that nutrients are needed in proper quantity, regardless of the *form* in which they are taken, should be an objective of food culture study.

Food Sociogram

In the United States, eating often assumes great social importance. In particular, the evening meal has been associated with family cohesiveness (the family that eats dinner together stays together), class snobbery (the long table with candelabra and waiters), and reward (the school athletic banquet, for example). Utilizing the unique role of the dinner meal, program participants can be helped to better understand the role of food in their society.

Whereas sociometric techniques have been recommended for use in groups to identify relationships between people, these techniques might also be employed to create an awareness of the importance of food. Participants should be asked to list the three people with whom they would *most* prefer to go to an expensive restaurant. These listings should be in descending order — that is, first choice, second choice, and third choice. Similarly, they should list three people with whom they would *least* like to go to such a restaurant. This listing should be in the same order as the previous — that is, the least, second least, and third least they would want to eat dinner with at an expensive restaurant.

The results of the listings can be placed in tabular form. Assuming, for the sake of space and brevity, that seven people are mentioned, the tables might be organized as follows:

Most Preferred

Choosers	First choice	Second choice	Third choice
John	Betty	Anita	Cindy
Frank	John	Paul	Todd
Anita	Todd	Cindy	Betty
Betty	Todd	Anita	Cindy
Cindy	Todd	Betty	Anita
Paul	John	Anita	Betty
Todd	John	Cindy	Anita

A similar table could be developed for the least preferred listing. The tables are then analyzed for any commonalities or distinctions that can be noted. For example, in the most preferred table several conclusions might be drawn:

1. John enjoys the company of females during dinner.
2. Frank enjoys the company of males during dinner.
3. Todd seems to possess some characteristic with which females enjoy being associated during dinner, since every female chose him as the one most preferred.
4. John seems to possess some characteristic with which males enjoy being associated during dinner, since every male chose him as the one most preferred.

Once such conclusions have been formulated, an analysis of the reasons behind them would help the group to better perceive the social aspects of foods. For instance, why is it that John enjoys sharing his dinner with women rather than with men? What characteristics do Todd and John possess that females and males want present during dinner? Why these characteristics over some others?

Hot Dogs and Pheasants

Due to numerous reasons, none of which seem necessary to cite here, there is a wide diversity in economic wealth, or lack of it, in the United States. There are very wealthy families and individuals, whose names the reader will easily recall, and indigents of whom no one ever heard. Obviously, some families

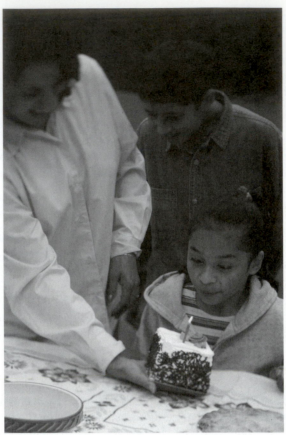

Source: Keith Brofsky/Brand X Pictures

can afford any foods they desire, while others can afford very little. The lesson of "hot dogs and pheasants" is to differentiate between undernourishment (not ingesting enough food and nutrients) and malnourishment (ingesting nutrients and food in inappropriate quantities). For example, a millionaire might be malnourished because of eating too much animal fat (meat) or too little vitamin C (citrus fruit); a welfare recipient might be undernourished because not enough food can be purchased with the food stamps he or she gets. The second lesson is that inexpensive foods may possess as much nutrient value as foods costing much more money.

Divide the class into groups of five members each. Assign each group a certain sum of play money with which they are to purchase foods and prepare meals for a family of four: father, mother, 15-year-old boy, and 5-year-old girl. The weekly food allowances might vary with the cost of living for individual communities, but the following are recommended:

1. An infinite amount of money.
2. Eighty dollars.
3. Sixty dollars.

4. Forty dollars.

5. Thirty dollars.

6. Twenty dollars.

Each group is then responsible for developing a nutritionally sound week's menu for the family. The development of this menu will require

1. The study of nutrients and their food sources.

2. An investigation of food prices by visiting food shops, supermarkets, fish stores, and so on.

3. The study of food preparation through reading cookbooks and, perhaps, interviewing worksite and school food service directors.

4. An investigation of recommended daily dietary allowances by sex, age, occupation, and so on.

Once the menus have been planned, they should be duplicated for the participants so that comparisons can be made and the objectives achieved.

Weight Control

The emphasis on weight control for reasons of appearance and health provides an impetus for the study of nutrition that should not be overlooked by the health educator. Obesity has been identified as one of the culprits in heart disease and hypertension, as well as being considered unattractive by many. For these reasons, people are concerned with their weight status.

However, some people are so overly concerned with body weight that they engage in extremely unhealthful and dangerous behavior. Anorexia nervosa is a condition in which this concern with being overweight is so exaggerated that the person eats so little that malnutrition develops. This condition can even become life threatening (the singer Karen Carpenter died of anorexia nervosa). Another similar condition is bulimia. With this condition, the person eats well enough—actually eats too much (binges)—but soon afterward purges the food by sticking a finger down the throat and purposefully vomiting.

Responsive health educators will conduct activities to aid participants in arriving at and maintaining a *healthy* weight. The activities in this section are designed for just such a purpose.

Alter Egoing

Used often in group therapy sessions, the alter ego technique allows a third party to say *for* one of the two people engaging in a discussion what that person may be thinking or feeling but unwilling or unable to express. For example, a role-playing situation might have two people discussing busing to achieve racial integration in schools. Player A might argue that busing his or her child across town would create inconvenience for the child and A, since both would have to wake up earlier than usual. Utilizing the alter ego opportunity, the instructor or another participant might interrupt the conversation to become player A and say, "Actually, I don't want my kid going to school with those blacks who really aren't serious about getting an education anyhow." Player B then responds to A as though A had made the alter ego statement—and the conversation continues.

Relative to nutrition (especially weight control), the health educator could establish a role-playing situation in which two or more participants discuss weight control. One discussant should play the role of group therapist assigned the responsibility of helping the other participants lose weight. As the role-playing situation progresses, any person not assigned a role may assume the alter ego of any discussant by standing behind him or her. When an observer does stand behind a discussant, the conversation stops and the alter ego speaks. After the alter ego statement is made, the conversation picks up and relates to that statement.

This activity usually begins with some superficial statement by a discussant such as, I know my excessive weight is unhealthy, and that's why I want to lose some. Eventually an observer will decide to alter ego and say something like, Actually, I can't get any dates looking like this and everyone makes fun of me. In this way the many facets of obesity and the means and motivations for weight control are discussed in an interesting manner.

Problem Analyzing

The following questionnaire needs only a brief introduction. If an overweight condition is seen as a problem, people can learn to identify factors tending to help the problem and those tending to worsen it. Once this analysis is made, recommendations for increasing the "helpers" and decreasing the "worseners" can be formulated. For example, Jane, who lives with her younger brother, younger sister, and mother, is 30 pounds overweight. She does most of the shopping and cooking for her family. Her brother and sister pressure her to buy sugared cereals and candies. That pressure would be one of the "worsening" factors, and Jane's control of what she buys (since she does the shopping) is one of the "helping" factors. Jane would complete the chart here to analyze this situation and devise strategies to change it. The questionnaire that follows asks questions designed for this end and, once completed individually, should be discussed in small groups.

Problem Analysis Questionnaire*

Part I: Problem Specification

Think about the problem of obesity. Respond to each of the items as fully as needed so that other groups will be able to understand the problem.

1. I understand the problem to be specifically that:

2. The following people are involved in the problem:

   They relate to the problem in the following manner:

3. I consider these other factors to be relevant to the problem:

4. I would choose the following aspect of the problem to be changed if it were in my power to do so (choose only one aspect):

---

*Reprinted from J. W. Pfeiffer and J. E. Jones (eds.), *A Handbook of Structured Experiences for Human Relations Training,* vol. II, San Diego, CA: Pfeiffer & Company, 1974. Used with permission.

Counterthrust

```
        /   a   /   b   /   c   /   d   /   e   /   f   /   g   /   h
5   /       /       /       /       /       /       /       /
4   _____
3   _____
2   _____
1   _____
Status quo_____
1   _____
2   _____
3   _____
4   _____
5   _____
        /   a   /   b   /   c   /   d   /   e   /   f   /   g   /   h
```

Thrust

Part II: Thrusting and Counterthrusting Forces

5. If you consider the present status of the problem to be a temporary balance of opposing forces, the following would be on your list of forces providing thrust toward change:

_____ a. _____

_____ b. _____

_____ c. _____

_____ d. _____

_____ e. _____

_____ f. _____

_____ g. _____

_____ h. _____

6. The following would be on your list of forces in counterthrust to change:

_____ a. _____

_____ b. _____

_____ c. _____

_____ d. _____

_____　e.　_____

_____　f.　_____

_____　g.　_____

_____　h.　_____

7. In the spaces to the left of the letters in item 5, quantify the forces on a range from one to five in the following manner:

　1 — It has almost nothing to do with the thrust toward change in the problem.

　2 — It has relatively little to do with the thrust toward change in the problem.

　3 — It is of moderate importance in the thrust toward change in the problem.

　4 — It is an important factor in the thrust toward change in the problem.

　5 — It is a major factor in the thrust toward change in the problem.

8. Fill in the spaces in front of the letters in item 6 to quantify the forces in counterthrust to change.

9. Diagram the forces of the thrust and counterthrust quantified in question 7 by drawing an arrow from the corresponding degree of force to the status quo line. For example, if you considered the first on your list of forces in item 5 to be rated a 3, draw your arrow from the 3 position in the left column of numbers indicating thrust up to the status quo line.

Part III: Strategy for Changing the Status Quo

Detail a strategy for decreasing two or more counterthrust elements from your list from item 6.

Weight Goal Telegramming

People tend to lose sight of their goals, especially when those goals are long-term. To help people achieve their weight-related goals, whether by increasing or decreasing, the following activity is suggested: Ask participants to write themselves a telegram on which appears the weight (more, less, or the same) that they would like to be in two months. Caution the group that these weight goals should be realistic. For instance, a loss of 100 pounds in two months might not only be unreasonable, but also unhealthful. The telegrams can then be mailed to participants two months hence to remind them of their goals, or they can be distributed in a subsequent group session.

Body Image and Self-Talk

Everyone has parts of his or her body, or personality, or limitations with which he or she is dissatisfied. Too many people focus on those aspects of themselves and, as a result, remain unhappy. However, concurrent with parts of ourselves that we would wish to change, there are parts of ourselves about which we are proud, happy, or satisfied. If we focused on those parts, we would achieve more satisfaction with ourselves and our lives. This does not mean we ignore those parts of ourselves that need improvement. Certainly, we should desire to continue to grow as people and become better. Still, to focus on the need for improvement while ignoring the many positive traits we have is dysfunctional. One way to help program participants to be more likely to remember their many positive traits is a technique called *self-talk*.

Self-talk can be used to convert negative thoughts to positive ones. For example, you might say to yourself, "I have too big a nose," and feel sorry for yourself as a result. Using self-talk in that example, you might say to yourself, "I have too big a nose, but very attractive blue eyes." This does not ignore the negative, but rather adds a positive to it—a positive that is as true as the negative we might have chosen to focus on.

Ask program participants to identify five parts of their bodies they think need improvement. For each part listed, have participants write a self-talk statement that identifies a positive aspect related to the negative one they listed:

1. Negative aspect: _____

   Positive aspect: _____

2. Negative aspect: _____

   Positive aspect: _____

3. Negative aspect: _____

   Positive aspect: _____

4. Negative aspect: _____

   Positive aspect: _____

5. Negative aspect: _____

   Positive aspect: _____

Program participants should be encouraged to work on improving those parts of their bodies that require attention, but not to forget those parts of their bodies about which they should feel good.

Food Association Recalling

Though some obesity is a result of physiological factors, much overweight is a consequence of overeating. As previously described, food tends to be associated with pleasant occasions. For instance, family gatherings at a Thanksgiving Day dinner, or Christmas dinner, or Passover Seder tend to be remembered as enjoyable experiences and may be subconsciously associated with food. Such an association, it is thought, can lead one to overeat as a reward; that is, the food is associated with pleasure, and one wants pleasure for something done well or to relieve some anxiety or frustration, so one eats food to provide such pleasure. To aid program participants to see food, in a conscious manner, as associated with pleasure and reward, the following activity is suggested.

Ask participants to remain seated with their eyes closed. They are instructed to imagine themselves as young as they can recall. The following directions are then recited by the health educator with pauses to allow listeners time to experience feelings long repressed:

1. What do you see? Objects? Furniture? People?
2. Look carefully at what you see. Notice shapes, sizes, colors, odors, sounds, voices.
3. Think of where you lived then. Smell it. Hear it. Observe it carefully.
4. Recall a Thanksgiving Day dinner there. Smell it. Taste it.

5. How do you feel? Are the memories pleasant? Is your mouth watering? Would you like to be there now?

A discussion should then be conducted that relates to the food associations the group possesses. Other holiday occasions associated with food should be discussed, as should everyday meals and the memories and feelings associated with them.

Healthful Eating

In addition to the sociological aspects of food and weight control concerns, health educators should be conduct experiences designed to educate people regarding the proper foods to eat. The following activities are selected for this purpose.

Food Guide Pyramid Centering (Cost and Turley 2000)

In the early 1980s Howard Gardner of Harvard University proposed a theory involving multiple intelligences — more particularly, seven different forms of intelligence. Later, Gardner added an eighth intelligence (Checkley 1997). The eight forms of intelligences hypothesized by Gardner are listed in Table 12.1 with an instructional strategy consistent with each of these forms of intelligence. Using Gardner's vision of intelligence, the health educator establishes eight learning centers, each based on one form of intelligence, that include instructional strategies for learning about the food guide pyramid. After a brief lecture about the food guide pyramid, the health educator instructs the participants to move from one learning center to another and, in 15 minutes, complete or participate in the task described at each center. In this way, program participants who learn in different ways, who have different intellectual skills, will each have a chance of success.

Food Inspectors

The health educator should be concerned with the health status of others as well as those enrolled in health education groups. One means of responding to concerns for all students or workers or patients relative to their food intake requires the appointment of "food inspectors." Program participants, after studying foods and nutrition, should be the inspectors. The function of the food inspectors should include

1. Observing food consumption and buying patterns in the cafeteria and lounges.
2. Making recommendations to appropriate personnel based on these observations.
3. Developing two handouts to be distributed to people in the cafeteria. One of these handouts will be given to people whose food tray evidences a healthful lunch and will apprise them of the healthful nature of their selection. The other should be given to those whose luncheon selections are not nutritionally balanced, and it will apprise them of that fact. Both handouts will include a description of the food pyramid (Figure 12.1).

Fighting Back/Reading Labels

For program participants to be informed decision makers regarding the foods they eat, they need to be able to read food labels. Using the food label from a breakfast cereal in Figure 12.2, show students how

TABLE 12.1

Types of Intelligence

CENTER	CHARACTERISTICS	ACTIVITY
Linguistic	This person likes to read, write, and tell stories.	Have the person create a story about the food guide pyramid.
Logical/ mathematical	This person likes to experiment, problem solve, and do math.	Have the person solve math problems related to the food guide pyramid.
Spatial	This person likes to draw, design, and create or imagine things.	Have the person draw the food guide pyramid as he or she sees it.
Musical	This person likes to sing, play instruments, and listen to music.	Have the person write a song to the tune of a nursery rhyme about the food guide pyramid.
Bodily/ kinesthetic	This person likes to move around, talk, touch things, and dance.	Have the person play a game of "food guide pyramid twister."
Interpersonal	This person likes to work with others, share ideas, and cooperate.	Have the person interview another person about eating habits.
Intrapersonal	This person likes to work alone on individual projects in his or her own space.	Have the person complete a worksheet on facts about the food guide pyramid.
Naturalist	This person likes to interact with the earth's natural resources.	Have the person draw conclusions about different types of food and their origins.

to identify important nutritional aspects of that cereal. For example, show them how to determine the average serving size, calories per serving and calories for the whole box, grams of fat and the type of fat included, grams of cholesterol, and the percentage of the daily value provided for selected vitamins and minerals and other food nutrients. In addition, the amount of ingredients relative to one another is shown on the label by listing them by content in the "ingredients" section.

Once students can read food labels, have them go to their local food markets and pretend to purchase nutritionally healthful foods for two days' meals and snacks. They should write down each food they would purchase and the nutritional rationale for that purchase. In addition, have them keep a record of foods they considered but decided not to "buy" and the reasons they steered away from those foods.

Factors other than a food's nutritional value influence food purchases. For example, how a food is packaged, where it is stored in the market, and the advertising of the food all affect how much of that food is purchased. While they are in the food market, participants should note where foods are stored (candies are usually at the eye level of children and where children can reach them), how they are

FIGURE 12.1
The Food Pyramid

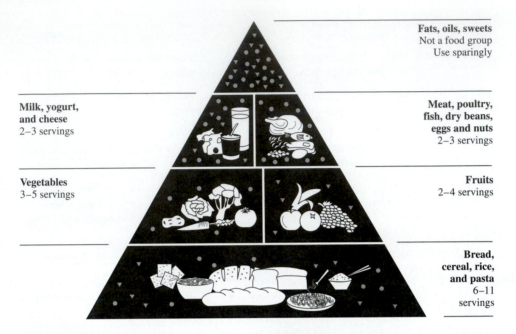

Fats, oils, sweets
Not a food group
Use sparingly

Milk, yogurt, and cheese
2–3 servings

Meat, poultry, fish, dry beans, eggs and nuts
2–3 servings

Vegetables
3–5 servings

Fruits
2–4 servings

Bread, cereal, rice, and pasta
6–11 servings

 1 cup of milk or yogurt; 1 1/2 oz. of natural cheese; 2 oz. of processed cheese
(2 to 3 servings)

 1/2 cup of chopped vegetables, cooked or raw; 1 cup of raw leafy vegetables; 3/4 cup of vegetable juice (3 to 5 servings)

 2 to 3 oz. of cooked lean meat, poultry or fish; 1/2 cup of cooked dried beans; 1 egg or 2 tbs. of peanut butter counts as 1 oz. of lean meat (2 to 3 servings)

 1 slice of bread; 1 oz. of ready-to-eat cereal; 1/2 cup of cooked cereal; 1/2 cup of rice or pasta (6 to 11 servings)

 1 medium apple, banana, or orange; 1/2 cup of chopped, cooked, or canned fruit; 3/4 cup of fruit juice (2 to 4 servings)

Source: U.S. Department of Agriculture and Department of Health and Human Services

packaged (some will be in colorful boxes, some will have sports stars on the box), and which items are on sale or discounted. They should also record which foods are near the checkout counter (these are "impulse buying" items that can catch one's attention and encourage a purchase even when that was not originally intended) and the names of the different products. The implications of these findings should be discussed in a group session.

FIGURE 12.2

The Nutrition Label

Serving Size

Is your serving the same size as the one on the label? If you eat double the serving size listed, you need to double the nutrient and calorie values. If you eat one-half the serving size shown here, cut the nutrient and calorie values in half.

Calories

Are you overweight? Cut back a little on calories! Look here to see how a serving of the food adds to your daily total. A 5'4", 138-lb. active woman needs about 2,200 calories each day. A 5'10", 174-lb. active man needs about 2,900. How about you?

Total Carbohydrate

When you cut down on fat, you can eat more carbohydrates. Carbohydrates are in foods like bread, potatoes, fruits, and vegetables. Choose these often! They give you more nutrients than sugars like soda pop and candy.

Dietary Fiber

Grandmother called it "roughage," but her advice to eat more is still up-to-date! That goes for both soluble and insoluble kinds of dietary fiber. Fruits, vegetables, whole-grain foods, beans, and peas are all good sources and can help reduce the risk of heart disease and cancer.

Protein

Most Americans get more protein than they need. Where there is animal protein, there is also fat and cholesterol. Eat small servings of lean meat, fish, and poultry. Use skim or low-fat milk, yogurt, and cheese. Try vegetable proteins like beans, grains, and cereals.

Vitamins & Minerals

Your goal here is 100% of each for the day. Don't count on one food to do it all. Let a combination of foods add up to a winning score.

Nutrition Facts
Serving Size 1/2 cup (114g)
Servings Per Container 4

Amount Per Serving

Calories 90   Calories from Fat 30

% Daily value*

Total Fat 3g	**5%**
Saturated Fat 0g	**0%**
Cholesterol 0mg	**0%**
Sodium 300mg	**13%**
Total Carbohydrate 13g	**4%**
Dietary Fiber 3g	**12%**
Sugars 3g	
Protein 3g	

Vitamin A 80%	•	Vitamin C 60%	
Calcium 4%	•	Iron 4%	

*Percent Daily Values are based on a 2,000 calorie diet. Your daily values may be higher or lower depending on your calorie needs:

		Calories	2,000	2,500
Total Fat	Less than		65g	80g
Sat Fat	Less than		20g	25g
Cholesterol	Less than		300mg	300mg
Sodium	Less than		2,400mg	2,400mg
Total Carbohydrate			300g	375g
Fiber			25g	30g

Calories per gram:
Fat 9 • Carbohydrate 4 • Protein 4

More nutrients may be listed on some labels.
Key Words: *Fat Free:* Less than 0.6 g of fat per serving: *Low Fat:* 3 g of fat or less per serving: *Lean:* Less than 10 g of fat, 4 g of saturated fat, and 96 mg. of cholesterol per serving: *Light (Lite):* 1/2 less calories or no more than 1/2 the fat of the higher-calorie, higher-fat version; or no more than 1/2 the sodium of the higher-sodium version; *Cholesterol Free:* Less than 2 mg. of cholesterol and 2 g or less of saturated fat per serving. To Make Health Claims About... The Food Must Be... Heart Disease and Fats: Low in fat, saturated fat and cholesterol; Blood Pressure and Sodium: Low in sodium; Heart Disease and Fruits, Vegetables, and Grain Products: A fruit, vegetable, or grain product low in fat, saturated fat and cholesterol, that contains at least 0.6 g soluble fiber, without fortification, per serving.

Total Fat

Aim low. Most people need to cut back on fat! Too much fat may contribute to heart disease and cancer. Try to limit your calories from fat. For a healthy heart, choose foods with a big difference between the total number of calories and the number of calories from fat.

Saturated Fat

A new kind of fat? No— saturated fat is part of the total fat in food. It is listed separately because it's the key player in raising blood cholesterol and your risk of heart disease. Eat less!

Cholesterol

Too much cholesterol—a second cousin to fat—can lead to heart disease. Challenge yourself to eat less than 300 mg each day.

Sodium

You call it "salt," the label calls it "sodium." Either way, it may add up to high blood pressure in some people. So keep your sodium intake low—2,400 to 3,000 mg or less each day.*

*The AHA recommends no more than 1,000 mg sodium per day for healthy adults.

Daily Value

Feel like you're drowning in numbers? Let the Daily Value be your guide. Daily Values are listed for people who eat 2,000 or 2,500 calories each day. If you eat more, your personal daily value may be higher than what's listed on the label. If you eat less, your personal daily value may be lower.

For fat, saturated fat, cholesterol, and sodium choose foods with low % Daily Value. For total carbohydrate, dietary fiber, vitamins and minerals, your daily value goal is to reach 100% of each.

g = grams
    (About 28 g = 1 ounce)
mg = milligrams
    (1,000 mg = 1 g)

Source: Food and Drug Administration, American Heart Association, 1993.

A trip to food markets in different neighborhoods might also be interesting. For example, program participants might find that different foods are available in communities made up of different ethnic or cultural populations, or that different products are sold at stores in communities of different socio-economic status.

Nutrition Labeling and Finagling *(Chavent 2002)*

This instructional strategy helps program participants to read food labels and use that knowledge to plan healthful diets. To begin, participants download guidelines for the listing of nutrition information on food labels. These guidelines are available from the U.S. Food and Drug Administration website (vm.cfsan.fda.gov/label.html). Participants are also taught how to calculate calories provided by the total fat, total carbohydrate, and protein per serving by multiplying the grams listed by the appropriate calories per gram (9, 4, and 4 calories, respectively). Participants are also made aware that "percentage daily value" indicates the percentage of the day's allowance for that nutrient, not the percentage of nutrient in a serving of food. Participants then analyze labels from food products they were instructed to bring in. Comparisons between foods used for comparable purposes are computed. For example, an analysis might be made between drinking orange juice or a soft drink when thirsty. Participants then develop a healthful, balanced diet that contains foods providing the percentage daily value of various nutrients. Participants can judge each other's diets based on the following criteria:

- Is the diet appealing?
- Do ingredients listed in descending order reflect sources of protein, fat, and carbohydrate?
- Are there sources of wholesome carbohydrates including whole grains, fruits, vegetables, or nonfat dairy ingredients?
- Is there at least one ingredient that is a good source of iron, calcium, vitamin C, or vitamin A?
- Is the percent of calories from fat per serving no more than 30 percent of the total calories per serving?

Eat Well Day

After the food inspectors have been functional for a while, an "eat well day" should be organized. If the eat well day was scheduled for a Friday, Monday through Thursday could be devoted to public address announcements and posters pertaining to the event and healthful eating practices. During the day, the food inspectors should be available in places where foods are purchased to remind people of the day and to help them select a balanced meal. The inspectors should be cautioned, however, not to coerce anyone to adopt good eating habits, but rather to attempt to educate people about such habits while they are choosing foods for lunch.

Food Investigating

There are other ways in which health educators and the participants enrolled in their programs can respond to nutritional needs:

1. Participants can be stationed by the cafeteria cash registers to record the lunches purchased. An analysis of the food bought can lead to recommendations relative to nutrition education needs and activities.

2. A sifting through food purchase requisitions completed by the food services director can aid participants in recognizing balanced meals, as well as the types of foods most preferred by the school, hospital, or worksite population.

3. An investigation of the refill needs of any food vending machines will tend to indicate the snack consumption habits of the population. (I refer to vending machines containing such things as milk, juice, apples, candy, soft drinks, or hot foods.)

These three activities will provide a picture of people's eating habits from which an educational program can be formulated. In this manner, nutritional activities will be particular to the needs of the population, rather than general in nature.

Selecting Lunch

Because the food services director must select foods to compose the cafeteria lunches sometime and somewhere, why not in the health education class with the aid of participants? An activity of this nature would allow the group to observe a dietitian on the job, as well as provide the dietitian with feedback on student or employee food likes and dislikes. The use of an overhead projector is recommended so that everyone can see the lunches as they develop.

Restauranting

The school, hospital, or place of work is not the only environment outside the home in which people select foods to eat. Restaurants nearby can provide menus that the group can use to practice selecting balanced meals. Restaurateurs can be interviewed, in class or at their establishments, relative to purchase orders. These purchase orders will indicate which foods are most often selected by the restaurant's clientele, since those foods will be the most often recorded. A comparison of any available data on differences in food selection for different meals (breakfast, lunch, and dinner) would also be valuable. In addition, whether the restaurant serves heart-healthy meals and marks them as such on the menu can be noted.

Infant's Letter

It has been said somewhere that one doesn't really learn a subject until one is required to teach it. To learn the role of nutrients in the body and the composition of a nutritionally balanced diet, participants can pretend to be teachers of newborn babies. Rather than educate these babies personally, however, letters should be composed. These letters should specify which foods the baby should refrain from eating, and a schedule of approximate weight and height increases the baby should experience. The information included should be scientifically accurate, so the letter necessitates some research.

Several uses can be made of this letter once it has been composed and its content validated as factual:

1. Copies can be mailed to local pediatricians and obstetricians in sufficient quantity for them to distribute to parents, or soon-to-be parents, of newborn infants.

2. Copies can be mailed to local hospitals and health clinics for distribution to parents of newborn babies.

3. Copies can be sent to homes of schoolchildren who indicate they have a new brother or sister.

4. Local newspapers can be asked to publish the letter in their letters-to-the-editor or health-related section.

Food Coaching

The use of sport to promote the study of nutrition seems worthwhile. One means of utilizing sport in this fashion is to develop a diet for athletes of a strenuous sport, such as track or basketball. The diet should relate to two particular time phases: everyday meals, and meals and snacks directly (several hours) before athletic competition. That protein is necessary for growth and repair of tissue and that carbohydrates are needed for energy are examples of considerations necessary for devising a nutritionally sound diet. Previous study of foods and nutrition will be necessary to develop appropriate diets.

After these diets have been composed, a panel of school, college, and/or professional coaches should present their views on athletic diets to the group, against which the participants will validate the diets they've developed. It should be mentioned that many coaches have misconceptions about nutrition. For example, some coaches still believe that athletes should eat a steak before a strenuously competitive event, although it is known that the consumption of carbohydrates approximately four hours before such an activity is more beneficial. However, even though some of the panel may present errors of fact, that in itself can be used to show how pervasive misconceptions about nutrition are, and to demonstrate the need for more research in the area.

Malnutrition Epidemic

Still another means of motivating and educating people about nutrition employs dramatization. The following handout should be distributed.

Attention

This notice is to announce a serious health problem in Fantasyland. It has been determined that there exists a *malnutrition epidemic* in our kingdom. Such signs and symptoms as the following have appeared:

1. Bleeding, weak gums and loose teeth.
2. Crooked, soft, and weak bones.
3. A lack of energy.
4. An excessively long time for tissue damage to repair.
5. A lack of usual growth.
6. Anemia.
7. Neurological disturbances.

This communiqué is asking for you to help save your homeland by suggesting to our Chancellor of Health remedies for this epidemic. Please write the Chancellor immediately.

Each person is then asked to write to Fantasyland's Chancellor of Health with recommendations for responding to the epidemic. The nutritional deficiencies represented by the signs and symptoms in the handout are listed here and numbered to correspond with the numbering in the handout:

1. Vitamin C deficiency.
2. Vitamin D deficiency.
3. Carbohydrate deficiency.
4. Protein deficiency.
5. Mineral deficiency (in particular, selenium, molybdenum, zinc, and chlorine) and protein deficiency.

6. Iron deficiency.

7. Vitamin B$_1$ deficiency.

Students should recommend to the Chancellor of Health a program that specifies

Step 1: The deficiencies evidenced by the signs and symptoms.

Step 2: The foods that can relieve these deficiencies.

Step 3: A description, in detail, of the educational program that the Fantasyland government should finance and conduct to get the kingdom's population to eat the foods identified in step 2.

Eating Disorders/Disordered Eating: A Self-Analysis

Anorexia nervosa and bulimia are two well-known eating disorders. It is estimated there are 1 million teenagers (not to mention adults) with an eating disorder, 90 percent of whom are female. Anorexia nervosa is a condition in which weight and dieting consume almost all of the person's time and thought. The anorexic seeks total control over her eating, such that more and more weight is lost until her health and even her life may be threatened. On the other hand, the bulimic binges on food only to purge afterward (by vomiting or use of a laxative). The questions that follow can be used as self-analysis to uncover an eating disorder. People with eating disorders will respond with a "yes" to most questions.

1. Do you prefer to eat alone?

2. Are you terrified of being overweight?

3. Do you constantly think about food?

4. Do you "binge" (overeat drastically) occasionally?

5. Are you highly knowledgeable about the calorie content of all the foods you eat?

6. Do you always feel "stuffed" after meals?

7. Are you constantly weighing yourself?

8. Do you eat a lot of "diet" foods?

9. Do you overexercise to burn all the calories you eat?

10. Do you take a long time to eat meals?

11. Are you frequently constipated?

12. Do you feel guilty when you eat sweet or fattening foods?

13. Do you feel the urge to throw up after eating?

14. Do you feel your life is controlled by food and eating?

If program participants respond "yes" to most of these questions, encourage them to seek professional help with their eating disorder.

Valuing Activities

As in other health content areas, values play a major role in determining nutritional behavior. In this section, several instructional strategies designed to help people identify and clarify their values related to choice of foods and nutritional habits are described. Osman (1973) has presented an excellent rationale for the inclusion of valuing activities in nutrition education:

Nutrition educators have done a commendable job in sorting out the reliable research and transmitting that information to their students. Some nutrition educators erroneously believe that since they have presented the facts of nutrition (especially if they have presented controversial points of view) they have fulfilled their didactic duties.

One of the ultimate objectives of education is to be able to make intelligent decisions based upon the best knowledge available, to live in congruence with what a person knows. Syllogistic reasoning would suggest that those who know the most should behave the best. Yet the world is filled with persons who know much better than they do. The overweight dietitian knows that excessive weight is harmful to her health but she still leads a hypokinetic-high-calorie life. Such behavior could hardly be described as "rational" or "intelligent" or as the kind of behavior that characterizes truly educated people. Perhaps knowledge is not as simplistically related to attitudes and behavior as educators once thought. We need to go beyond just disseminating knowledge. Even the Basic Four and conceptual approaches have recently been criticized as being "inadequate to accomplish the desired results in nutrition education."

Facts and concepts can still leave students cold; they seem abstract and impersonal. What is needed is a personal "you-centered" approach based, in part, on the here and now of reality. The scientific approach needs to be tempered with a values-level application of the specific facts and general concepts. The values level is characterized by lifting and transforming both information and concepts to a personal "you-centered" level. This level adds meaning and relevancy to the facts, thereby increasing the possibility of their application to the student's life.

We need to assist students in clarifying what all the content and concepts mean to them at that point in their lives. As [the accompanying] figure suggests, facts and concepts provide a base for effective thinking, but it is our values, in the final analysis, that ultimately determine our behavior. In short, facts are needed to inform our values.

Values are like stars that guide our lives. Some people freely choose to follow certain values, others choose different (life patterns) that have meaning for their lives at that point in time.

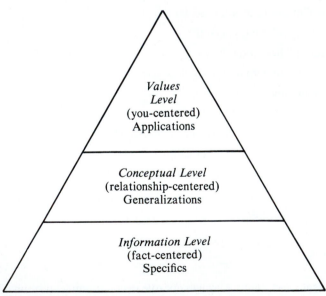

From Jack Osman, "Teaching Nutrition with a Focus on Values" in *Nutrition News,* April 1973, vol. 36 no. 2. Courtesy of National Dairy Council®.

Students should be educated as to the alternative nutritional values open to them. Students need to choose freely those nutritional values which have meaning for them at that point in their lives. Some educators, however, feel that the only values worth mentioning in a classroom are the ones that can be stamped in, indoctrinated, moralized, inculcated, or rammed down kids' throats.

Often in life, things (situations, circumstances, problems, conflicts) obfuscate or cloud our vision of the choices open to us. We can no longer see clearly those values that guide our lives. At times like this we need someone to blow away the clouds. Instead of teaching his own values, the teacher should assist students in the process of seeing and following their own values.

Values Grid

One variation of the values grid presented in Chapter 7 concerns itself with opinions and values choices and can be applied to nutrition. From responses of participants on the following grid, discussions can branch off to such varied topics as how to shop wisely (both nutritionally and financially), how all

	Strongly Agree	Agree	Disagree	Strongly Disagree
Generally, people eat nutritionally balanced meals.				
Generally, people feel that health foods are reasonably priced.				
Most people are well familiarized with the government's food stamp program.				
People generally spend too much money on food.				
People are generally frustrated trying to be treated fairly in the marketplace.				
People generally appreciate the foods prepared for them by their schools or work-sites in terms of their nutritional quality.				
People generally recognize the value of milk and drink several glasses each day.				
Most people take advantage of unit pricing in their shopping practices.				
People generally have very little problem judging the validity of advertisements for foods.				
People generally rely on the government to protect their foods.				

family members can be involved in food selection and meal preparation, and the merits of arguments presented by health food advocates.

Ask participants to mark an X to the right of each statement in the box that best expresses their opinion. After everyone has done this, organize small-group discussions about the topics of *how* each participant responded to the statements and the *reasoning process* used to arrive at that response.

Values Ranking

Asking participants to rank order their preferences related to nutrition will help them to identify values of which they may not have been aware. Below appear several groupings that can be employed in this exercise.

1. Taste	1. Meat	1. Pizza
2. Texture	2. Fish	2. Hamburger
3. Color	3. Poultry	3. Welsh rabbit
1. To be strong	1. Oranges	1. Eggs
2. To be slim	2. Potato chips	2. Milk
3. To be alert	3. Yogurt	3. Liver

Values List

Another valuing activity that can confront program participants with discrepancies between what they know is good for them and how they act is the values list. In this exercise people are asked to list the 20 foods they eat most often. After they have listed these foods, recite the following instructions:

1. Place the letter *T* next to those foods that are good for your teeth, and the letter *B* next to those foods harmful to your teeth.
2. Place the letter *C* next to those foods that are good for your circulatory system and heart, and the letter *N* next to those foods that are not.
3. Place the letter *H* next to those foods that are generally healthful, and the letters *NH* next to those that are not.
4. Place the letter *Y* next to those five foods that you eat most often.
5. Place the letter *L* next to those five foods that you like the most.
6. Using only the foods on your list, compose three well-balanced meals — breakfast, lunch, and dinner.

Then read and discuss the following questions:

1. Do you most often eat the foods that are healthful for you, or those that are not?
2. Are all of the nutrients included in your diet or are some missing?
3. Which foods not on your list of 20 do you think you should add?
4. Which foods on your list do you think you should eliminate?
5. How else might we analyze your list?

Values Voting

A more direct manner of ascertaining participants' values related to foods is to ask them to vote *yes, no,* or *maybe* on statements that indicate these values. Discussion regarding why they voted as they did should then be conducted. Here are some value statements related to nutrition:

1. In order to have children, people should have to pass a test demonstrating their knowledge of nutrition.
2. Everyone should refrain from eating meats, fish, and poultry and become vegetarians.
3. Foods sold at supermarkets should not be allowed to contain such harmful products as additives.
4. Everyone should supplement his or her diet with vitamin tablets.
5. Schools should not be allowed to have vending machines that sell such foods as soft drinks or candy.
6. Health education should have nutrition as a required part.

Another means of values voting requires participants to complete the following handout:

How important are the following factors to you regarding the store in which you buy your food?

Factor	Very Important	Marginally Important	Not Important
Price			
Product name			
Unit price label			
Personality of employees			
Advertising			
Bright lighting			
Coupons given			
Number of other shoppers			

Values Questions

Questions and discussion of responses to them can be a very effective way of identifying and clarifying values. Some questions that can be used for this purpose are given here:

1. Do people in your family eat together? If so, which meals?
2. If people eat together in your family, does age affect whether they eat together? For example, do teenagers or the family breadwinner not join the others?

3. Which meals does your family usually enjoy the most? Why these meals?

4. Which stores do family members shop in? Why these stores rather than some others?

5. Do family members snack? If so, what foods do they most enjoy for snacks? Why these foods?

6. Have any of the stores in which you shop for food done anything to educate you regarding the most healthful foods to purchase? What have they done? Has it changed your buying habits?

7. Do you think food coupons affect the way people purchase food? How? Do they affect your food buying habits? How?

8. Do you know what you should be eating? Do you eat these foods? In the right quantities? Do others in your family?

9. Have you tried to educate other family members about nutrition? Why or why not? Has it been effective?

10. At which restaurants do you most enjoy eating? What is it about these restaurants that you like so much?

11. What have you eaten today? Were your choices healthful? Were they satisfying?

Summary

Nutrition education need not be dull and tedious. The activities presented in this chapter are motivating and educationally sound. These activities, through their requirement for participants to be actively involved in their conduct, can result in greater learning and increased interest in foods and nutrition. It is believed that such learning and interest will result in improved nutritional behavior by people who have participated in these learning experiences.

CHAPTER THIRTEEN

Instructional Strategies for Aging, Spirituality, and Death

This chapter concerns itself with aging, spirituality, and death education. Instructional strategies that can help program participants appreciate and better the life of the elderly, that can help them better manage their own elderly lives, and that can confront them with their own mortality are presented. These topics—aging, spirituality, and death—are often taught together and are therefore presented here together. However, it should be realized that even the very young need to concern themselves with death. Their pets die, their older relatives die, and their schoolmates sometimes die. As we get older, our experience with death becomes more pervasive, but all age groups can be helped to better their lives by appreciating their mortality.

The Aged and Aging

Certainly one aspect of health education must be the study of the aged and the aging process. Since the nature of life is the content of health education, to neglect the latter stages of life is to do a disservice to those engaged in the study—namely program participants. In addition, the study of the aged and of the aging process will lead program participants to insights into their own lives through understanding the aged's disappointments, joys, feelings about things left undone, accomplishments of which they are proud, and so on. To help in this study, the following activities are suggested.

Aged Visitors

One means of studying the aged is to talk with them. A valuable, touching, and enjoyable experience is to invite to class, and spend a session or two with, several elderly people. The visitors can be residents of a nursing home, members of a golden-age club, or relatives of people in the group. Questions and topics for discussion should be developed by the participants prior to the visitors' arrival and screened by a representative for the invited guests to ensure that the aged will appreciate the items proposed. For instance, questions pertaining to the imminence of death for the aged and questions related to feelings about dying might be very much out of place for some groups and perfectly acceptable to others.

The experience of such visits will serve both the participants and the aged well. The group will develop a greater appreciation of life by viewing it from "the other end," and the aged will be brought closer to life by socializing with others and contributing to their education.

Adoptions

As a follow-up to group sessions in which the aged visit — or as a separate activity altogether — participants can "adopt" an aged person. This adoption, of course, is not of a legal or binding nature but represents a commitment on the part of the participant to visit with the elderly person, keep that person in touch with the world, invite the adopted one to his or her home for a visit, and so on. Obviously, the advantages of this activity are similar to those already delineated, with the added opportunity for closer contact and a more intimate relationship.

Phone Pal

Like having a pen pal with whom one exchanges letters on a periodic basis, participants can choose phone pals. Phone pals should be residents of a nursing home or retirement home to whom participants make telephone calls. Such calls should be devoted to establishing a relationship between the participant and the aged to improve the understanding of life for each. Several steps should be followed to set up the phone pal activity:

Step 1:   The health educator should ask administrators of local nursing and retirement homes whether they would cooperate in such an activity.

Step 2:   Those administrators approving of the project should identify certain of the aged as prospective phone pals.

Step 3:   The prospective phone pals should be approached by the appropriate nursing home staff member to solicit their participation.

Step 4:   Participants should select a phone pal from a list of the aged willing to participate.

Step 5:   Participants should telephone the nursing home and arrange for personal visits with their phone pals.

Step 6:   During the visit the phone pals should decide the time of day and days of the week (two or three) when the telephone calls should be placed. During these visits, telephone numbers of the phone pals should be exchanged.

Step 7:   The activity is then conducted until one or both of the callers decide it should be abandoned. The disengagement of pals should be conducted with the prior knowledge of the health educator to allow him or her some input into the process. In this manner, a sense of rejection on the part of the elderly may be avoided.

Visits

Either elderly people can be asked to visit the group, or the group can visit the elderly. Such visits might consist of a walk, talk, or other informal activity. However, more planned activities can be arranged, such as the performing of skits, the organization of arts and crafts sessions, or the sharing of gifts made by program participants.

Sensory Deprivation Simulation Exercises

The activities that follow are designed to bring to the young and healthy a sensitivity to what it might be like to be old and suffering from some common sensory deficits reported by the elderly (Briggs 1977):

Although this photograph depicts a young girl, all program participants, regardless of age, can learn a great deal about aging and the aged by serving as phone pals. Of course the questions asked and the objectives of this instructional strategy will vary depending on the age and other characteristics of the learners.

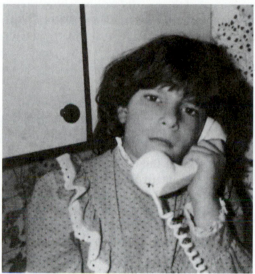

Source: Jerrold S. Greenberg

Arthritis (reported by 33 out of 100 elderly): Using cellophane tape, tape participants' fingers together in various combinations; for example, tape the thumb and index finger together and the fourth and fifth fingers together. Wrap elastic bandages around the knees to simulate stiff knees. Have participants perform simple tasks and then share their experiences of what it might be like to be old and have arthritis.

Visual handicaps (reported by 15 out of 100 elderly): Take sunglasses or laboratory protective glasses and smear Vaseline on them until you simulate visual loss. Have participants wear the glasses and perform simple tasks such as reading a menu or a newspaper or locating the phone number of a pharmacy (if there is one) that will deliver prescriptions to the elderly. Have them record and share their reactions.

Hearing loss (reported by 22 out of 100 elderly): Place a cotton ball in the participants' exterior ear canals. For a more pronounced effect, have them also wear headphones or earmuffs. Have them listen to the TV or radio at a low level, or try to carry on a conversation with someone who has no hearing loss and must shout at them to be heard. Again, have them share their feelings.

This article is reprinted with permission from *Health Education,* September/October, 1977, 37–38. *Health Education* is a publication of the American Alliance for Health, Physical Education, Recreation and Dance, 1900 Association Drive, Reston, VA 22091.

Loss of touch: Cover the participants' fingers with rubber cement and, after it dries, have them try to thread a needle.

Loss of smell: Have participants taste various foods while pinching their nostrils shut.

Multiplicity (polymorbidity): Many elderly people suffer from several aging insults. They may have hearing loss, arthritis, and visual handicaps. To help participants understand multiplicity and what it might be like, have several of them perform tasks with various combinations of the earlier simulations. For example, one person can simulate finger arthritis, visual loss, and loss of touch and smell, then go to the cafeteria and buy a carton of milk. Upon returning, have the person share some of his or her feelings during the experience as an older person with sensory deprivation. Be sure to exercise necessary safety precautions when participants perform such simulations.

Keeping the Elderly Active

Ask participants to answer fully the following question about a parent, grandparent, or other elderly person: Does this elderly person regularly, occasionally, or never engage in each of the following activities?

Going grocery shopping	Reading newspapers
Going to the beauty shop or barber	Reading books or magazines
Attending movies or concerts	Sewing or gardening
Participating in clubs	Painting, sculpting, working with wood
Attending sports events	Listening to or playing music
Visiting	Watching television
Telephoning or writing to friends	Walking or exercising
Engaging in religious activities	Doing volunteer work
Cooking	

Collect, compile, and analyze responses. Give the participants an idea of the range of activities among older people. Hold a discussion of people's reactions to older people. Suggest ways in which participants can help enlarge the range of activities of older people.

Eldercize

The Andean village of Vilcabamba in Ecuador and the community of Abkhagia in Georgia share an unusual reputation. They are places where people supposedly live longer and remain more vigorous in old age than is the case in most places. What factors contribute to the unusual longevity of people in these communities, where men and women who are well beyond 100 years of age are common? Clearly genetics play a role, as do nutrition and several other factors. One of these is physical activity. These communities are located in remote and mountainous regions and tend to be agricultural. That means daily living requires significant climbing and descending steep slopes and vigorous activity.

There is a lesson to be learned here. Our country's elders don't hike to get where they want to go. Rather, they take a bus or drive their cars. They don't tend the fields, but rather water their potted plants. They tend to be far less active than the centenarians just described. To remedy this situation, the health educator can organize exercise programs for elders. Table 13.1 presents recommended physical activities accompanied by frequency and duration guidelines. Remember, though, the importance of a brief warmup and cooldown when engaging in physical activities.

The elderly can, and should be encouraged to, maintain an active lifestyle. Regular exercise, including stretching, is important in preparation for such a lifestyle.

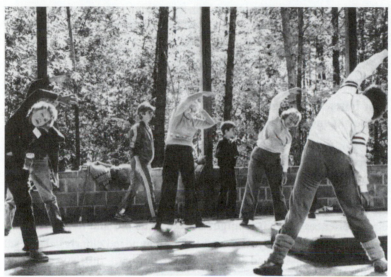

Source: Daniel Leviton

TABLE 13.1
Good Physical Activities for the Elderly*

ACTIVITY	HOW OFTEN	DURATION
Walking	3 times per week	¾ hour
Swimming	3 times per week	½ hour
Dancing	2 times per week	Sets of 20 minutes with intervals of rest
Stretching/calisthenics	Every day	10–15 minutes
Golf	2 or 3 times per week	As long as necessary to complete 9 or 18 holes
Horseshoe pitching	According to desire	½ hour
Shuffleboard	According to desire	1 hour
Bocce	According to desire	1 hour
Croquet	According to desire	1 hour

From Jerrold S. Greenberg, George B. Dintiman, and Barbee Myers Oakes. *Physical Fitness and Wellness,* 2nd ed. Boston, MA: Allyn and Bacon, 1998, p. 385. Reprinted by permission.

Elderly Myths

This activity is designed to explore the many myths that surround the elderly and life during the later years. The health educator should distribute copies of the following questionnaire.

Instructions: Place a *T* to the left of each of the statements here that you believe to be true, and an *F* next to each you believe to be false.

_____ 1. Over 20 percent of Americans over 80 years old live in institutions.

_____ 2. The majority of the elderly have serious health problems.

_____ 3. Not having enough money is a problem for the elderly.

_____ 4. Poor housing is a problem for the elderly.

_____ 5. Insufficient medical care is a problem for the elderly.

_____ 6. Loneliness is a problem for the elderly.

_____ 7. The elderly are not very interested in sex.

_____ 8. The focus of the elderly on the past is unhealthy.

_____ 9. Older people are generally not efficient at work and should retire.

_____ 10. Older workers are absent from the job more often than younger workers.

Program participants are instructed to administer the questionnaire to people they know and to bring completed questionnaires to the next health education session. Then the total average number of *True* and *False* responses for each item should be calculated. Since all 10 of the items on the questionnaire represent untruths (myths) about the elderly, the group will get insight into the view most people have regarding old age—that is, stereotypes that are unfounded. If there are sufficient numbers of participants (approximately 75), the belief in stereotypes regarding the elderly can be computed by age, gender, ethnicity, years of education, and marital status of the respondents.

Elder Interviews

Another way to help students dispel myths about the lives of the elderly and, in particular, what their lives were like years ago, is to have them conduct interviews. Instruct program participants to arrange to interview an elderly person—a relative, a friend, or a neighbor. Interviews can be audiotape recorded or videotaped if students want to preserve them. This might be the case if the interviewee is a relative or someone dear to them. Several questions that might be asked are listed here, but students should be encouraged to add to this list according to their interests:

1. What restrictions were placed on you by your parents and at what age were these restrictions removed?

2. At what age did you first date? What did you usually do on dates? Where did you go? How did you get there? When were you expected to return?

3. What was the first job you had that earned you money? Was it difficult to get this job? How much did you earn?

4. How did you get around? How old were you when you first drove an automobile?

5. What were the world wars like? What did you do during the wars? What did your relatives and friends do?

6. What did you do for recreation? Did you participate in sports? Did you go to the movies?

7. What were the media like when you were growing up? The radio? The newspapers and magazines? When did you first watch television? When did you first own a television set?

8. Who were the celebrities during your youth? Show business celebrities? Sports stars? Politicians?

9. What was considered outrageous during your early years?

10. When did you first fall in love? How did you manifest your love? What did your family think about the person you married? What was important in choosing a marital partner?

Retirement Brainstorming

Retirement has both advantages and disadvantages. This learning activity will help participants better appreciate this fact. The instructor should tape two sheets of newsprint to the wall, one titled "Advantages of Retirement" and the other "Disadvantages of Retirement." Participants are then called on in alphabetical order and must give an advantage and a disadvantage of retirement that has not been given before. If someone can't think of a new one, that person is disqualified, and the next is called on. The last person to be able to add to the list is the winner. The instructor should review the list after the activity is over to summarize what the group saw as advantages and disadvantages of retirement. A discussion should then ensue regarding participants' feelings about retirement. For example, are they looking forward to it or apprehensive about it? Are they planning for their retirement? Could they plan for it better? Add other discussion questions to help participants make more sense out of their potential retirement or that of someone close to them.

Spiritual Health

As one ages, the desire to feel connected to those who came before and those who will follow, either through a belief in a supreme being or a reverence of nature, becomes more prominent. Younger people also are concerned with spirituality as they try to relate to their environment and those within it. The instructional activities in this section confront the issue of spiritual health in a manner that activates program participants.

The Spiritual Scavenger Hunt (Wood and Holander (2002)

The health educator starts this activity by describing constructs related to spiritual health, including connectedness, meaning and purpose in life, sacrifice for others, joy for living, and love. Then the spiritual scavenger hunt worksheet is distributed to program participants (see Table 13.2). Participants are instructed to mingle with other participants for 20 minutes and place the initials, in the appropriate boxes on the handout, of those they meet who can be described by that box's description. Once participants have obtained as many initials as they can, begin with the first box on the matrix and inquire how this statement pertains to spirituality. Move through each statement in the matrix explaining how each is related to spirituality.

Spiritual Sloganing (Wood and Hollander 2002)

Spiritual sloganing can be used as a concluding activity in spirituality health education. Program participants are asked to develop a slogan that represents their concept of spiritual health. The slogan must

TABLE 13.2
Spiritual Scavenger Hunt Worksheet

SPIRITUAL SCAVENGER HUNT				
Has seen a ghost	Practices meditation	Smiled at a stranger today	Told someone "I love you" today	Attended a religious service over the past week
Has turned to a higher power for support	Spent time communing with nature over the last week	Has forgiven someone over the past week	Believes spirituality can be used to treat illness	Knows who Albert Schweitzer is
Has taken steps to simplify his/her life recently	Has spent time with family/or close friends recently	Has experienced a miracle	Spends time in self-reflection	Has read a book about spirituality
Has committed an act of random kindness recently	Recently experienced a loss	Knows who Mahatma Ghandi is	Has had a near-death experience	Has challenged himself/herself recently

meet the following criteria: (1) It must be short enough to fit on the front of a T-shirt. (2) It must represent their current feelings and beliefs about spiritual health. Participants write their slogans on index cards and then pass their slogans to the participant on their right. Slogans keep being passed until they are returned to their authors. As participants read others' slogans, they are to record any that are particularly meaningful to them, as well as any common themes they can identify. A group discussion is then conducted to summarize what has been learned about spirituality and spiritual health. Table 13.3 lists slogans one health educator's group members created.

Spiritual Drawings

An alternative instructional strategy to spiritual sloganing is spiritual drawings. In this activity, instead of developing a slogan, program participants draw pictures of constructs related to spirituality or spiritual health. Some participants might draw a picture of a family, others of a religious activity, and still others of a nature scene. The pictures are passed to the participants to the right until they are returned to their artists. As participants receive and analyze each drawing, they write their impressions on the back of the drawing. When the artist has his or her drawing returned, the comments on the back are read. The group then discusses the reactions of others to their drawings and the congruence of these comments to what the artists intended to express. The health educator lists the various expressions of spirituality and spiritual health that artists sought to express as a summary of how these constructs can be and are conceptualized by different people.

TABLE 13.3
Previous Student Slogans

A Rainbow of Spiritual Guidance

Biggie Size Your Spirituality

Count Your Blessings—Not Your Money

Love Is All You Need

Love Is Letting Go of Fear

Lead the Children

Have Faith

A Recipe for Life—God, Love, Purpose, and Hope

We Are All People United by One God, Regardless of What We Call Him

Forgive and Forget

Together We All Achieve

Blessed and Beyond

Looking Back on Hurt to Move Ahead in Healing for Life

Spirituality Is in Everyone

Find Your Own Way

God First

Searching for a Better Tomorrow

LIFE: Bigger Than All of Us—As Small as Each of Us

Health Is in Your Spirit

Spring Into Health: Forgiveness, Recreation, Love, and Team Spirit

Do You Have S.O.U.L.: Spirit Overrules Your Life

Know Who You Are, Accept Who You Are, and Be Happy

Share, Care, and Spread Spirituality Everywhere

Choose Your Battles

Body, Mind, and Soul—Make a Person Whole

Your Spirit Leads You; Without a Strong Leader, How Can Health Follow?

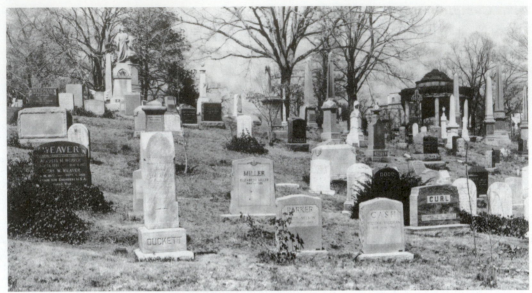

Source: The Diamondback, University of Maryland

Death and Dying

An educational setting is a unique environment, in which people are brought together to learn. It seems reasonable to assume that by the act of forming these people into a group for learning, something is planned that could not be offered to them individually at their home. What better reason for gathering people together than to provide an environment conducive to their interaction? And what better topic to talk about than something that is interesting, perplexing, confusing, and upsetting, that has been suppressed and repressed all our lives? Such a topic is death.

Seldom are people provided the opportunity to vent feelings about death. Parents don't initiate such discussions, and in fact shy away from answering children's questions about death. Cartoon programs on television depict death in a bizarre manner. "Heroes and villains alike are shot with rifles, crushed by gigantic boulders, blown to pieces by dynamite, bombarded with cannon balls, and pushed off cliffs, only to jump to their feet (after the laughter stops) to be killed again" (Dumont and Foss 1972, 35). Even hospitals segregate their morgue from the eyes of the public and patients, isolate dying patients (even though some research findings indicate that dying patients are better able to cope with their status if in contact with others not in such a condition), and often prohibit staff from referring to ward-mates who have died.

With a realization that death is a subject not responded to anywhere in our society, though present in our mental functioning at all times, it seems appropriate for health educators to organize activities that result in a study of death and dying and that allow for the venting of feelings regarding one's own death. The instructional activities that follow are designed to help the health educator with this responsibility.

Musical Perspectives on Death (*Fetro 2001*)

There are many different perspectives on death, and program participants can be helped to realize that by participating in the "musical perspective on death" instructional strategy. Participants are asked to

TABLE 13.4
Self-Assessment of Perspectives on Death and Dying

Think about your personal perspective on death and dying. Indicate what percentage of your personal perspective relates to each of the five perspectives on death and dying. Note: The sum of the five perspectives should equal 100%.

Ecological	_____
Humanistic	_____
Religious	_____
Reincarnation	_____
Life after life	_____
Total	100%

write their definitions of death. Some may see death as an end, others as a beginning. Some may see it as a transformation from one form to another. The health educator then states that there is no one definition of or perspective on death, and people's experiences lead them to their own definitions and perspectives. Participants then discuss what experiences led them to their perspectives. The health educator next distributes Table 13.4 and clarifies each perspective listed on the handout, starting with a musical selection. The following musical selections can be used:

- Ecological perspective: "Where Have All the Flowers Gone," Kingston Trio; "Dust in the Wind," Kansas).
- Humanistic perspective: "The Rose," Bette Midler; "Memories," Barbra Streisand.
- Religious perspective: "Turn, Turn, Turn," The Byrds; "Amazing Grace," Judy Collins.
- Reincarnation perspective: "Galileo," Indigo Girls; "And When I Die," Blood, Sweat, and Tears.
- Life after life perspective: "Everybody's Talking," Harry Nilsson; "Coming Out of the Dark," Gloria Estefan.

Participants identify the degree to which they ascribe to these various perspectives, and the health educator collects and tabulates the group perspective in Table 13.5.

Run for Your Life

A television series titled *Run for Your Life* had as its theme the predicted near-death of its star character. This character was told at the series outset that he had a terminal illness and had a year or two of life remaining. He decided to cram a lifetime of adventure into his two remaining years, and the show followed its star about the world as he sped around tracks with his racing car, made deep-sea dives and sky dives, and fell repeatedly in love.

Using a similar theme, participants can be asked to role-play being placed in a like position: being told that they are terminally ill. Once placed in that role, they are asked to describe how they would spend their time. An analysis of these descriptions might involve the following queries:

TABLE 13.5
Summary of Personal Perspectives on Death and Dying

PERSPECTIVE ON DEATH AND DYING					
	Ecological	Humanistic	Religious	Rein-carnation	Life after Life
Mean Score for Each Perspective					
Dominant Perspective					
Number indicating 100% of One Perspective					
Number Indicating 0% on One or More Perspectives					

1. At what places did you choose to spend your time? Why there?
2. With whom did you choose to spend your time? Why?
3. Whom did you exclude from spending time with that you usually do? Why?
4. What did you spend your time doing? Why? Do you *presently* spend your time in this way?
5. What can be concluded from these answers to the questions?

The results of this activity will evidence two factors in particular: (1) people differ in their values, as indicated by the priorities they set for their most precious commodity, time; and (2) some people tend to spend a significant amount of their time doing the things they feel are important, at places enjoyable to them, with people with whom they like to spend time—whereas others do not. With this activity, the threat of death can be used as a positive force to make more sense out of life.

Death Completions

To allow people the opportunity to show their feelings about death, they can be asked to complete the following sentences, which will then be discussed in small groups:

1. Death is _____.
2. I would like to die at _____.
3. I don't want to live past _____.
4. I would like to have at my bedside when I die _____.
5. When I die, I will be proud that when I was living I _____.
6. My greatest fear about death is _____.
7. When I die, I'll be glad that when I was living I didn't _____.
8. If I were to die today, my biggest regret would be _____.

9. When I die, I will be glad to get away from _____.

10. When I die, I want people to say _____.

Possessions

It has often been said that one's view of death determines how one lives. Those believing in life after death, for instance, can be expected to live in such a way as to improve their likelihood of a good afterlife. Those not believing in life after death might behave hedonistically, to get pleasure out of life now rather than to postpone a great deal of pleasure for a later existence. One aspect of death sometimes neglected by health educators relates to life's possessions. Possessions, and what one decides to do with these upon one's death, can reveal much about one's life. To investigate this relationship, ask the group to respond to the following questions:

1. Which 10 things that you own do you most cherish?

2. Why are these so dear to you?

3. Which of these do you expect to own 20 years from now?

4. Which of these have you already owned for several (two) years?

5. Which *three* of the possessions you cited are most cherished by you? Why?

6. What do you want to happen to these 10 possessions when you die?

This activity will require participants to reevaluate the importance of things they own and how they behave regarding these items. For example, do they treat others' possessions casually, while expecting their own possessions to be handled with care? Are they more concerned with things than with people? The answers to these questions and others can be used by participants to draw conclusions about how they behave and how they would like to behave—which can then be integrated into their patterns of living.

Living Will

A living will is a contract between a dying person on the one hand, and his or her loved ones and physicians on the other. This will requests that no heroic life-sustaining attempts be made to endlessly prolong one's life, but rather that one be allowed to die with dignity and in peace when the time comes. The development of a living will is a procedure in which participants can be asked to participate. As a result of this experience, they will have developed greater insight into the question of when one should be allowed to die. The right-to-life and right-to-die argument will inevitably enter into a discussion accompanying the development of the living will. Such questions as the following should be considered:

1. How expensive is it to use life-sustaining technology to prolong the life of a hopelessly ill patient? Who pays for these procedures?

2. Who should determine when to "pull the plug"?

3. Is such a contract legally binding?

4. Does a person have the right to die if he or she so chooses? If yes, then should suicide be permitted?

Last Will

As a follow-up to the previous exercise, participants should be asked to list as many of their possessions as come to mind. After this list is complete, they should write a last will and testament, in which they designate what is to be done with their possessions. The same objectives will be achieved as in the possessions exercise.

Interruption

One concern often expressed about death is that it interrupts the achievement of one's goals for life—that is, people feel that they will die with goals left unaccomplished. These goals can vary from person to person, but the feeling of interruption by death is fairly common. An activity to help participants recognize this feeling in themselves and to organize their lives in ways in which this feeling is taken into account is the "interruption" exercise.

Ask participants to complete a chart that requires them to establish goals for each decade of their lives as follows:

Decade	Goal
0–10	_____
11–20	_____
21–30	_____
31–40	_____
41–50	_____
51–60	_____
61–70	_____
71–80	_____

When the chart is completed, the instructor asks the following:

1. Rank these goals in order of importance.
2. Cross out the goals already achieved.
3. If you were to die 10 years from now, which goals would not have been achieved?
4. Of the unaccomplished goals, if you died 10 years from now, how many are in the top four?
5. Can these goals be reorganized so that those more important to you (as indicated by your rankings) can be achieved earlier in your life? If so, which?
6. Are there goals you would like to add? If so, where would you place them in terms of importance? Where would you place them in terms of decades of your life?

Euthanasia/Assisted Suicide

To force participants to face the issue of when not to sustain life, present to them a handout on which appears the following critical incident (Wittner 1974):*

Ken and Cheryl Bater had been married just four months when they found out for sure that she was pregnant. Ken picked her up at the doctor's office that afternoon, and before the dinner dishes were washed they had chosen two names—Claudia, for a girl; Todd, if it turned out to be a boy. Then the teenage newlyweds made long-term plans as they happily faced the responsibilities of parenthood.

---

*Reprinted from *Today's Health,* March 1974 by special permission. Copyright © 1974 Family Media, Inc. All rights reserved.

They opened their first savings account. Ken cut his beer budget in half. Cheryl began preparing the house. Their lives were now wrapped up in anticipation of that day in mid-November when the baby would arrive.

Everything went well until one October afternoon when Ken's foreman called him off the assembly line to the phone. "Just listen," Cheryl ordered, her voice edged with tears. "I'm going to the hospital in a taxi. I think the baby might be coming early." No, she couldn't be positive. "But Ken, you've got to meet me there," she said. "And hurry, please."

Todd was born 90 minutes later—six weeks premature—weighing barely four pounds. He was weak, and it was immediately obvious that he had serious respiratory problems. The doctor could not get him to breathe on his own.

A few years ago Todd would have died at birth. But now, even at the modest-sized, midwestern hospital where the drama of Cheryl and Ken and Todd unfolded, new techniques and equipment have dramatically reversed the odds of survival for babies with acute problems.

Todd was rushed from the delivery room to the intensive-care nursery and placed in an incubator with an infant respirator attached. This machine actually breathes for the baby until his own lungs can take over the job.

"Don't worry, we'll pull the little fella through," John Filipelli, M.D., assured Ken and Cheryl. But what the pediatrician did not tell them was that there was a significant chance that Todd had suffered lasting brain damage as a result of the oxygen deficiency he experienced just after birth.

In a few days, Cheryl went home. But Todd remained in the hospital, still under intensive care, on and off the respirator. One week stretched to two and then four. Still, the infant did not fully respond. His weight hovered around five pounds. Each new breathing crisis increased the likelihood that his brain would sustain permanent damage from the lack of oxygen.

Nurses on the 3 P.M. to 11 P.M. shift, the hours when Ken and Cheryl visited, were becoming increasingly concerned, both for the young parents whom they watched sadly gaze at their struggling son, and for the baby himself.

"Poor kids," a floor nurse said after the couple had left one day in November.

"I wonder how much they know—I bet if they knew that they might wind up with just half a child, they wouldn't want us to keep putting him back on the respirator every time he has a failure."

"If it were up to me," said the nurse checking the gauges, "the next time we take him off, if he can't make it on his own, I would just let him go."

What would you do?

The health educator should then form small groups to discuss what each person's reaction would be in the case described. After 20 minutes of such discussion, the following handout, which completes the story, should be distributed.

The medical staff has been calling on Frank Reidy for eight years. He took the job as the first staff chaplain at the hospital only after being assured by the administration that he was to be "an ethical consultant to the medical staff as well as performing the usual handholding service and dispensing the death notices." In fact, he still has a copy of the letter with these words underlined. An ordained Lutheran minister, Chaplain Reidy has earned a reputation for asking the kind of direct questions that doctors and hospital administrators often find painful. (The chaplain, the doctor, and the Baters are all real people, and the events described here really happened in a regional hospital somewhere in the Midwest. Their names have been changed to protect their privacy and legal rights.)

Picking up the telephone in his office near the waiting room, Frank Reidy immediately recognized the voice of the nurse on the other end. "You sound upset, Barbara. What's up? . . . Of course, I'll be up in a minute. By the way, who's the doctor? . . . Oh sure, I know John Filipelli. Okay, well I'm on my way."

As the chaplain rounded the last corner on his way toward the nurseries, he was deep in thought. "Frank? . . . Is that you?" The voice that interrupted him from behind belonged to John Filipelli. They talked about the Baters' baby.

"Before you make any decision about the baby, I think you have to be sure that you have eliminated any prejudices you have," Chaplain Reidy was telling Dr. Filipelli. "Once you are sure that you have done all you can, you should try to get into it from the parents' point of view — and even from the baby's. First, though: Are you sure that you haven't kept the child alive this long out of some sense of guilt on your part?"

"No, no. There's nothing like that," the pediatrician answered quickly. Then a pause. "At least nothing about the baby. At the start though, when I first met the parents, I might have gone a little too strong in assuring them that the kid would be okay. I feel badly about that now, sure. But I don't think 'guilty' is the word. Still, now that I stop to really think about it, I guess something like that *could* have influenced me to push just a little harder to keep the baby alive — against better judgment. Another thing, too, is that the longer the baby is up there the bigger the bill gets. I suppose that insurance will pay most of it, but it must be over $5,000 by now. I guess what I am saying is that it becomes even harder to pull the plug after we all have put so much into it. Yet the longer I keep putting him on the respirator, the less the chances are that they will have an intact baby in the end. The chances of brain damage are already awfully high, to say nothing of his physical problems which haven't stabilized."

The doctor was almost talking to himself now. His head bent, staring into the cold, stagnant cup of coffee in front of him, his thoughts trailed into silence. Suddenly he looked up, remembering where he was and relieved to see that he and the chaplain were still alone in the snack bar. No strangers were close enough to have overheard his self-doubt.

"How much do you know about the parents?" Reidy asked. "Have you talked to them honestly about all this?"

"Oh come off it, Frank," the doctor exploded. "They're kids themselves. You can't ask them to make this kind of decision. What do you want me to do — walk up to them and say, 'Okay, what do we do: kill your child or give him back to you as a vegetable?' Heck, every time they go into the nursery, they look scared stiff," the doctor rebutted.

"Maybe they wouldn't be so scared if they knew what was going on, if you hadn't tried to protect them from the start. Are you sure that part of the problem isn't that you are copping out of facing them? Don't forget: It's *their* child, and they are the ones who are getting up to their necks in debt.

"By the way, do you actually know how important money is to them?" The minister's questions were jolting.

"Maybe they have more money than you do. And one other thing that's probably important: Is there any reason why the mother can't carry another child? If there is, you know they are going to try everything to save this one, no matter how badly damaged it is."

The doctor stood and slowly walked across the room to a window overlooking a dreary parking lot. For nearly a full minute he watched the patterns of raindrops splashing below. "Look, Frank," he finally said, "You've been a big help. You always are. I need a few minutes to sort some of this out alone. Then I want to call her doctor and see if he can give me answers to some of those questions. Why don't you tell the nurses that we talked and ask them to page me when the parents come in this afternoon. Then I may want you to talk to them after I have seen them. Okay?"

"If you need me I'll be in my office or up on the dialysis unit. There's a tough one up there today, too," the chaplain said. "Do you know what you are going to tell the parents?"

"I'm going to tell them that I think we should switch the respirator from 'control' to 'assist' if Todd has to go back on it again. The machine will help him keep himself alive, but it won't force him to breathe if he wants to stop. At least that's what I think we should do," Dr. Filipelli said.

After Ken and Cheryl Bater heard John Filipelli's recommendation, they indeed wanted to talk to Frank Reidy. The chaplain assured them that their decision to follow the doctor's suggestion was morally sound and that they had done all they could. They waited at the hospital through the next several hours — long enough to again meet with Frank Reidy when he told them that Todd was dead.

Eyes were moist inside and outside the intensive-care nursery that afternoon as everyone worked through another of those hard decisions — the kind that have called for bioethics to come into being in medical centers everywhere.

Valuing Activities

Emerging health concerns such as death, dying, spirituality, the aged, and the aging process lend themselves very well to valuing activities. By definition, emerging health topics are new or have been given recent emphasis. Because of this newness, very few right or wrong answers can be provided to people studying issues related to these topics. Consequently, an exploration of values underlying proposed alternative solutions to these issues seems appropriate. The activities to follow are designed for this purpose.

Values Ranking

The following groups of terms can be rank ordered and the rankings discussed in small groups:

1. Old	1. Family	1. Dying
2. Young	2. Independence	2. Dead
3. Middle-aged	3. Friends	3. Pain

1. Abortion any time mother decides to.
2. Abortion with physician's approval only.
3. Abortion never.

If you were old and ill which would you prefer?

1. Living in a nursing home.
2. Living in a hospital.
3. Living with a relative.

If you were dying, which would you prefer?

1. Letting nature take its own course.
2. Letting physicians keep you alive by any means.
3. Letting a close relative decide when physicians should pull the plug.

When you die, which would you prefer?

1. Burial.
2. Cremation.
3. Body donated to science.

If you were to donate one of your organs upon death to another, which organ would it be?

1. Heart.
2. Eyes.
3. Kidneys.

Survival

The following game will require participants to discuss the value of life without ever having to identify it as such. Participants should be divided into small groups of from four to six members. One group will imagine that they are *physicians,* another that they are *politicians,* another that they are *teachers,* another that they are *clergy,* and the last that they are *teenagers.* Each group will receive these instructions:

> It is anticipated that a nuclear holocaust is imminent. Many deaths will occur, but luckily some bomb shelters have been equipped to provide safety for a select few. Since only 100 people can live in these shelters, all but these 100 will die. It is your group's task to establish criteria for selecting which 100 people will be allowed to inhabit the bomb shelters.

> *Don't forget the role you are playing.*

After each group has determined the criteria they would use, have these listed on the chalkboard. Next, have a member of each group present the reasoning that group used in establishing these criteria. After all such presentations, drop the role-playing and have the total group review each of the criteria on the board and decide whether or not they should keep it. At the conclusion of this exercise, the following questions can be used to bring ethical issues into greater focus:

1. Who has the right to determine who shall live and who shall die?
2. When other than a nuclear bombing might such a decision be necessary?
3. In each of these situations, who should make the decision?
4. What should be considered in making each of these decisions?
5. How should this country be preparing *now* for dealing with such ethical issues in the future?

Values Listings

This exercise asks participants to list the 15 people with whom they most like to spend time. Once this list is complete, the following directions should be given:

1. Place an *O* next to anyone older than 50.
2. Place a *Y* next to anyone younger than 10.
3. Place a *D* next to five people most likely to die first.
4. Place a *T* next to the five people you would most trust in a life-and-death situation.
5. Think of your three most valuable material possessions. Place a *G* next to the three people to whom you would give one of these possessions if you were to die today.
6. If you were told you were dying and could say goodbye to only five of the people on your list, whom would they be? Place the letter *M* next to these people.

The following questions will afford the participants in this exercise the opportunity for introspection:

1. After following the instructions, did you think of people who weren't on your list but you would now like to include? Who are they? Why did you originally leave them off?
2. Do you enjoy spending time with younger people, people your own age, or those older? Why?
3. Relative to the people most likely to die first:
   a. Are they the oldest on your list?
   b. Do you now want to spend more time with them?
   c. What do you want to do with them before they die?

d. Do you think they would guess that you would include them on such a list? Should you tell them you did?

4. If you were dying in a hospital, would you want any of the five people you designated as the ones you most trust to decide when to pull the plug? Or is there someone else you would rather assign that responsibility?

5. How would you feel giving one of your most valued possessions to the people you designated with a *G now* rather than when you are dying? Would the meaning behind the gift be more valuable to you than the possession itself?

6. What have you learned from having participated in this exercise?

Values Behavior

To confront people with the inconsistency between their professed values and their behavior relative to emerging health concerns discussed in this chapter, they should complete the following handouts:

A. Briefly describe what you believe to be the typical day of a senior citizen resident of a nursing home. _____

_____

_____

_____

_____

Identify three things about this typical day that you would not like were you this senior citizen.
1. _____
2. _____
3. _____
What could you do for such a resident to help make one of these three things less troublesome?

_____

_____

Are you going to do it? _____ When? _____

B. Do you believe legislation should allow for abortions, or do you believe legislation should disallow abortions? Check one: _____ allow _____ disallow. Which branch or branches of your state government would be responsible for such legislation? _____

_____

_____

Have you communicated your opinions to your elected representative in this branch of government? Check one: _____ yes _____ no
Are you going to? _____ When? _____

C. If you were to die right now, is there something you would regret never having done? _____
If so, what is it? _____

_____

Is there something you would regret not having told someone? What? Who? _____

_____

Are you going to do that thing soon? _____ When? _____
Are you going to tell that person? _____ When? _____

Values Statements

As stated earlier, unfinished sentences can be used to explore values. The following sentence stems can be employed to consider values related to emerging health concerns.

1. Death _____
2. Dying _____
3. Living _____
4. Free choice _____
5. The aged _____
6. The aging process _____
7. Nursing homes _____
8. Euthanasia _____
9. I want to die when _____
10. Abortion is _____
11. When I die I'll miss _____
12. Ethics means _____
13. Sex for the aged _____
14. Social Security payments _____
15. The "plug" should be pulled when _____

Summary

The purpose of this chapter has been twofold: first, to present instructional strategies for health concerns of recent emphasis (the aged and aging, spirituality, and death and dying); and second, to illustrate how new health education topics can easily be adapted to the learner-centered approach to health instruction. Regardless of the content being considered, a more interesting, exciting, and meaningful approach to that content is to actively involve the learner. This chapter has demonstrated that this involvement is possible when it is consciously sought.

CHAPTER FOURTEEN

Instructional Strategies for Personal Health

The dichotomy between mind and body, too often separated by some traditional health educators, is being increasingly questioned. With a better understanding of psychosomatic illnesses, recent work with biofeedback training, scientific verification of many of the claims of the Eastern yogis, and the suspicion that conditions previously thought of as mental illnesses may have physiological bases (for example, schizophrenia and depression), we are coming to recognize that the mind and body affect each other in many ways not previously understood or even suspected. Unfortunately, most health education programs still separate the study of physical health from other health components.

Rather than separate the mind from the body, this chapter combines the two. A good example is the area of stress management, since it has been clearly demonstrated to have physical and psychological components. Once it experiences a stressor, the mind will interpret a threat and change the body to deal with the threat. The change in the body can, if it occurs chronically or goes unabated, result in one of a number of psychosomatic ailments (for example, tension headaches, backache, coronary heart disease, or stroke).

In addition to stress management, which was discussed in Chapter 8, we consider in this chapter other topical areas like communicable diseases (such as AIDS), physical fitness, dental health, consumer health, and genetics. As in other chapters, valuing activities are included that pertain specifically to personal health education.

We begin with instructional activities relevant to the understanding of communicable diseases.

Communicable Diseases

Disease Bag

The study of communicable diseases has often been conducted in such a fashion that the relationship of the diseases to the program participants has remained obscure. Since everyone has been both a carrier and a receiver, the opportunity to relate the investigation of communicable diseases to their lives should be pursued. How to do this?

Request participants to bring 3 × 5 index cards on which they have written the name of a communicable disease they had at some time. Each person should write only one disease on each card but bring as many cards as needed to represent the different communicable diseases he or she has contracted. A listing of the different diseases should be made and distributed to each member, who then will be responsible for researching various related components of the disease:

1. Means of transmission.
2. Causes.
3. Signs and/or symptoms.
4. Treatment.
5. Time of incapacity.

The researching of these diseases should consist of interviewing parents who have cared for victims of the condition in question, talking with physicians, reading appropriate material, and/or assembling participants' memories of the times they were afflicted with the disease.

After a week devoted to the research just described, the health educator should play "disease bag" with the group. All of the index cards are placed in a paper bag, which is shaken several times to mix its contents. The group is then randomly divided into two teams, which compete against each other, with the team accumulating the most points the winner of the game. Alternating teams, and with each team having a turn, the health educator reaches into the disease bag for a disease (index card). The person whose turn it is must provide the five researched aspects of that disease: means of transmission, causes, signs and/or symptoms, treatment, and time of incapacity. For each of the five aspects accurately answered (in the judgment of the health educator or a panel of experts), the team is awarded five points. After everyone has had a chance, the game ends.

If the health educator should pull a disease from the bag that has already been discussed, the disease should be used again. In this manner learning will be reinforced through repetition.

Policy Study

Although the incidence of communicable diseases has decreased with the advancement of science and the development of vaccines, organizations still must be concerned with policies governing persons contracting such diseases. Given the concern regarding HIV/AIDS, this is of particular importance. This activity requires program participants to consider several important questions regarding their organization's policies pertaining to people associated with the organization—for example, workers, pupils, patients, or community laypeople. Such questions as the following should be posed and answered:

1. Which diseases does the organization policy refer to as *communicable?*
2. Who is the organization's representative who is notified when someone has contracted a communicable disease?
3. What, if any, procedures are employed by the organization's staff to minimize the spread of this disease to others in the organization?
4. What relationship, if any, exists between the local health department and the organization relative to preventing and responding to communicable diseases?
5. At what point in the development of the disease is the afflicted person required to be excluded from the organization's facilities?
6. At what point may the afflicted person return to the organization's facilities? Are there any special procedures for returning to which the afflicted person must adhere?

Numerous people might be interviewed to obtain answers to these questions: the organization's health director, the nurse, the administrators, the health educator, and so on. Or these people might be invited to visit and address the group. Another procedure that could be used to answer these questions would entail the gathering and careful review of the organization's written policy statements on communicable disease. If such an activity discovers a lack of appropriate written materials, the program participants might recommend the development of such materials to the management of the organization, or even write the policy themselves.

Simulated Epidemic

An interesting means of illustrating the concept of contagion has been described in the instructor's guide to a health text (CRM 1972, 87):

> The students could act as epidemiologists in a simulated epidemic. The instructor can illustrate the concept and pattern of infection spread by applying a substance that is illuminated only under a black light on the right hand of one unknown student prior to class. (Such a substance is known as *tracer powder.*) When class has begun, ask everyone to walk around and shake hands with three people they don't know. The idea is to spread the substance from the original student to as many others as possible. Determine who is "infected" by shining the black light on each person's hand. Have the "noninfected" members of the class interrogate the "afflicted" members and locate the original source of infection.

This activity is most appropriate and timely given the concern regarding HIV/AIDS and the spread of sexually transmitted infections (for example, syphilis, gonorrhea, chlamydia), provided participants understand the difference between direct contact and casual contact.

Health Inspectors

In this activity, program participants become "health inspectors." The total group is divided into smaller groups of six to eight people. Each group is assigned a site to inspect for the potential spread of communicable diseases. For example, one group may have the cafeteria, while another group may have the bathrooms. Participants then brainstorm behaviors and environmental factors that can result in the spread of disease. They might come up with shaking hands, touching the eyes, sneezing, poor ventilation, drinking out of the same cup, sharing towels or combs, or not washing after using the bathroom. The next week is devoted to group members watching their areas for evidence of potential disease-spreading behaviors or environmental factors and reporting to the larger group what they have found.

Noncommunicable Diseases

Family Tree of Life and Death (Dintiman and Greenberg 1983, 423)

Heredity plays a major role in both the probability of people's contracting certain diseases as well as their longevity. The "family tree of life and death" can be used to bring this fact home. The family tree (see Figure 14.1) should be handed out to each participant, who is then assigned the task of finding out the date of birth, date of death, cause of death, and the age of death for each relative listed on the tree. The health educator should be sensitive to those who have been adopted by advising them either to work with another person, to refrain from the activity, or to make some other accommodation. Once completed, the tree is analyzed. The following questions are the focus of that analysis:

1. What was the average age of death among relatives who died of natural causes?
   a. Number of relatives dying from natural causes: _____

FIGURE 14.1

Family tree

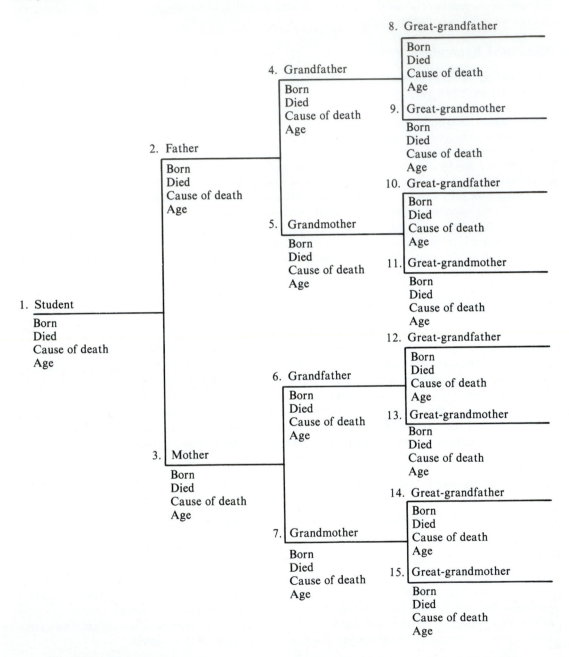

From George B. Dintiman and Jerrold S. Greenberg. *Health through Discovery,* 2d ed. New York: Random House, 1989, p. 378.

b. Total years lived of these relatives (add all years): _____

c. Average age of relatives dying from natural causes (divide the answer in *b* by the answer in *a*): _____

2. List the chronic and degenerative diseases causing death in your family.

3. What diseases appear more than once in your hereditary line?

4. Are any of these diseases hereditary?

5. What preventive action can you take to reduce the probability of acquiring this disease?

6. What will you do to decrease the probability of contracting this disease?

Risko

The most deadly pervasive noncommunicable disease threat is coronary heart disease. To help program participants determine their chances of contracting coronary heart disease, have them play Risko. Divide the large group into smaller groups of 5 to 10 people. Have each person score his or her chances of heart disease by following the accompanying directions. After participants have determined their risk, have them brainstorm in their small groups ways in which each person's risk can be minimized.

Cancer Paneling

Invite a panel to join the group to present various aspects of cancer etiology, cancer detection, cancer prevention, and cancer therapy. The panel might include representatives of the local chapter of the American Cancer Society, the county or city health department, or a local university's medical school; a university professor or researcher from one of the sciences that are related to cancer (for example, biology, chemistry, or ecology); a member of the clergy who counsels cancer patients; and a person who has contracted cancer, who might appear with his or her relatives who are also having to manage the effects of the disease. Allow sufficient time for both brief presentations and for program participants to ask all of the questions they may have.

Physical Fitness

While relaxation skills (see Chapter 8) help to relax the body, exercising the body will also help prevent the early onset of diseases and add to the quality of life. Physical fitness is the condition of the body relative to muscular strength and endurance, cardiorespiratory endurance, flexibility, and agility and balance (Greenberg, Dintiman, and Myers-Oakes 1998).

Harvard Step Test

Asking program participants to take the Harvard Step Test (Brouha 1943) is an excellent way of demonstrating several points about the circulatory system. It can be used to introduce pulse taking or to demonstrate the need for the heart to send more blood around the body during strenuous work or to introduce the topic of physical fitness. All that is needed is an 18-inch bench or step and a wristwatch with a second hand. The participants are told to step up and down 30 times a minute. Each time, the participant should step all the way up on the bench with the body erect. The health educator should keep a cadence so that each person takes the same number of steps as each other person. Stepping should be

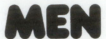

Find the column for your age group. Everyone starts with a score of 10 points. Work down the page *adding* points to your score or *subtracting* points from your score.

		54 OR YOUNGER	55 OR OLDER

1. WEIGHT

Locate your weight category in the table below. If you are in . . .

		54 OR YOUNGER	55 OR OLDER
	STARTING SCORE	**10**	STARTING SCORE **10**
☐ weight category A		SUBTRACT 2	SUBTRACT 2
☐ weight category B		SUBTRACT 1	ADD 0
☐ weight category C		ADD 1	ADD 1
☐ weight category D		ADD 2	ADD 3
		EQUALS ☐	**EQUALS** ☐

2. SYSTOLIC BLOOD PRESSURE

Use the "first" or "higher" number from your most recent blood pressure measurement. If you do not know your blood pressure, estimate it by using the letter for your weight category. If your blood pressure is . . .

		54 OR YOUNGER	55 OR OLDER
A 119 or less		SUBTRACT 1	SUBTRACT 5
B between 120 and 139		ADD 0	SUBTRACT 2
C between 140 and 159		ADD 0	ADD 1
D 160 or greater		ADD 1	ADD 4
		EQUALS ☐	**EQUALS** ☐

3. BLOOD CHOLESTEROL LEVEL

Use the number from your most recent blood cholesterol test. If you do not know your blood cholesterol, estimate it by using the letter for your weight category. If your blood cholesterol is . . .

		54 OR YOUNGER	55 OR OLDER
A 199 or less		SUBTRACT 2	SUBTRACT 1
B between 200 and 224		SUBTRACT 1	SUBTRACT 1
C between 225 and 249		ADD 0	ADD 0
D 250 or higher		ADD 1	ADD 0
		EQUALS ☐	**EQUALS** ☐

4. CIGARETTE SMOKING

If you . . .

(If you smoke a pipe, but not cigarettes, use the same score adjustment as those cigarette smokers who smoke less than a pack a day.)

		54 OR YOUNGER	55 OR OLDER
☐ do not smoke		SUBTRACT 1	SUBTRACT 2
☐ smoke less than a pack a day		ADD 0	SUBTRACT 1
☐ smoke a pack a day		ADD 1	ADD 0
☐ smoke more than a pack a day		ADD 2	ADD 3
		FINAL SCORE EQUALS ☐	**FINAL SCORE EQUALS** ☐

WEIGHT TABLE FOR MEN
Look for your height (without shoes) in the far left column and then read across to find the category into which your weight (in indoor clothing) would fall.

YOUR HEIGHT FT IN	WEIGHT CATEGORY (lbs.)			
	A	B	C	D
5 1	up to 123	124–148	149–173	174 plus
5 2	up to 126	127–152	153–178	179 plus
5 3	up to 129	130–156	157–182	183 plus
5 4	up to 132	133–160	161–186	187 plus
5 5	up to 135	136–163	164–190	191 plus
5 6	up to 139	140–168	169–196	197 plus
5 7	up to 144	145–174	175–203	204 plus
5 8	up to 148	149–179	180–209	210 plus
5 9	up to 152	153–184	185–214	215 plus
5 10	up to 157	158–190	191–221	222 plus
5 11	up to 161	162–194	195–227	228 plus
6 0	up to 165	166–199	200–232	233 plus
6 1	up to 170	171–205	206–239	240 plus
6 2	up to 175	176–211	212–246	247 plus
6 3	up to 180	181–217	218–253	254 plus
6 4	up to 185	186–223	224–260	261 plus
6 5	up to 190	191–229	230–267	268 plus
6 6	up to 195	196–235	236–274	275 plus
ESTIMATE OF SYSTOLIC BLOOD PRESSURE	119 or less	120 to 139	140 to 159	160 or more
ESTIMATE OF BLOOD CHOLESTEROL	199 or less	200 to 224	225 to 249	250 or more

Because both blood pressure and blood cholesterol are related to weight, an estimate of these risk factors for each weight category is printed at the bottom of the table.

WOMEN

Find the column for your age group. Everyone starts with a score of 10 points. Work down the page *adding* points to your score or *subtracting* points from your score.

	54 OR YOUNGER	55 OR OLDER
	STARTING SCORE **10**	STARTING SCORE **10**

1. WEIGHT

Locate your weight category in the table below. If you are in . . .

		54 OR YOUNGER	55 OR OLDER
	weight category A	SUBTRACT 2	SUBTRACT 2
	weight category B	SUBTRACT 1	SUBTRACT 1
	weight category C	ADD 1	ADD 0
	weight category D	ADD 2	ADD 1
	EQUALS		

2. SYSTOLIC BLOOD PRESSURE

Use the "first" or "higher" number from your most recent blood pressure measurement. If you do not know your blood pressure, estimate it by using the letter for your weight category. If your blood pressure is . . .

		54 OR YOUNGER	55 OR OLDER
A	119 or less	SUBTRACT 2	SUBTRACT 3
B	between 120 and 139	SUBTRACT 1	ADD 0
C	between 140 and 159	ADD 0	ADD 3
D	160 or greater	ADD 1	ADD 6
	EQUALS		

3. BLOOD CHOLESTEROL LEVEL

Use the number from your most recent blood cholesterol test. If you do not know your blood cholesterol, estimate it by using the letter for your weight category. If your blood cholesterol is . . .

		54 OR YOUNGER	55 OR OLDER
A	199 or less	SUBTRACT 1	SUBTRACT 3
B	between 200 and 224	ADD 0	SUBTRACT 1
C	between 225 and 249	ADD 0	ADD 1
D	250 or higher	ADD 1	ADD 3
	EQUALS		

4. CIGARETTE SMOKING

If you . . .

		54 OR YOUNGER	55 OR OLDER
	do not smoke	SUBTRACT 1	SUBTRACT 2
	smoke less than a pack a day	ADD 0	SUBTRACT 1
	smoke a pack a day	ADD 1	ADD 1
	smoke more than a pack a day	ADD 2	ADD 4
	EQUALS		

5. ESTROGEN USE

*Birth control pills and hormone drugs contain estrogen. A few examples are: *Premarin *Ogan *Menstranol *Provera *Evex *Menest *Estinyl *Meurium*

• Have you ever taken estrogen for five or more years in a row?
• Are you age 35 years or older and are now taking estrogen?

		54 OR YOUNGER	55 OR OLDER
	No to both questions	ADD 0	ADD 0
	Yes to one or both questions	ADD 1	ADD 3

	54 OR YOUNGER	55 OR OLDER
FINAL SCORE EQUALS		

WEIGHT TABLE FOR WOMEN
Look for your height (without shoes) in the far left column and then read across to find the category into which your weight (in indoor clothing) would fall.

YOUR HEIGHT FT IN	A	B	C	D
4 8	up to 101	102–122	123–143	144 plus
4 9	up to 103	104–125	126–146	147 plus
4 10	up to 106	107–128	129–150	151 plus
4 11	up to 109	110–132	133–154	155 plus
5 0	up to 112	113–136	137–158	159 plus
5 1	up to 115	116–139	140–162	163 plus
5 2	up to 119	120–144	145–168	169 plus
5 3	up to 122	123–148	149–172	173 plus
5 4	up to 127	128–154	155–179	180 plus
5 5	up to 131	132–158	159–185	186 plus
5 6	up to 135	136–163	164–190	191 plus
5 7	up to 139	140–168	169–196	197 plus
5 8	up to 143	144–173	174–202	203 plus
5 9	up to 147	148–178	179–207	208 plus
5 10	up to 151	152–182	183–213	214 plus
5 11	up to 155	156–187	188–218	219 plus
6 0	up to 159	160–191	192–224	225 plus
6 1	up to 163	164–196	197–229	230 plus
ESTIMATE OF SYSTOLIC BLOOD PRESSURE	119 or less	120 to 139	140 to 159	160 or more
ESTIMATE OF BLOOD CHOLESTEROL	199 or less	200 to 224	225 to 249	250 or more

Because both blood pressure and blood cholesterol are related to weight, an estimate of these risk factors for each weight category is printed at the bottom of the table.

WHAT YOUR SCORE MEANS

0–4

You have one of the lowest risks of Heart Disease for your age and sex.

5–9

You have a low. to moderate risk of Heart Disease for your age and sex but there is some room for improvement.

10–14

You have a moderate to high risk of Heart Disease for your age and sex, with considerable room for improvement on some factors.

15–19

You have a high risk of developing Heart Disease for your age and sex with a great deal of room for improvement on all factors.

20 & over

You have a very high risk of developing Heart Disease for your age and sex and should take immediate action on all risk factors.

WARNING

* If you have diabetes, gout or a family history of heart disease, your actual risk will be greater than indicated by this appraisal.
* If you do not know your current blood pressure or blood cholesterol level, you should visit your physician or health center to have them measured. Then figure your score again for a more accurate determination of your risk.
* If you are overweight, have high blood pressure or high blood cholesterol, or smoke cigarettes, your long-term risk of heart disease is increased even if your risk in the next several years is low.

© Reproduced with permission. *Risko.* American Heart Association.

It's surprising that some people seem to care more about maintaining the fitness of their cars than they do about maintaining the fitness of their bodies. Like a car, the body needs adequate fuel (food) and sufficient rest and needs to be well tuned. Health educators can help program participants recognize these needs and provide instruction on how to satisfy them.

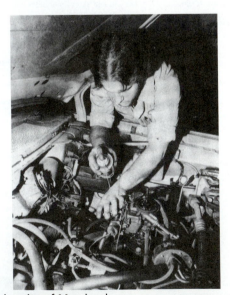

Source: The Diamondback, University of Maryland

done in four counts, so that the cadence should be, "Left—up—left—down." The stepping should continue for four minutes unless the person wants to stop earlier due to exhaustion. After the four minutes are up, participants should sit in chairs and have their pulses taken for 30 seconds, beginning at one, two, and three minutes after the stepping ceases. It is best to pair people initially and do the exercise twice. The first time, one partner exercises, and the other takes the pulse readings, and then they switch roles. After the pulse readings are recorded, a physical efficiency index is computed utilizing the following formula:

$$PEI = \frac{\text{Duration of exercise in seconds} \times 100}{2 \times \text{sum of pulse counts in recovery}}$$

A PEI of 60 or less indicates poor physical condition, whereas a score of 81 or higher indicates excellent physical condition.

The Agility Run

Motor skills include the abilities to engage in various physical activities: speed, power, balance, agility, reaction time, and coordination. Agility, being such a key component of motor skills, might be one you are particularly interested in assessing for your program's participants. To do so, you can use the agility run.

To begin, mark off a course as shown in Figure 14.2. Use chairs or cones 10 feet apart from one another where the four squares are marked. Start participants lying on the floor on their stomachs with their hands placed on the floor just under their shoulders. At the signal, they are to jump to their feet and follow the course, completing it as quickly as possible. Their score is the time to the nearest tenth of a second that it takes to complete the course.

FIGURE 14.2
Illinois Agility Run

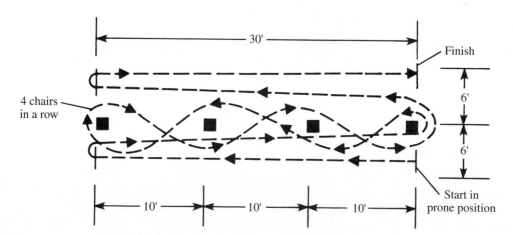

From T. K. Cureton. *Physical Fitness Workbook*, p. 24. Champaign, IL: Stipes Publishing Company, 1944. Reprinted with permission.

Participating in team sports, whether organized or just "pickup" games, is an excellent way to keep fit.

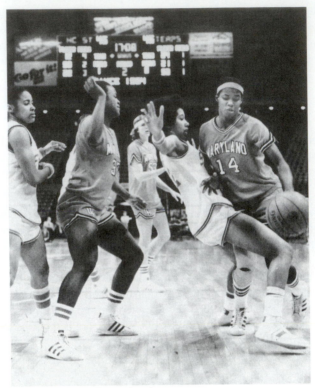

Source: The Diamondback, University of Maryland

This activity is interesting and educational in that the participants often feel a sense of competition (either between them and other participants or against the clock) and learn about a part of themselves that usually remains a mystery.

Completing the course in 17 seconds or sooner indicates an above-average agility; between 17.5 and 21.5 seconds indicates an average agility; and a time of 22 seconds or longer indicates a below-average agility.

Flexibility Assessment

Another component of physical fitness that is vital in terms of preventing injury and being able to function efficiently is flexibility. Whenever I think of flexibility, I'm reminded of the doctoral student who, upset that I corrected all the spelling errors in the first draft of her dissertation, told me, "It's a small mind that can spell a word only one way!" Well, the flexibility referred to in this section is the ability to move the body throughout a range of motion and concerns the stretching of the muscles and tissues around skeletal joints.

FIGURE 14.3
Shoulder Reach

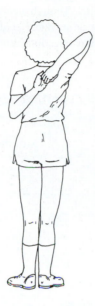

Flexibility of program participants can be measured at various locations within the body: for example, at the shoulder, hip, or back. The instructional strategy presented here will show you how to measure flexibility at the shoulder because the only equipment required is a ruler, and it can be challenging to students.

Have participants stand against a pole or a projecting corner, raise their right arms, and reach down behind their backs as far as they can. At the same time, they should reach up from behind with their left hands and try to overlap the palms of their right hands (see Figure 14.3). Have a partner measure the overlap, or by how much an overlap is missed, to the nearest half-inch. If there is an overlap, a + sign is placed in front of the amount of the overlap. If the fingers are short of touching, a minus sign is placed in front of the amount of the gap. If the fingers of one hand just barely touch those of the other, the score is a zero. Have participants then repeat the assessment with the arms reversed.

To interpret the score (the amount of overlap or the amount of the gap if an overlap is not possible), use the following scale. The first figure is with the right arm up; the second figure is with the left are up.

For Men
Above average	=	6 and higher — 3 and higher
Average	=	Plus 4–plus 5 — 0–plus 2
Below average	=	Below plus 4 — Below 0

For Women
Above average	=	7 and higher — 6 and higher
Average	=	Plus 5–plus 6 — 0–plus 5
Below average	=	Below plus 5 — Below 0

Sleep Study

Another part of being physically fit is acquiring enough sleep so the body is rested and has sufficiently recovered from the previous day's activities. Though health educators talk about the importance of sleep, little if any significant part of a unit on physical health is devoted to this subject. It is true that sleep is an area of investigation in which many questions remain unanswered. However, it is known that,

DAILY SLEEP CHART							
Name_____ Monday's date_____							
1. Time to sleep	1.	1.	1.	1.	1.	1.	1.
2. Time woke up	2.	2.	2.	2.	2.	2.	2.
Hours of sleep	____hrs.	____hrs.	____hrs.	____hrs.	____hrs.	____hrs.	____hrs.
Check one:							
When woke up							
1. Felt tired	1. ____	1. ____	1. ____	1. ____	1. ____	1. ____	1. ____
2. Felt OK	2. ____	2. ____	2. ____	2. ____	2. ____	2. ____	2. ____
3. Felt great	3. ____	3. ____	3. ____	3. ____	3. ____	3. ____	3. ____

for youth, sleep is associated with the release of the growth hormone (luteinizing hormone), and with the secretion of testosterone in males during puberty. It is known that during sleep, the high level of hormonal secretions aids cell division, thus restoring worn tissue; cells of the skin multiply twice as fast; and the heart rate slows, thereby affording the heart muscle a rest. Sleep is also associated with psychological wellness (for example, it reduces irritability).

It is further recognized that sleep occurs more readily under some conditions than others. It is suggested that one sleep in a familiar and comfortable environment that is quiet and of moderate temperature; that this environment contain little lighting, be well ventilated, and be nonodorous; and that the sleeper wear loose-fitting clothing, use lightweight blankets, and refrain from the ingestion of stimulants (like caffeine) prior to sleep.

With such knowledge, health educators should be concerned with helping people obtain good sleep and the benefits thereof. The accompanying chart (Schmitt 1976) has been successfully used to investigate the effects of sleeping behavior.

When the responses on this chart were analyzed, it was concluded that long sleepers (more than 10 hours) profited more from their sleep than did short sleepers (fewer than 7.5 hours).

CHECK THOSE SPACES THAT APPLY:							
Conditions	Mon.	Tues.	Wed.	Thurs.	Fri.	Sat.	Sun.
1. Temperature (hot, cold, OK)							
2. Too noisy							
3. Too much light							
4. Ate before going to bed							
5. Restful time before bed							
6. Tight night clothes							
7. Could hear TV							
8. Plenty of fresh air							
9. Awakened by noise or person							
10. Drank coffee or cola before bed							

From Raymond H. Schmitt, "Sleep: An Instructional Unit." Unpublished paper, April 1976. Reprinted by permission of the author.

RESULTS OF SLEEP CHARTING			
	Felt Tired	OK	Felt Great
Long sleepers	1 student	10 students	7 students
Short sleepers	10 students	4 students	1 student

Relaxation exercises (progressive relaxation, autogenic training, or meditation) can then be practiced as aids to initiating sleep and eliminating feelings of sleeplessness.

Consumer Health

One health education content area that is too often overlooked is consumer health. Given the societal interest in health lately and the vast economic resources—both personal and governmental—flowing into health promotion, it is not surprising that product manufacturers are advertising their products as health enhancing. Program participants can be helped to better evaluate these claims through the following activities.

Price Sense

It isn't always the case that the higher-priced product is the most effective or the most healthful. To make this point, ask program participants to bring in two different brands of the following products, whose effectiveness they have inquired about from the pharmacist at the drugstore where they were purchased:

Aspirin	Cough syrup	Mouthwash
Eye drops	Acne medicine	Laxatives
Vitamins	Cough drops	Contact lens cleaner

In groups of five students each, have participants compare the two different brands of each product by responding to the following questions:

1. How do these products differ in price?
2. How do these products differ in effectiveness?
3. How do these products differ in their ingredients?
4. How do these products differ in your familiarity with them? That is, have you seen them advertised?
5. How do these products differ in their containers? In their labels?
6. Do these products make different appeals to the consumer, either through their advertising or through their packaging or labeling?
7. Do the dosages of the active ingredient in these products differ?
8. Do these products appeal to one gender in particular?

Once these questions are answered in the small groups, a recorder from each group reports the results to the larger group. It is often found that although products do not differ in their effectiveness, they are priced differently. For example, even though a brand of aspirin may have the same amount of acetyl-salicylate as another brand, one may be more heavily advertised or packaged in a container more costly than the other and, as a result, may be priced higher.

Gender Advertising and Appealing

Health products are often directed at one gender or another. This appeal is made based upon the perceived interest of men and women (as perceived by the product manufacturers). Too often these per-ceived interests perpetuate gender stereotypes and are actually insulting. To demonstrate this, instruct program participants to bring to the group session several different current magazines, some that they know are obviously published for men (for example, *Esquire*) and some that they know are published

When the group works together, such as in analyzing or creating magazine ads, their verbal expression and body language reflect their concern and interest. This interest may be more difficult to elicit with lecture or other student-inactive learning strategies.

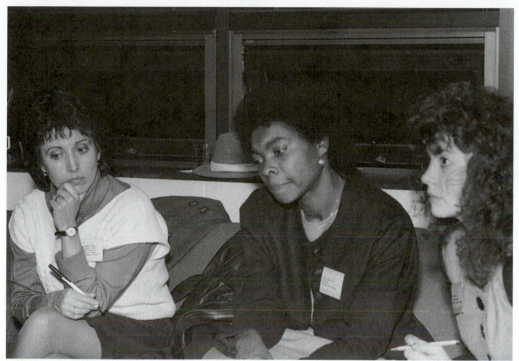

Source: Dr. Robert Gold

for women (for example, *Cosmopolitan*). Prior to bringing these magazines in, each participant is to identify advertisements directed at women and those directed at men. For example, ads for nylon stockings are not meant for men, and ads for aftershave are not directed at women. Students should add up the number of these ads and note where in the magazine they appear.

Form groups of eight students, with males and females in each group. In these groups, participants present what they have found: the number of ads for women and the number for men, the types of products advertised to women and the types advertised to men, the stereotype being perpetuated, and so on.

Next, have one female in the group agree to use a facial cream advertised in one of the magazines. She is to wash one side of her face with this facial cream and the other side with soap and water for two weeks (without informing anyone which side is which). After two weeks, reform the groups, and ask each participant to feel both sides of the face of the volunteer and to judge it for smoothness, softness, and the other claims made by the original ad. Add up the votes to determine if using the facial cream makes any difference.

An alternative procedure would be to ask another female in the class to use soap and water *and* facial cream on one side of her face and *only* facial cream on the other. Or ask a man in the group who shaves to use a different razor blade on different sides of his face and to have the smoothness of his face judged.

Creating Ad Appeals

Advertisers appeal to the needs and interests of the market; alternatively, they create needs and interests. You can turn your program participants into ad agents at a high-powered marketing firm—at least figuratively—by having them form small groups (marketing firms) of six members each. Present them with a product for which you want to commission their firm to develop an ad campaign. The product could be any of the following:

1. An automobile.
2. A soft drink to compete with Coca Cola and Pepsi.
3. A weight loss diet.
4. Any other product typically advertised that can have many different appeals.

Just make sure that each group (ad firm) is assigned the *same* product to advertise as each other group. However, each group is to employ a *different appeal* in its ad. The approaches the groups are to take in their ads can be any of the following:

1. Appeal to pride.
2. Appeal to sex.
3. Appeal to the need to be recognized.
4. Appeal to the need to be different.
5. Appeal to the need to be one of the group.
6. Appeal to the need to be associated with famous people.
7. Appeal to the need to follow authority.
8. Appeal to fear.

If videotaping and playback equipment are available, have each group videotape its ad. Then play the ads for the larger group as they try to guess to what need or interest the ad is appealing. If video equipment is not available, have groups make ads for magazines, photocopy them, and distribute copies to each class participant. As with the videotapes, the larger group is to guess to what need or interest the ad is appealing.

Once the ads have been processed as described, the homework assignment is to have participants randomly choose any three magazine advertisements (they should close their eyes and turn to pages and point at a spot until three ads are selected) and identify the appeal being made in those ads.

Other Personal Health Content

Other areas of concern regarding personal health education should not be overlooked. The topical areas of dental health, genetic counseling, laboratory experimentation, and the senses are used here to demonstrate instructional strategies that can be developed in these areas. However, space limitations require that other topical areas be excluded. Consider these activities as merely illustrative of what can be done with personal health education sessions.

Dental Health

The following dental health education activities were written to be utilized in a learner-centered health education situation and to require minimal, if any, instructor interpretation and direction. Each activity is worded as it could appear on an activity card to be available to the program participant in a self-instructional setting. Of course, activities may need to be rewritten as the health educator considers the specifics of his or her own temperament, program participants, circumstances, and expectations.

1. Collect and construct a bulletin board of dental products and/or advertisements of dental products.

2. How much did you eat yesterday? List all the food you ate yesterday. Using nutrition books, look up the sugar content in each of the foods on your list. For some of the foods, you may have to note approximate measures. Measure out the total amount of sugar you ate, and put it into a bottle labeled with your name. Many chances for tooth damage?

3. Set up a dental care supply counter. Role-play a shopping trip to purchase a toothbrush, a tube of toothpaste, and a package of dental floss. Do you know all of the facts you need to make wise selections? If not, ask the health education instructor.

4. Prepare pictures, posters, and/or collages regarding the importance of brushing and flossing, flossing and brushing techniques, good nutrition, visiting your dentist.

5. Construct a chain of decay. Each factor that contributes to the decay process can be written or pictured on an individual link made of construction paper. Other pictures or words can be added to show how each link can be broken to limit decay.

6. Construct a calendar. Make the picture for each month pertain to dental health. (This would make a nice gift for someone.)

7. Write a TV commercial or short play recommending periodic professional dental exams.

8. Make up your own dental health dictionary. Record and define any word new to you connected with teeth, mouth, nutrition, general health. From all of these dictionaries, compile a dental health dictionary to be placed in a library.

9. Prepare a dental health quiz, and interview several people to determine ideas people have about modern dental health.

10. Design a bulletin board of snack foods (fruits, raw vegetables, nuts, milk, juices, and so on) to substitute for sweet snacks.

11. Plan and have a party, using such snacks as fresh fruits, dried fruits, raw vegetables, juices, milk, punches, and so on, instead of the usual party foods.

12. Out of toothpaste? Mix your own: Combine equal parts of finely powered table salt and baking soda. Add a few drops of peppermint flavoring, if available.

13. Construct a traveling dental health wagon to carry dental health messages to other groups, other schools, other worksites. Decide how you are going to present these messages. Some suggestions include plays, puppet shows, demonstrations.

Genetic Counseling

The alter ego technique is an excellent means of introducing the topic of genetic counseling and inherited diseases. Distribute the following role-playing descriptions on index cards to participants who will be acting these parts.

Betty: You are a young black woman, age 24. You come from a large family and have always wanted three children. You married Tom three years ago when you both agreed that children were a vital ingredient of a good marriage. You have sickle-cell trait but did not know it until just now.

Tom: You are a young black man, age 26. You love your wife, Betty, and want all of her life's desires to be fulfilled. You love children in general and want to have three. You are active in social issues and believe that liberalized abortion and attempts at population control are means devised by those wishing to limit the number of blacks in the United States. You have sickle-cell trait but did not know it until now.

Ellen: You are a white physician who is in the process of explaining to Betty and Tom the implications of having children for a husband and wife who both have sickle-cell trait.

Lance: You are the town's director of social services. In that role you supervise Medicaid, Medicare, and welfare departments. You were brought to this town because the taxpayers wanted fewer people to need social services, thereby decreasing their tax payments.

The participants should then be asked to imagine that Betty and Tom are in a meeting with Ellen and Lance, at which they are to be told about their sickle-cell trait, the implications of this condition, and the town's desire that they not conceive children. Betty and Tom should explain their wishes and present their arguments for having children in spite of the fact that they both have sickle-cell trait. At any time, another person can kneel behind any of the role players and speak for that person. The one kneeling will be the alter ego of the role player, expressing what he or she believes is not being said but is being felt by that role player. At the conclusion of the role-playing incident, the group will vote whether they think Betty or Tom should conceive children or not.

Several topics, which will result in much learning, may be presented during this activity:

1. Sickle-cell disease.
2. Abortion.
3. Genetic counseling.
4. Adoption.
5. Social and personal responsibility.
6. Amniocentesis and chorionic villi sampling.

Playing the Mad Scientist

An ingenious health educator can develop a not so spectacular activity into one that will long be remembered by each participant. An example of this is the health educator who can, with a little Shakespeare within, help people to behave as mad scientists. Simple experiments can be used for this purpose, two of which are described here, but the important aspect of this activity is the zaniness underlying it. Participants should be asked to wear long shirts, smocks, raincoats, or whatever can serve as a laboratory coat. In addition, they should be encouraged to bring in any accoutrements such as white cotton balls for gray hair or toy eyeglasses. Some could walk with a limp, while others might talk with an accent. In any case, most will have fun and, if the experiments are organized properly, much learning will occur.

An experiment that can be used in the mad scientist activity is one in which each person inoculates petri dishes from swabs from various areas of his/her body (throat, ears, and so on). The dish is then placed in a warm area and, if an uninoculated dish is placed alongside, the bacterial growth can be clearly observed after several days.

Another experiment that illustrates the importance of proper food handling can be conducted by boiling peeled potatoes and inoculating them with microorganisms by touching them with dirty hands or utensils. Then place the potatoes in sterile containers, keep the containers in a warm place, and observe the growth of microorganisms. Uninoculated potatoes should be used as a sterile control.

Sense Appreciation

One aspect of personal health often overlooked in health education is the development of the appreciation of one's senses. The best way to accomplish this objective is to require people to concentrate on one sense or to eliminate one sense in order to appreciate its importance. There are several ways to do this:

1. Have participants close their eyes, place their extended arms out to their sides and then, by bending their elbows, touch the tips of their noses.
2. Have participants close their eyes, taste various foods, and guess what they just tasted.
3. Play pin the tail on the donkey.
4. Have participants bend down to pick something up while standing on one foot only.
5. Have participants close their eyes, feel some object, and guess what they just felt.
6. Open the windows of the room, then have the participants close their eyes and listen to and identify as many different sounds as they can.

Valuing Activities

Included here are some examples of how values clarification may be applied to the study of personal health content.

Values Statements

Program participants can be asked to complete unfinished sentences, like the following, which will manifest their values regarding personal health:

My body _____

Bathing _____

Flossing my teeth _____

Sneezing _____

Measles _____

An ill friend_____

Sleeping is_____

Amniocentesis_____

Circadian rhythms_____

Flu vaccine _____

Values Voting

The following questions can be posed by the instructor with the participants' voting *yes* or *no* on each. Discussion should be allowed to interrupt the voting at any time.

How many of you would have a heart transplant if that was needed to lengthen your life?

How many of you think that women live longer than men because of different lifestyles?

How many of you take vitamins daily?

How many of you get regular physical examinations?

How many of you would have a second child if your first child was born genetically ill?

How many of you stay away from other people when you have a cold?

How many of you brush and floss your teeth daily?

How many of you get enough sleep?

How many of you feel better in the morning than later in the day?

How many of you often feel tense?

Consistency Check

The consistency check is an interesting way to consider the degree to which people behave consistently with their thoughts and/or feelings. Ask people to fill out this handout:

You have an important test to take but you wake up that morning with a 101° fever. Relative to attending class,

What are you thinking you should do?_____

How do you feel? _____

What would you usually do? _____

How consistent is your behavior with your thoughts and/or feelings? _____

Here are other leading statements that can be considered similarly:

1. It's a Saturday, and when you awaken you notice it is only 8 A.M. (A decision regarding the choice of whether you go back to sleep or wake up.)

2. You are contemplating flossing your teeth, but you would rather watch television.

3. You are in a car with someone who is smoking a cigarette.

4. One of your friends is making fun of someone who practices transcendental meditation twice daily.

5. An instructor is doing something that is unhealthful.

6. You have sickle-cell trait and want to marry someone who also has sickle-cell trait.

7. A friend of yours is having an epileptic seizure.

8. A close friend is told by a physician that he or she has terminal cancer.

Values Continuum

For each of these questions, ask participants to place themselves on the continuum.

Always   Never

1. I brush my teeth daily.
2. I floss my teeth daily.
3. Physical health is more important than mental health.
4. Appearance is more important than health.
5. Schools and worksites are concerned with students' and employees' health.
6. My health education instructor is healthy.
7. It's as important to smell good as to be healthy.
8. I use a deodorant.
9. I use hair spray.
10. Epileptics who have seizures should be allowed to participate in sports.
11. People with sickle-cell trait should be allowed to marry.
12. Married couples who have a history of mental retardation in either family should have children.
13. Children not inoculated against childhood diseases should be allowed to attend school.
14. I wash my hands before eating anything.
15. Candy machines should be allowed in school or office buildings.
16. People with HIV should be allowed to marry.

Values Sheet

The purpose of this activity is to explore personal health behavior and to relate personal values to that behavior. Participants are given a handout on which is presented a statement for their consideration. After the statement is read they are to answer the questions below it. Here is an example of a values sheet that concerns itself with physical health behavior:

Each of us has habits that can be considered healthful, and each of us has habits that are unhealthful. Considering your *physical* health: What three habits of yours can you think of that are unhealthful?

1. _____
2. _____
3. _____

Why do you do these things?

1. _____
2. _____
3. _____

What are the consequences of continuing these unhealthful behaviors?

1. _____
2. _____
3. _____

Filling in Blanks

Still another means of exploring the values behind unhealthful behaviors is to fill in blanks of sentences designed for this purpose. Once the value is identified, other more healthful behaviors may be substituted that will meet the same needs. An example of the standard sentences that can be used for this purpose is

> I (unhealthful behavior) because it (why you do it). The value underlying this behavior is (the value). A more healthy way of achieving this need would be (healthful behavior). I (will or will not)(the new behavior) by (date).

These completed sentences might appear as

> I smoke cigarettes because it makes me appear grown up. The value underlying this behavior is independence. A more healthy way of achieving this need would be earning money at a job after school. I will get a job by two weeks from today.

Participants should be asked to keep a record of these completed sentences in a personal diary, and to note which timetables have been met and which have not. In this way, they will be required to assume responsibility for their own health-related behavior.

Giving Up

This activity can be used to achieve several health education objectives: It can help participants to experience the difficulty one has in quitting smoking; it can help them appreciate the difficulty of living one's life with a handicap that prohibits particular behaviors (for example, no contact sports for a child with a plastic heart-valve insert); or it can be used to demonstrate the relative values of the maintenance of physical health versus short-term gratification. When it is used for this latter purpose, participants are asked to give up, for one week, something *important to them.* Some may choose not to watch television for a week, others not to eat snacks between meals that week, or still others to refrain from sports activities that week. Whatever is given up, however, must be valued by the person giving it up. At the conclusion of that week, participants are asked to consider the following:

1. How difficult was it giving up something you valued? Explain.
2. How did you feel the first time you were able to, once again, do the thing you gave up?
3. How did you feel when you did it?

4. Did you substitute anything during the week for the thing you gave up? If yes, what was it?

5. Do you value the thing you gave up more now than before you gave it up?

6. Are there some people who can never, for whatever reason, do the thing you gave up? (For instance, people who are blind can never watch television.)

7. How do you think they feel?

8. What could you do for such a person if you knew one?

9. What other conditions result in having to give things up?

10. Do people with such conditions find other things to value? Or do they find other activities to manifest their values?

The Patient

An activity that will help people explore the consequences of uncontrolled communicable diseases and to examine the values involved in the decision-making process related to such diseases involves their responding in small groups to the following handout (Engs et al. 1975, 125–126):*

> You are a highly trained group called County Medical Helpers. Each of you has been specifically trained to administer first aid, recognize communicable diseases, and set up appointments for the doctor. Your primary responsibilities are to visit the residents of your county and identify those people who need medical assistance.
>
> The people in your rural community are poor and uneducated.
>
> There is only one traveling doctor who visits once a week. He makes the final diagnosis and treatment. The day before his regular visit you are informed that the doctor will have enough time to see only five patients. You are to bring them to the church basement, which is used for the doctor's office. Your group has identified 10 people who need medical assistance. Your job is to select the five who will see the doctor.
>
> 1. Mary, age 79, severe cold, chronic cough, possible pneumonia.
>
> 2. John, age 15, suspected tuberculosis.
>
> 3. Bobby, age 9, sudden fever, weakness, coughing, aching pain in back and extremities, possible influenza.
>
> 4. Susan, age 19, home from college, symptoms indicate polio or mononucleosis.
>
> 5. Sam, age 24, syphilis.
>
> 6. Linda, age 43, infectious hepatitis.
>
> 7. Mary, age 5, trachoma.
>
> 8. Virginia, age 7, smallpox.
>
> 9. Charles, age 54, HIV.
>
> 10. Butch, age 29, polio.

The following questions then give focus to a discussion of this activity:

1. Did all group members agree on the five patients who were to see the doctor?

2. What considerations were given to your choices?

---

*From Engs et al., *Health Games Students Play,* © 1975 by Kendall/Hunt Publishing Company. Used with permission.

3. Which five did your group select and why?

4. What are the consequences for the patients not selected?

5. What might have been done to prevent these 10 people from acquiring their diseases?

Summary

This chapter concerned itself with personal health education instructional strategies. You saw how such topics as communicable diseases, noncommunicable diseases, physical fitness, consumer health, and other personal health topics (for example, dental health and genetics) can be taught in an interesting manner, one that actively involves learners in the educational process. The result will be enhanced learning of the content.

The strategies presented in this chapter are but a smattering of possible learner-centered instructional activities for personal health education. You should feel limited only by your own imagination and willingness to consult other sources for additional ideas. Personal health need not be the dull, tedious, and uninteresting subject that too many health educators turn it into. *You* can do better! Just remember to involve your program's participants along the way.

PART FOUR

CONCLUSION

At the end of a book of this sort several requirements present themselves. First, a summary seems in order. Second, the reasons for describing over 200 learner-centered instructional strategies need to be reiterated. And third, encouragement for the type of health education advocated in this book can be offered. All of these tasks will be accomplished in this closing chapter.

Health Education in Summary

As conducted in its traditional form, health education consists of objectives, content, learning experiences, and instructional materials designed to encourage the adoption of behaviors on the part of program participants — behaviors predetermined to be healthful. Health education takes place in schools, in places of work, in medical care settings such as hospitals and health maintenance organizations, and in other community settings. Health education is concerned with *health,* which we defined as a quality of life that is a function of social health, mental health, emotional health, spiritual health, and physical health. In addition to health, health education is concerned with *wellness,* which we defined as the integration of the five components of health, and with *high-level wellness,* which we defined as the integration and *balance* of the five health components. The rationale for health education pertains to the current societal emphasis on the rising cost of health care, the fear regarding the spread of HIV/AIDS, the achievement of the nation's health objectives, a feeling of social responsibility to help people be healthy, a suspected cost benefit associated with preventing unnecessary use of the health care system so as to decrease health insurance premiums and to increase productivity, and an added benefit that recruiters can point to when attempting to convince people to join a community or place of work.

Health education as advocated in this book is defined as a process in which the goal is to free people so that they may make health-related decisions based on their needs and interests as long as these decisions do not adversely affect others. To offer this newer form of health education requires freeing people of such enslaving factors as low self-esteem, high alienation, feelings of inferiority and loneliness, values confusion, an excessive external locus of control, and poor health-related knowledge and skills. This form of health education raises several ethical issues that the health educator must consider. For example, is it ethical to predetermine how people ought to behave — even if we call that behavior healthy — and then program them through learning experiences to behave that way? What is the health educator's responsibility when observing other health educators behaving unethically? To provide guidance on these and other professional ethical issues, the Code of Ethics for the Health Education Profession was presented.

We also considered evaluation of health education, in particular *what* is being evaluated. In the traditional form of health education, behavioral change is the goal and is therefore the focus of evaluation. In the newer form of health education advocated in this book, the focus of the evaluation process becomes the *way* in which learners have arrived at their decisions, rather than their actual decisions. These evaluation foci stem from the objectives that differ in these two forms of health education. In one case the objectives are to get people to adopt healthful behaviors, whereas in the other form it is to free people to make their own decisions. Furthermore, we differentiated between outcome evaluation and process evaluation and described the difficulty of measuring long-range objectives in health education when the effects of instruction may be like seeds that take root but whose fruit isn't evident until some time later.

In addition, we discussed service-learning as one means of responding to the pervasive health needs of communities and underserved populations. Service-learning was described as a way to allow learners to apply what they learn in health education by participating in community service activities. Learners thereby learn health education content more completely, and the community benefits from the service provided. Suggestions for conducting service-learning were presented, including several different ways to direct learners to reflect on the meaning of their community service activities.

Last, to help health educators more easily adopt the Health Education as Freeing concept into their professional practice, over 200 instructional strategies that allow for the learner to become actively involved in his or her own learning were presented.

Learning Experiences in This Book

Each of the over 200 instructional strategies presented in this book requires students of health education to become active in the learning process. In a sense, the learners become partners with the health educator, both seeking a goal that pertains to a better quality of life through being healthier. Many of the activities presented may require the participation of people not immediately associated with the particular health education setting (for example, the use of the aged in school health education classes) or may require an environment other than the particular setting for the activity being conducted (for example, outdoor sense appreciation activities). In this manner, program participants will better appreciate that they are but a part of a larger group of people, community, school, workplace, or medical care facility. This sense of attachment to other things and people in their environments will develop in program participants the attitude of concern and caring that health education should include as one of its most important objectives. For not only is the health of the individual learner of importance, but the health of the whole organization or community is of importance as well. None of us can be as healthy as we might be if the places where we go to school, where we work, where we obtain health care, or where we live are not as health enhancing as they might be.

This recommended form of health education significantly changes the role of the health educator. Students are involved in the instructional activities presented in this book by requiring them to uncover information, draw inferences, identify feelings, or discover insights by their own actions. The role of the health educator, then, is transposed from one of being active (lecturing) to one of helping others be meaningfully active (process leader, facilitator of learning, or whatever other name suits the fancy of those who create pedagogical titles). This change in role creates a health educator who will serve as a resource for the learners, working *with* them instead of *on* them.

It should be noted, though, that while the activities included in this book are interesting and motivating for students, this is not justification alone for incorporating them into the reader's health education program. The additional, and even more important, consideration is that they contribute to the achievement of objectives in health education. Cognizant of this concern, I have related each learning experience to the health education objective that experience is designed to achieve. The reader should have clear in his or her own mind the reason for choosing a learning experience. Too often in the past, such activities have been used without the health educator being able to justify, educationally, their use.

The Hope for the Future

Several years back, a book of this sort would not have been published. Health instruction, and education in general, was not considered fun. That is, learning was serious business consisting of hard work and extreme sacrifice. The fact that the reader is now holding this book attests to the direction in which all of education is moving — health education along with the rest. The movement is toward the participation of people in a learning process whose objectives relate to people knowing themselves, others, and their environments better than has routinely been the case. It is my hope that, in some way, this book contributes to that movement.

Getting There

Health educators interested in adopting learner-centered health instruction might want to consider trying one or two of the activities in this book prior to adopting this approach in total. Different health educators and different participant–personality mixes might necessitate local adaptations of the activities herein proposed. An initial, slow phasing in of these activities and of this approach to health education is therefore recommended.

In addition, health educators should not be afraid of consulting with colleagues who have previously employed learner-centered forms of education. Trial and error are only necessary where others have not tried before. Profit from the mistakes of others; don't repeat their mistakes. Program participants can also be good sources of feedback to the health educator who is attempting to adopt a new form of education.

Last, colleges and universities often offer courses in humanistic education and/or methods of instruction in which health educators can enroll. The health educator desiring to become more proficient should consult local colleges about such courses. Similar courses may be offered as a workshop sponsored by the in-service component of a local school district or by community health departments and agencies. Often experts in values clarification and/or humanistic education are brought to town with the goal of introducing such approaches to education. Local newspapers usually announce such visits, so paying attention to newspapers is a good means of becoming aware of these opportunities.

To the Reader

It would be remiss of me to conclude such a book without a personal comment to the reader. Writing this book has been fun, profitable (I hope), and personally and professionally rewarding. However, only the reader can make the time spent on this project worthwhile. Only the employment of the activities included in this book, and the manifestation of concern for the program participants I have attempted to convey, will make the time spent (mine in writing and yours in reading) a useful, rather than wasteful, enterprise. As a football coach might say: The ball's in your hands — run with it.

Use the book in good health.

CODE OF ETHICS FOR THE
HEALTH EDUCATION PROFESSION

Preamble

The health education profession is dedicated to excellence in the practice of promoting individual, family, organizational, and community health. Guided by common ideals, health educators are responsible for upholding the integrity and ethics of the profession as they face the daily challenges of making decisions. By acknowledging the value of diversity in society and embracing a cross-cultural approach, health educators support the worth, dignity, potential, and uniqueness of all people.

The code of ethics provides a framework of shared values within which health education is practiced. The code of ethics is grounded in fundamental ethical principles that underlie all health care services: respect for autonomy, promotion of social justice, active promotion of good, and avoidance of harm. The responsibility of each health educator is to aspire to the highest possible standards of conduct and to encourage the ethical behavior of all those with whom they work.

Regardless of job title, professional affiliation, work setting, or population served, health educa-tors abide by these guidelines when making professional decisions.

Article I: Responsibility to the Public

A health educator's ultimate responsibility is to educate people for the purpose of promoting, maintaining, and improving individual, family, and community health. When a conflict of interest arises among individuals, groups, organizations, agencies, or institutions, health educators must consider all issues and give priority to those that promote wellness and quality of living through principles of self-determination and freedom of choice for the individual.

Section 1: Health educators support the right of individuals to make informed decisions regarding health, as long as such decisions pose no threat to the health of others.

Section 2: Health educators encourage actions and social policies that support and facilitate the best balance of benefits over harm for all affected parties.

Section 3: Health educators accurately communicate the potential benefits and consequences of

---

Capwell, E., Smith, B., Shirreffs, J., Olsen, L. *Development of a Unified Code of Ethics for the Health Education Profession.* Westerville, OH: Coalition of National Health Education Organizations, November 14, 1999.

the services and programs with which they are associated.

Section 4: Health educators accept the responsibility to act on issues that can adversely affect the health of individuals, families, and communities.

Section 5: Health educators are truthful about their qualifications and the limitations of their expertise and provide services consistent with their competencies.

Section 6: Health educators protect the privacy and dignity of individuals.

Section 7: Health educators actively involve individuals, groups, and communities in the entire educational process so that all aspects of the process are clearly understood by those who may be affected.

Section 8: Health educators respect and acknowledge the rights of others to hold diverse values, attitudes, and opinions.

Section 9: Health educators provide services equitably to all people.

Article II: Responsibility to the Profession

Health educators are responsible for their professional behavior, for the reputation of their profession, and for promoting ethical conduct among their colleagues.

Section 1: Health educators maintain, improve, and expand their professional competence through continued study and education; membership, participation, and leadership in professional organizations; and involvement in issues related to the health of the public.

Section 2: Health educators model and encourage nondiscriminatory standards of behavior in their interactions with others.

Section 3: Health educators encourage and accept responsible critical discourse to protect and enhance the profession.

Section 4: Health educators contribute to the development of the profession by sharing the processes and outcomes of their work.

Section 5: Health educators are aware of possible professional conflicts of interest, exercise integrity in conflict situations, and do not manipulate or violate the rights of others.

Section 6: Health educators give appropriate recognition to others for their professional contributions and achievements.

Article III: Responsibility to Employers

Health educators recognize the boundaries of their professional competence and are accountable for their professional activities and actions.

Section 1: Health educators accurately represent their qualifications and the qualifications of others whom they recommend.

Section 2: Health educators use appropriate standards, theories, and guidelines as criteria when carrying out their professional responsibilities.

Section 3: Health educators accurately represent potential service and program outcomes to employers.

Section 4: Health educators anticipate and disclose competing commitments, conflicts of interest, and endorsement of products.

Section 5: Health educators openly communicate to employers expectations or job-related assignments that conflict with their professional ethics.

Section 6: Health educators maintain competence in their areas of professional practice.

Article IV: Responsibility in the Delivery of Health Education

Health educators promote integrity in the delivery of health education. They respect the rights, dignity, confidentiality, and worth of all people by adapting strategies and methods to the needs of diverse populations and communities.

Section 1: Health educators are sensitive to social and cultural diversity and are in accord with the law when planning and implementing programs.

Section 2: Health educators are informed of the latest advances in theory, research, and practice, and use strategies and methods that are grounded in and contribute to development of professional standards, theories, guidelines, statistics, and experience.

Section 3: Health educators are committed to rigorous evaluation of both program effectiveness and the methods used to achieve results.

Section 4: Health educators empower individuals to adopt healthy lifestyles through informed choice rather than by coercion or intimidation.

Section 5: Health educators communicate the potential outcomes of proposed services, strategies, and pending decisions to all individuals who will be affected.

Article V: Responsibility in Research and Evaluation

Health educators contribute to the health of the population and to the profession through research and evaluation activities. When planning and conducting research or evaluation, health educators do so in accordance with federal and state laws and regulations, organizational and institutional policies, and professional standards.

Section 1: Health educators support principles and practices of research and evaluation that do no harm to individuals, groups, society, or the environment.

Section 2: Health educators ensure that participation in research is voluntary and is based on the informed consent of the participants.

Section 3: Health educators respect the privacy, rights, and dignity of research participants, and honor commitments made to those participants.

Section 4: Health educators treat all information obtained from participants as confidential unless otherwise required by law.

Section 5: Health educators take credit, including authorship, only for work they have actually performed and give credit to the contributions of others.

Section 6: Health educators who serve as research or evaluation consultants discuss their results only with those to whom they are providing service, unless maintaining such confidentiality would jeopardize the health or safety of others.

Section 7: Health educators report the results of their research and evaluation objectively, accurately, and in a timely fashion.

Article VI: Responsibility in Professional Preparation

Those involved in the preparation and training of health educators have an obligation to accord learners the same respect and treatment given other groups by providing quality education that benefits the profession and the public.

Section 1: Health educators select students for professional preparation programs based on equal opportunity for all and the individual's academic performance, abilities, and potential contribution to the profession and the public's health.

Section 2: Health educators strive to make the educational environment and culture conducive to the health of all involved and free from sexual harassment and all forms of discrimination.

Section 3: Health educators involved in professional preparation and professional development engage in careful preparation; present material that is accurate, up-to-date, and timely; provide reasonable and timely feedback; state clear and reasonable expectations; and conduct fair assessments and evaluations of learners.

Section 4: Health educators provide objective and accurate counseling to learners about career opportunities, development, and advancement, and assist learners to secure professional employment.

Section 5: Health educators provide adequate supervision and meaningful opportunities for the professional development of learners.

TOLL-FREE NUMBERS
FOR HEALTH INFORMATION

Advocacy Center for the Elderly and Disabled
(800) 662-7705 (within Louisiana)
210 O'Keefe Ave., Suite 700
New Orleans, LA 70112

Akron Regional Poison Control Center
Children's Hospital Medical Center of Akron
(800) 362-9922 (within Ohio)
281 Locust St.
Akron, OH 44308

Alabama Department of Health
AIDS Program
(800) 228-0469 (within Alabama)
State Office Building, Room 662
434 Monroe St.
Montgomery, AL 36130

Alabama Poison Center
(800) 462-0800 (within Alabama)
809 University Blvd., E
Tuscaloosa, AL 35401

AL-ANON Family Group Headquarters
(800) 344-2666
1372 Broadway
New York, NY 10018-0862

Alcoholism and Drug Addiction Treatment
Center
(800) 382-4357
McDonald Center
Scripps Memorial Hospital
9904 Genesee Ave.
La Jolla, CA 92037

Alcohol Rehab for the Elderly
(800) 354-7089
(800) 344-0824 (within Illinois)
P.O. Box 267
Hopedale, IL 61747

Alzheimer's Association
(800) 621-0379
(800) 572-6037 (within Illinois)
70 E. Lake St., #600
Chicago, IL 60601

AMC Cancer Information Line
(800) 525-3777
1600 Pierce St.
Denver, CO 80214

American Academy of Allergy and Immunology
(800) 822-2762

This information is reprinted with permission from the *Journal of Health Education.* The *Journal of Health Education* is a publication of the American Alliance for Health, Physical Education, Recreation and Dance, 1900 Association Drive, Reston, Virginia 22091.

611 East Wells St.
Milwaukee, WI 53202

American Academy of Pediatrics (AAP)
(800) 433-9016
(800) 421-0589 (within Illinois)
141 NW Point Rd.
P.O. Box 927
Elk Grove, IL 60007

American Cancer Society
National Office
(800) ACS-2345 (within each state with a
divisional office)
1599 Clifton Rd. N.E.
Atlanta, GA 30329

American College of Legal Medicine
(800) 433-9137
P.O. Box 3190
Maple Glen, PA 19002

American College of Physicians
(800) 523-1546
Independence Mall West
6th St. at Race
Philadelphia, PA 19104

American Council of the Blind (ACB)
National Legislative Hotline
(800) 424-8666
1010 Vermont Ave., N.W., Suite 1100
Washington, DC 20005

American Council on Transplantation
(800) ACT-GIVE
P.O. Box 1709
Alexandria, VA 22313-1709

American Diabetes Association
(800) 232-3472
1660 Duke St.
Alexandria, VA 22314

American Foundation for the Blind
(800) 232-5463
15 W. 16th St.
New York, NY 10011

American Kidney Fund
(800) 638-8299
(800) 492-8361 (within Maryland)
6110 Executive Blvd., Suite 1010
Rockville, MD 20852

American Leprosy Missions
(800) 543-3131
1 Broadway
Elmwood Park, NJ 07407

American Liver Foundation
(800) 223-0179
1425 Pompton Avenue
Cedar Grove, NJ 07009

American Mental Health Counselors Association
(AMHCA)
(800) 326-2642
5999 Stevenson Ave.
Alexandria, VA 22304

American Paralysis Association
(800) 225-0292
P.O. Box 187
Short Hills, NJ 07078

American Parkinson Disease Association
(800) 223-2732
116 John St., Suite 417
New York, NY 10038

American Schizophrenia Association
(800) 783-3801
900 N. Federal Highway
Boca Raton, FL 33432
(See also: Huxley Institute for Biosocial
Research)

American Social Health Association
(800) 227-8922 (National STD Hotline)
(800) 342-AIDS (National AIDS Hotline)
(800) 344-SIDA (Spanish)
(800) AIDS-TTY (Hearing Impaired)
P.O. Box 13827
Research Triangle Park, NC 27709

American Society for Psychoprophylaxis in
Obstetrics (ASPO/LAMAZE)

(800) 368-4404
1840 Wilson Blvd., Suite 204
Arlington, VA 22201

American Society of Plastic and Reconstructive
Surgeons
(800) 635-0635
444 E. Algonquin Rd.
Arlington Heights, IL 60005

American Trauma Society
(800) 556-7890 (outside Maryland)
1400 Mercantile Lane, Suite 188
Landover, MD 20785

Amyotrophic Lateral Sclerosis Association
(ALSA)
(800) 782-4747
21021 Ventura Blvd.
Woodland Hills, CA 91364

Anchorage Poison Center
Providence Hospital
(800) 478-3193 (within Alaska)
P.O. Box 196604
Anchorage, AK 99519-0604

Arizona Department of Health
Office of Health Education
(800) 334-1540 (within Arizona)
431 North 24th St.
Phoenix, AZ 85008

Arizona Poison and Drug Information Center
University of Arizona
(800) 362-0101 (within Arizona)
Arizona Health Sciences Center
Tucson, AZ 85724

Arkansas Department of Health
AIDS Activities
(800) 445-7720 (within Arkansas)
4815 West Markham
Little Rock, AR 72205

Arthritis Foundation
(800) 283-7800
1314 Spring St. N.W.
Atlanta, GA 30309

Association of Surgical Technologisis
(800) 637-7433
8307 Shaffer Parkway
Littleton, CO 80127

Be Healthy, Inc.
Positive Pregnancy and Parenting Fitness
(800) 433-5523
51 Saltrock Road
Baltic, CT 06330

Better Hearing Institute
(800) 424-8576
Box 1840
Washington, DC 20013

Blind Children's Center
(800) 222-3566
(800) 222-3567 (within California)
4120 Marathon St.
P.O. Box 29159
Los Angeles, CA 90029-0159

Blodgett Regional Poison Center
Blodgett Medical Center
(800) 632-2727 (within Michigan)
1840 Wealthy St., S.E.
Grand Rapids, MI 49506

Blue Ridge Poison Center
Box 67 Blue Ridge Hospital
University of Virginia
(800) 451-1428
Charlottesville, VA 22901

Bulimia Anorexia Self-Help (B.A.S.H.)
(800) BASH-STL
(800) 762-3334 (24 hours)
6125 Clayton Ave., Suite 215
St. Louis, MO 63139-3295

California Department of Health
Office of AIDS
(800) 367-2347 (within Northern California)
P.O. Box 160146
Sacramento, CA 95816

California Self-Help Center
(800) 222-LINK (within California)

2349 Franz Hall
405 Hilgard Ave.
Los Angeles, CA 90024

California Teratogen Registry
University of California at San Diego
(800) 532-3749 (within California)
Department of Pediatrics, H-814-B
225 Dickinson St.
San Diego, CA 92103

Cancer Information Service
(800) 4-CANCER (in various states and regions)
(800) 524-1234 (within Hawaii)
(800) 638-6070 (within Alaska)
Office of Cancer Communications, NCI, NIH
Bldg. 31, Rm. 10A24
9000 Rockville Pike
Bethesda, MD 20892

Cardinal Glennon Children's Hospital Regional
Poison Center
(800) 392-9111 (within Missouri)
1465 S. Grand Blvd.
St. Louis, MO 63104

Center for Self-Help
Riverwood Center
(800) 336-0341 (within Michigan)
P.O. Box 547
Benton Harbor, MI 49022-0547

Central and Southern Illinois Regional Poison
Resource Center
St. John's Hospital
(800) 252-2022 (within Illinois)
800 E. Carpenter St.
Springfield, IL 62769

Central New York Poison Control Center
Upstate Medical Center
(800) 252-5655 (within New York)
750 E. Adams St.
Syracuse, NY 13210

Central Ohio Poison Control Center
Children's Hospital
(800) 682-7625 (within Ohio)

700 Children's Dr.
Columbus, OH 43205

Central Washington Poison Center
Yakima Valley Memorial Hospital
(800) 572-9176 (within Washington)
2811 Tieton Dr.
Yakima, WA 98902

Chicago and Northeastern Illinois Regional
Poison Control Center
Rush-Presbyterian-St. Luke's Medical Center
(800) 942-5969 (within Illinois)
1753 W. Congress Pkwy.
Chicago, IL 60612

Child Help USA
(800) 422-4453
6463 Independence Ave.
Woodland Hills, CA 91367

Children's Hospice International
(800) 242-4453
1101 King Street, #131
Alexandria, VA 22314

Children's Hospital of Alabama Poison
Control Center
(800) 292-6678 (within Alabama)
1600 Seventh Ave., S.
Birmingham, AL 35233

Children's Hospital of Michigan
Poison Control Center
(800) 462-6642 (within Michigan)
3901 Beaubien Blvd.
Detroit, MI 48201

Cleft Palate Foundation
(800) 242-5338
1218 Grandview Ave.
Pittsburgh, PA 15211

Clinical Genetic Services Center, Michigan
Henry Ford Hospital
Medical Genetics and Birth Defects Center
(800) 421-7946 (within Michigan)
2799 West Grand Blvd.
Detroit, MI 48202

Clinical Genetic Services Center, Oregon
Emanuel Hospital
Department of Medical Genetics
(800) 452-7032 Ext. 4726 (within Oregon)
2801 North Gantenbein Ave.
Portland, OR 97227

Clinical Genetic Services Center, Pennsylvania
Pennsylvania Hospital
Division of Perinatology
(800) 336-5633
Spruce Building
8th and Spruce Sts.
Philadelphia, PA 19107

Commission on Professional and Hospital
Activities
(800) 521-6210
(800) 828-6762 (within Michigan)
1968 Green Road
Ann Arbor, MI 48106

Consumer Health Information Resource Institute
(800) 821-6671
3030 Baltimore
Kansas City, MO 64108

Consumer Product Safety Commission (CPSC)
(800) 638-2772 (Product Safety Line)
(800) 638-8270 (TTY National)
(800) 492-8104 (TTY Maryland)
Washington, DC 20207

Contact Lens Manufacturers Association
(800) 343-5367
2000 M St. N.W.
Washington, DC 20036

Cooley's Anemia Foundation
(800) 221-3571
105 East 22nd St.
New York, NY 10010

Cornelia De Lange Syndrome Foundation
(800) 223-8355
(Birth defects information)
60 Dyer Ave.
Collinsville, CT 06022

Covenant House
(800) 999-9999
(Homeless youth-various locations in U.S. and
Canada)
460 West 41st St.
New York, NY 10036

Cystic Fibrosis Foundation
(800) 344-4823
6931 Arlington Rd.
Bethesda, MD 20814

Deafness Research Foundation
(800) 535-3323
9 E. 38th St., 7th Fl.
New York, NY 10016

Devereux Foundation
(800) 345-1292
(Treatment of emotionally, developmentally, and
mentally handicapped)
19 S. Waterloo Rd.
Devon, PA 19333

Device Experience Network
Division of Product Surveillance
Office of Compliance and Surveillance
Center for Devices and Radiological Health
(FDA)
(800) 638-6725
FDA HFZ-343
8757 Georgia Ave.
Silver Spring, MD 20910

Duke University Poison Control Center
Duke University Medical Center
(800) 672-1697 (within North Carolina)
Durham, NC 27710

Edna Gladney Center
(800) 433-2922
(800) 772-2740 (within Texas)
(Maternity home and infant placement agency)
2300 Hemphill
Fort Worth, TX 76110

Emergency Planning and Community Right-to-
Know Hotline

Environmental Protection Agency
(800) 535-0202
401 M St. S.W.
Washington, DC 20460

Encore
(800) 932-0912 (within Pennsylvania)
(Drug and alcohol information)
Health and Welfare Building
6th & Commonwealth
Harrisburg, PA 17120

Endometriosis Association
(800) 992-ENDO
P.O. Box 92187
Milwaukee, WI 53202

Epilepsy Foundation of America
(800) EFA-1000 (outside Maryland)
4351 Garden City Dr., Suite 406
Landover, MD 20785

Facial Plastic Surgery Information Service
(800) 332-FACE (USA)
(800) 523-FACE (Canada)
1101 Vermont Ave., N.W., Suite 304
Washington, DC 20005

Familial Polyposis Registry
Cleveland Clinic Foundation
Dept. of Colorectal Surgery
(800) 321-5398
Cleveland, OH 44106

Family Pharmaceuticals of America
(800) 922-3444
966 Houston Northcutt Blvd.
Mt. Pleasant, SC 29465-1288

Family Survival Project for Brain Damaged
Adults
(800) 445-8106 (within California)
425 Bush St., Suite 500
San Francisco, CA 94108

Florida Department of Health-Rehabilitation
State Aids Hotline
(800) FLA-AIDS (within Florida)
1317 Winewood Blvd.

Bldg. 6, Room 453
Tallahassee, FL 32399

Florida Poison Information Center at the Tampa
General Hospital
(800) 282-3171 (within Florida)
P.O. Box 1289
Tampa, FL 33601

Food Safety and Inspection Service
Meat and Poultry Hotline
(800) 535-4555
Department of Agriculture, Room 1165-S
Washington, DC 20250

Foster Parents Plan, Inc.
(800) 556-7918
155 Plan Way
Warwick, RI 02886

Foundation Center
(800) 424-9836
79 5th Ave. at 16th St.
New York, NY 10003

Fragile X Foundation
(800) 835-2246, x58
P.O. Box 300233
Denver, CO 80220

Fresno Regional Poison Control Center of Fresno
Community Hospital and Medical Center
(800) 346-5922
Fresno & R Sts.
Fresno, CA 93715

Georgia Department of Human Resources
AID ATLANTA
(800) 876-9944 (AIDS Information Line)
1132 W. Peachtree St., N.E., Suite 112
Atlanta, GA 30309

Georgia Poison Control Center
Grady Memorial Hospital
(800) 282-5846 (within Georgia)
80 Butler St., S.E.
Atlanta, GA 30335-3801

Great Lakes Poison Center
Bronson Methodist Hospital

(800) 442-4112 (within Area Code 616)
252 E. Lovell St.
Kalamazoo, MI 49001

Guide Dog Foundation for the Blind
(800) 548-4337
371 E. Jericho Turnpike
Smithtown, NY 11787

Hawaii Poison Center
Kapiolani-Children's Medical Center
(800) 362-3585 (within Hawaii)
1319 Punahou St.
Honolulu, HI 96826

Health Resources and Services Administration
Bureau of Health Maintenance Organizations and
Resources
Office of Health Facilities
(800) 492-0359 (English & Spanish, within
Maryland)
(800) 638-0742 (English & Spanish, outside
Maryland)
5600 Fishers Lane
Rockville, MD 20857

Healthy Mothers, Healthy Babies Coalition
(800) 533-8811
409 12th St. S.W.
Washington, DC 20024-2188

Hearing Helpline
(800) 424-8576
P.O. Box 1840
Washington, DC 20013

Helpline
(800) 346-2211 (within New York)
22 West Third St.
Corning, NY 14830

Higher Education and Adult Training for People
with Handicaps Resource Center
(800) 544-3284
1 Dupont Circle
Washington, DC 20036-1193

Hospice Education Institute
(800) 331-1620

5 Essex Square, Suite 3-B
Essex, CT 06426-0713

Human Growth Foundation
(800) 451-6434
(Child growth abnormalities)
7777 Leesburg Pike, Suite 202S
Falls Church, VA 22043

Huntington's Disease Society of America
(800) 345-4372
140 W. 22nd St., 6th Fl.
New York, NY 10011-2420

Huxley Institute for Biosocial Research
(800) 847-3802
900 North Federal Highway
Boca Raton, FL 33432
(See also: American Schizophrenia Association)

Idaho Poison Control Center
St. Alphonsus Regional Medical Center
(800) 632-8000 (within Idaho)
1055 N. Curtis Rd.
Boise, ID 83704

Illinois Department of Health
Health Education
(State AIDS Hotline)
(800) 243-2438 (within Illinois)
525 West Jefferson
Springfield, IL 62761

Illinois Teratogen Information Service
(800) 252-4847 (within Illinois)
836 West Wellington
Chicago, IL 60657

Indiana Department of Aging and Community
Services
(800) 545-7764 (within Indiana)
251 N. Illinois St.
P.O. Box 7083
Indianapolis, IN 46207-7083

Indiana Poison Center
Methodist Hospital of Indiana
(800) 382-9097 (within Indiana)

1701 N. Senate Blvd.
Indianapolis, IN 46206

Information Center for Individuals with
Disabilities
(800) 462-5015 (within Massachusetts)
20 Park Plaza, Room 330
Boston, MA 02116

Institute of Logopedics
(800) 835-1043
(Programs for multiply handicapped children)
2400 Jardine Dr.
Wichita, KS 67219

Intermountain Regional Poison Control Center
(800) 456-7707 (within Utah)
50 N. Medical Dr., Bldg. 528
Salt Lake City, UT 84132

Job Accommodation Network
(800) 526-7234
(800) 526-4698 (within West Virginia)
West Virginia University
809 Allen Hall
P.O. Box 6122
Morgantown, WV 26506-6122

Joseph and Rose Kennedy Institute of Ethics
National Reference Center for Bioethics
Literature
(800) MED-ETHX
Georgetown University
Washington, DC 20057

Just Say No International
(800) 258-2766
1777 North California Blvd.
Walnut Creek, CA 94596

Juvenile Diabetes Foundation (JDF)
(800) 223-1138
432 Park Ave. S., 16th Floor
New York, NY 10016

Kansas Department of Health and Environment
Office of Health Education
(State AIDS Hotline)
(800) 232-0040 (within Kansas)

Mills Building, Suite 605
Topeka, KS 66612

Kansas Department on Aging
(800) 432-3535 (within Kansas)
Docking State Office Building, 122-S
915 S.W. Harrison
Topeka, KS 66612-1500

Kentucky Department for Health Services
AIDS Health Education
(800) 654-AIDS (within Kentucky)
275 Main St.
Frankfort, KY 40621

Kentucky Regional Poison Center of Kosair
Children's Hospital
(800) 722-5725 (within Kentucky)
P.O. Box 35070
Louisville, KY 40232-5070

Kevin Collins Foundation for Missing Children
(800) 272-0012
Box 590473
San Francisco, CA 94159

Kidsrights
(800) 892-5437
3700 Progress Blvd.
Mount Dora, FL 32757

Living Bank
(800) 528-2971
P.O. Box 6725
Houston, TX 77265

Lorain Community Hospital
Poison Control Center
(800) 821-8972
3700 Kolbe Rd.
Lorain, OH 44053

Los Angeles County Medical Association
Regional Poison Center
(800) 825-2722
(800) 777-6476
1925 Wilshire Blvd.
Los Angeles, CA 90057

Louisiana Office of Prevention Medicine and
Public Health Services
State AIDS Hotline
(800) 992-4379 (within Louisiana)
325 Loyola Ave., Room 615
New Orleans, LA 70012

Lupus Foundation of America
(800) 558-0121
1717 Massachusetts Ave, N.W., Suite 203
Washington, DC 20036

Maine Bureau of Health
Office on AIDS
(800) 851-AIDS (within Maine)
State House, Station 11
Augusta, ME 04333

Maine Poison Control Center at Maine Medical
Center
(800) 442-6305 (within Maine)
22 Bramhall St.
Portland, ME 04102

Mary Bridge Poison Center
Mary Bridge Children's Health Center
(800) 542-6319 (within Washington)
P.O. Box 5299
1317 South K St.
Tacoma, WA 98405-0987

Maryland AIDS Hotline
(800) 638-6252 (within Maryland)
201 West Preston St.
Baltimore, MD 21201

Maryland Poison Center
University of Maryland School of Pharmacy
(800) 492-2414 (within Maryland)
20 N. Pine St.
Baltimore, MD 21201

Massachusetts Department of Public Health
AIDS Health Education
(800) 235-2331 (within Massachusetts)
150 Tremont St.
Boston, MA 02111

Massachusetts Nutrition Resource Center
(800) 322-7203 (within Massachusetts)

150 Tremont St.
Boston, MA 02111

Massachusetts Poison Control System
(800) 682-9211 (within Massachusetts)
300 Longwood Ave.
Boston, MA 02115

McKennen Hospital Poison Center
(800) 952-0123 (within South Dakota)
(800) 843-0505 (within Iowa, Minnesota,
Nebraska)
P.O. Box 5045
800 E. 21st St.
Sioux Falls, SD 57117-5045

Medic Alert Foundation International
(800) ID-ALERT
(800) 344-3226
2323 Colorado
Turlock, CA 95381-1009

Medical and Chirurgical Faculty of the State of
Maryland Library
(800) 492-1056 (within Maryland)
1211 Cathedral St.
Baltimore, MD 21201

Metro-Help
National Runaway Switchboard
(800) 621-4000
(800) 621-3230 (within Illinois)
3080 N. Lincoln Ave.
Chicago, IL 60657
(See also: Runaway Hotline)

Michigan Department of Health
Special Office on AIDS Prevention
(800) 872-AIDS (within Michigan)
3423 N. Logan
Lansing, MI 48909

Michigan Self-Help Clearinghouse
(800) 752-5858 (within Michigan)
109 West Michigan Ave., Suite 900
Lansing, MI 48933

Mid-America Poison Center
University of Kansas Medical Center
(800) 332-6633 (within Kansas)

39th & Rainbow Blvd.
Kansas City, KS 66103

Mid-Atlantic AIDS Regional Education and
Training Center
(800) 332-UMAB x2382
University of Maryland at Baltimore
520 West Lombard St.
Baltimore, MD 21201

Mid-Plains Poison Control Center
Children's Memorial Hospital
(800) 642-9999 (within Nebraska)
(800) 228-9515 (Colorado, Iowa, Kansas,
Missouri, South Dakota, Wyoming)
8301 Dodge St.
Omaha, NE 68114

Minnesota Department of Health
AIDS Program
(800) 752-4281 (within Minnesota)
717 E. Delaware St.
Minneapolis, MN 55440

Minnesota Regional Poison Center
St. Paul-Ramsey Medical Center
(800) 222-1222 (within Minnesota)
640 Jackson St.
St. Paul, MN 55101

Missing Children Help Center
(800) USA-KIDS (outside Florida)
410 Ware Blvd., #400
Tampa, FL 33619

Mississippi Department of Health
AIDS Education Program
(800) 826-2961 (within Mississippi)
P.O. Box 1700
Jackson, MS 39215

Myasthenia Gravis Foundation
(800) 541-5454
53 West Jackson Blvd., Suite 1352
Chicago, IL 60604

Names Project
(800) USA-NAME
P.O. Box 14573
San Francisco, CA 94114

National Abortion Federation
(800) 772-9100
900 Pennsylvania Ave., SE
Washington, DC 20003

National AIDS Hotline
Centers for Disease Control
(800) 342-AIDS
(800) 344-SIDA (Spanish)
(800) AIDS-TTY (Hearing Impaired)
Atlanta, GA 30333

National AIDS Information Clearinghouse
(800) 458-5231 (for publications)
P.O. Box 6003
Rockville, MD 20850

National Alliance of Blind Students
(800) 424-8666
1010 Vermont Ave., N.W., Suite 1100
Washington, DC 20005

National Association for Hearing and
Speech Action
(800) 638-8255 (outside Maryland)
10801 Rockville Pike
Rockville, MD 20852

National Association for Sickle-Cell Disease
(800) 421-8453
4221 Wilshire Blvd., Suite 360
Los Angeles, CA 90010-3505

National Association for the Education of Young
Children
(800) 424-2460
1834 Connecticut Ave. N.W.
Washington, DC 20009-5786

National Asthma Center
(800) 222-5864
3800 E. Colfax Ave.
Denver, CO 80206

National Center for Missing and Exploited
Children
(800) 843-5678
1835 K Street N.W., Suite 700
Washington, DC 20006

National Center for Youth with Disabilities
(NCYD)
(800) 333-NCYD
University of Minnesota
Box 721-UMHC
Harvard Street at East River Road
Minneapolis, MN 55455

National Child Abuse Hotline
(800) 422-4453
Box 630
Hollywood, CA 90028

National Child Safety Council
(800) 222-1464
P.O. Box 1368
Jackson, MI 49204

National Cocaine Hotline
(800) 262-2463
P.O. Box 100
Summit, NJ 07901

National Council on Alcoholism
(800) NCA-CALL
12 West 21st St., Suite 700
New York, NY 10010

National Council on Child Abuse
(800) 222-2000
1155 Connecticut Ave. N.W., Suite 300
Washington, DC 20036

National Domestic Violence Hotline
Michigan Coalition Against Domestic Violence
(800) 333-SAFE
P.O. Box 7032
Huntington Woods, MI 48070

National Down Syndrome Congress
(800) 232-NDSC
1800 Dempster Street
Park Ridge, IL 60068-1146

National Down Syndrome Society
(800) 221-4602
666 Broadway
New York, NY 10012

National Drug Information and Referral Line
National Institute on Drug Abuse
(800) 662-HELP
5600 Fishers Lane
Rockville, MD 20857

National Eye Care Project
(800) 222-EYES
(Free eye exams for the elderly)
P.O. Box 9688
San Francisco, CA 94101-9688

National Foundation for Depressive Illness
(800) 248-4344
245 Seventh Ave.
New York, NY 10001

National Foundation for Ileitis and Colitis
(800) 343-3637
444 Park Avenue South
New York, NY 10016

National Gay and Lesbian Crisis Line Fund for
Human Dignity
(800) SOS-GAYS
666 Broadway, 4th Fl., Room 410
New York, NY 10012

National Headache Foundation
(800) 843-2256
(800) 523-8858 (within Illinois)
5252 North Western Ave.
Chicago, IL 60625

National Head Injury Foundation
(800) 444-6443
333 Turnpike Rd.
Southboro, MA 01772

National Health Information Center
(800) 336-4797
P.O. Box 1133
Washington, DC 20013-1133

National Hearing Aid Society
Hearing Aid Helpline
(800) 521-5247
20361 Middlebelt
Livonia, MI 48152

National Highway Traffic Safety Administration
Auto Safety Hotline
(800) 424-9393
400 7th St. S.W.
Washington, DC 20590

National Hospice Organization
(800) 658-8898
1901 North Moore St., Suite 901
Arlington, VA 22209

National Information Center for Children and
Youth with Handicaps
(800) 999-5599
P.O. Box 1492
Washington, DC 20013

National Information Center for Orphan Drugs &
Rare Diseases
(800) 336-4797
P.O. Box 1133
Washington, DC 20002

National Information System for Health Related
Services
(800) 922-9234
(800) 922-1107 (within South Carolina)
University of South Carolina
Benson Building
Columbia, SC 29208

National Jewish Hospital and Research Center
LUNGLINE
(800) 222-5864
3800 East Colfax Ave.
Denver, CO 80206
(See also: National Asthma Center)

National Kidney Foundation
(800) 622-9010
30 East 33rd St.
New York, NY 10016

National Library of Medicine
(800) 638-8480
8600 Rockville Pike
Bethesda, MD 20894

National Library Services for the Blind and
Physically Handicapped
Library of Congress
(800) 424-8567
1291 Taylor St. N.W.
Washington, DC 20542

National Multiple Sclerosis Society (NMSS)
(800) 624-8236
205 E. 42nd St.
New York, NY 10017

National Native American AIDS Prevention
Center
Indian AIDS Hotline
(800) 283-AIDS
6239 College Ave., Suite 201
Oakland, CA 94618

National Neurofibromatosis Foundation
(800) 323-7938
141 Fifth Avenue, Suite 7-S
New York, NY 10010

National Organization for Rare Disorders
(800) 999-6673
P.O. Box 8923
New Fairfield, CT 06812

National Organization on Disability (NOD)
(800) 248-ABLE
910 16th St., NW, Suite 600
Washington, DC 20006

National Osteopathic Foundation (NOF)
(800) 621-1773
142 E. Ontario St.
Chicago, IL 60611

National Parents' Resource Institute for Drug
Education (PRIDE)
(800) 241-7946
Hurt Building, #210
50 Hurt Plaza
Atlanta, GA 30303

National Parkinson Foundation
(800) 327-4545
(800) 433-7022 (within Florida)

1501 N.W. 9th Ave.
Miami, FL 33136

National Pesticide Telecommunications Network
(800) 858-7378
3601 4th St.
Lubbock, TX 79430

National Rehabilitation Information Center
(800) 34-NARIC
8455 Colesville Rd., Suite 935
Silver Spring, MD 20910

National Retinitis Pigmentosa Foundation
(800) 638-2300
1401 Mount Royal Avenue, 4th Fl.
Baltimore, MD 21217
(See also: R P Foundation Fighting Blindness)

National Reye's Syndrome Foundation, Inc.
(800) 233-7393
(800) 231-7393 (within Ohio)
P.O. Box 829
Bryan, OH 43506

National Runaway Switchboard
(800) 621-4000
3080 North Lincoln
Chicago, IL 60657

National Safety Council
(800) 621-7619
444 North Michigan Ave.
Chicago, IL 60611

National Second Surgical Opinion Program
(800) 638-6833
(800) 492-6603 (within Maryland)
200 Independence Ave., S.W.
Washington, DC 20201

National Sheriffs' Association
(800) 424-7827
(AIDS Project Information)
1450 Duke St.
Alexandria, VA 22314

National Spinal Cord Injury Association
(800) 962-9629
600 W. Cummings Park, Suite 2000
Woburn, MA 01801

National Sudden Infant Death Syndrome
Foundation
(800) 221-SIDS (outside Maryland)
10500 Little Patuxant Parkway
Columbia, MD 21044

National Tuberous Sclerosis Association
(800) 225-6872
4351 Garden City Drive, Suite 660
Landover, MD 20785

Nebraska Department of Health
AIDS Prevention Program
(800) 742-AIDS (within Nebraska)
P.O. Box 95007
Lincoln, NE 68509

New England Headache Treatment Program
(800) 245-0088
778 Longridge Road
Stamford, CT 06902

New Hampshire Poison Information Center
(800) 562-8236 (within New Hampshire)
2 Maynard St.
Hanover, NH 03756

New Jersey Department of Health
AIDS Division
(800) 624-2377 (within New Jersey)
C.N. 360, 363 West State St.
Trenton, NJ 08625

New Jersey Poison Information and Education
System
(800) 962-1253 (within New Jersey)
201 Lyons Ave.
Newark, NJ 07112

New Jersey Self-Help Clearinghouse
(800) 367-6274 (within New Jersey)
St. Clare's-Riverside Medical Center
Pocono Road
Denville, NJ 07834

New Mexico Poison and Drug Information
Center
(800) 432-6866 (within New Mexico)
University of New Mexico
Albuquerque, NM 87131

New York State Department of Health
AIDS Institute
(800) 962-5065 (within New York)
1315 Empire State Plaza, 25th Floor, Room 2580
Albany, NY 12237

New York State Office for the Aging
Senior Citizens' Hot Line
(800) 342-9871 (within New York)
Empire State Plaza
Agency Bldg. 2
Albany, NY 12223

North Carolina Department of Human Resources
CARELINE
(800) 662-7030 (within North Carolina)
325 N. Salisbury St.
Raleigh, NC 27611

North Dakota Department of Health
AIDS Project
(800) 742-2180 (within North Dakota)
State Capitol Bldg.
Bismark, ND 58505

North Dakota Poison Information Center
St. Luke's Hospitals
(800) 732-2200 (within North Dakota)
5th St. N. & Mills Ave.
Fargo, ND 58122

North Texas Poison Center
(800) 441-0040 (within Texas)
P.O. Box 35926
Dallas, TX 75235

Northwest Regional Poison Center
Saint Vincent Health Center
(800) 822-3232
232 W. 25th St.
Erie, PA 16544

Occupational Hearing Service
Dial A Hearing Screen Test
(800) 222-3277
(800) 345-3277 (within Pennsylvania)
P.O. Box 1880
Media, PA 19063

Office of Drug and Alcohol Programs
Encore

(800) 932-0912 (within Pennsylvania)
Health & Welfare Bldg., Rm. 929
6th & Commonwealth
Harrisburg, PA 17120

Ohio Department of Health
AIDS Activity Unit
(800) 322-AIDS (within Ohio)
35 E. Chestnut St., 7th Floor
Columbus, OH 43266

Oklahoma Poison Control Center
Oklahoma Children's Memorial Hospital
(800) 522-4611 (within Oklahoma)
P.O. Box 26307
940 N.E. 10th
Oklahoma City, OK 73126

Oregon Drug and Alcohol Information Center
(800) 237-7808
(800) 452-7032 (within Oregon)
100 N. Cook
Portland, OR 97227

Oregon Poison Center
Oregon Health Sciences University
(800) 452-7165 (within Oregon)
3181 S.W. Sam Jackson Park Rd.
Portland, OR 97201

Orton Dyslexia Society
(800) ABCD-123 (outside Maryland)
724 York Rd.
Baltimore, MD 21204

PMS Access
(800) 222-4PMS
(Information on premenstrual syndrome)
P.O. Box 9326
Madison, WI 53715

Palmetto Poison Center
University of South Carolina College of Pharmacy
(800) 922-1117 (within South Carolina)
Columbia, SC 29208

Parents Anonymous (PA)
(800) 421-0353
(800) 352-0386 (within California)

7120 Franklin Avenue
Los Angeles, CA 90046

Parkinson's Education Program USA
(800) 344-7872
1800 Park Newport, #302
Newport Beach, CA 92660

Pennsylvania Department of Health
(800) 932-0912 (within Pennsylvania)
Health & Welfare Bldg., Rm. 929
6th & Commonwealth
Harrisburg, PA 17120
(See also: Office of Drug and Alcohol Programs)
(See also: Encore)

Pennsylvania Department of Health
State AIDS Hotline
(800) 662-6080 (within Pennsylvania)
P.O. Box 90
Harrisburg, PA 17108

People's Medical Society
(800) 624-8773
462 Walnut St.
Allentown, PA 18102

Pharmacy Management Services, Incorporated
(800) 237-7676 (Pharmacy Assistance Services)
(Retrovir Prescription Program for AIDS patients)
3311 Queen Palm Drive
P.O. Box 20248
Tampa, FL 33622-0248

Practitioner Reporting System
(800) 638-6725 (Defect reporting)
(Reporting of product defects)
12601 Twinbrook Parkway
Rockville, MD 20852

Pride Institute
(800) 54-PRIDE (Medical services, spiritual and
pastoral counseling, funeral assistance)
(Inpatient facility treating alcohol- and/or
drug-dependent lesbians and gay men)
14400 Martin Dr.
Eden Prairie, MN 55344

Project Inform
(800) 334-7422 (within California)
(800) 822-7422 (outside California)
(Information on experimental drugs for AIDS,
ARC, and HIV infection)
347 Delores St., Suite 301
San Francisco, CA 94110

Project Share
(800) 537-3788
7830 Old Georgetown Road, Suite 204
Bethesda, MD 20814

Recording for the Blind (RFB)
(800) 221-4792 (outside New Jersey)
20 Rozel Road
Princeton, NJ 08540

Recovery of Male Potency
(800) 835-7667
27211 Lahser Road, Suite 208
Southfield, MI 48034

Regional Poison Control System and Cincinnati
Drug and Poison Information Center
University of Cincinnati Medical Center
(800) 872-5111 (regional)
231 Bethesda Ave., M.L. 144
Cincinnati, OH 45267-0144

Resolve
(800) 662-1016
(Infertility information)
5 Water St.
Arlington, MA 02174

Rocky Mountain Poison Center
(800) 332-3073 (within Colorado)
(800) 525-5042 (within Montana)
(800) 442-2702 (within Wyoming)
645 Bannock St.
Denver, CO 80204-4507

R P Foundation Fighting Blindness
(800) 638-2300
1401 Mt. Royal Ave., 4th Floor
Baltimore, MD 21217
(See also: National Retinitis Pigmentosa
Foundation)

Runaway Hotline
(800) 231-6946
(800) 392-3552 (within Texas)
P.O. Box 12428
Austin, TX 78711
(See also: Metro-Help, National Runaway
Switchboard)

San Francisco AIDS Foundation
(800) 367-2437 (within Northern California)
P.O. Box 6182
25 Van Ness Ave., Suite 660
San Francisco, CA 94102-6182

San Francisco Bay Area Regional Poison Center
San Francisco General Hospital
(800) 523-2222
1001 Potrero Ave., Rm. 1E86
San Francisco, California 94110

Santa Clara Valley Medical Center Regional
Poison Center
(800) 662-9886 (within California)
751 S. Bascom Ave.
San Jose, CA 95128

Sarcoidosis Family AID and Research
Foundation
(800) 223-6429
760 Clinton Ave.
Newark, NJ 07108

Seattle Poison Center
Children's Hospital and Medical Center
(800) 732-6985 (within Washington)
4800 Sand Point Way N.E.
P.O. Box C5371
Seattle, WA 98105-0371

The Self-Help Center
(800) 322-6274 (within Illinois)
1600 Dodge Ave.
Evanston, IL 60201

Shriners Hospital Referral Line
(800) 237-5055
(Free orthopedic or burn care for children)
2900 Rocky Point Drive
Tampa, FL 33607

Simon Foundation
(800) 237-4666
(Incontinence information)
P.O. Box 815
Wilmette, IL 60091

South Carolina Department of Health
AIDS Project
(800) 322-AIDS (within South Carolina)
2600 Bull St.
Columbia, SC 29201

South Dakota Department of Health
AIDS Program
(800) 472-2180 (within South Dakota)
523 East Capital
Pierre, SD 57501

South Dakota Tie-Line
(800) 592-1865 (within South Dakota)
(Statewide information and referral system)
State Capitol
Pierre, SD 57501

Spina Bifida Association of America
(800) 621-3141
1700 Rockville Pike, Suite 540
Rockville, MD 20852

Spokane Poison Center
(800) 572-5842 (within Washington)
(800) 541-5624 (within N. Idaho and
W. Montana)
South 715 Cowley
Spokane, WA 99202

Statewide Poison Control Drug Information
Center
University of Arkansas for Medical Sciences
(800) 482-8948 (within Arkansas)
4301 W. Markham St.
Little Rock, AR 72205

St. Luke's Midland Poison Control Center
(800) 592-1889
305 S. State St.
Aberdeen, SD 57401

Sturge-Weber Foundation
(800) 627-5482
P.O. Box 460931
Aurora, CO 80015

Task Force on Education for the Handicapped,
Inc. (TFEH)
Indiana Parent Training Program (IPTP)
Indiana Educational Surrogate Parent Program
(ISPP)
(800) 332-4433 (within Indiana)
833 Northside Blvd., Building 1
South Bend, IN 46617

Tennessee Department of Health and Environment
(800) 342-3145 (within Tennessee)
(Medicaid information)
344 Cordell Hull Building
Nashville, TN 37219

Tennessee Department of Health and Environment
State AIDS Hotline
(800) 342-AIDS (within Tennessee)
C2-227 Cordell Hull Building
Nashville, TN 37219

Terri Gotthelf Lupus Research Institute
(800) 82-LUPUS
50 Washington St., 10th Floor
South Norwalk, CT 06854

Tidewater Poison Center
(800) 552-6337 (within Virginia)
150 Kingsley Lane
Norfolk, VA 23505

Tourette Syndrome Association (TSA)
(800) 237-0717
42-40 Bell Blvd.
Bayside, NY 11361

Triad Poison Center
Moses H. Cone Memorial Hospital
(800) 722-2222 (within North Carolina)
1200 N. Elm St.
Greensboro, NC 27401-1020

Tripod Grapevine
(800) 352-8888
(800) 346-8888 (within California)

(Hearing-impaired children)
2901 North Keystone St.
Burbank, CA 91504

United Cerebral Palsy Associations
(800) USA-1UCP
7 Penn Plaza, Suite 804
New York, NY 10001

University of Florida
College of Pharmacy
Drug Information and Pharmacy Resource Center
(800) 342-1106 (within Florida)
J. Hillis Miller Health Center, Box J-4
Gainesville, FL 32610

University of Iowa Hospitals and Clinics Poison
Control Center
(800) 272-6477 (within Iowa)
Iowa City, IA 52242

University of Wisconsin-Madison
Wisconsin Clinical Cancer Center
Department of Human Oncology
(800) 422-6237
1300 University Ave., 7C
Madison, WI 53706

Utah Department of Health
Baby Your Baby Hotline
(800) 826-9662 (within Utah)
288 North 1460 West
P.O. Box 2500
Salt Lake City, UT 84116

Utah Department of Health
State AIDS Hotline
(800) 537-1046 (within Utah)
288 North, 1460 West
P.O. Box 16660
Salt Lake City, UT 84116

Variety Club Poison and Drug Information Center
Iowa Methodist Medical Center
(800) 362-2327 (within Iowa)
1200 Pleasant St.
Des Moines, IA 50309

Vermont Department of Health
(800) 642-3323 (within Vermont)

60 Main Street
P.O. Box 70
Burlington, VT 05402

Vermont Department of Health
AIDS Education
(800) 882-AIDS (within Vermont)
60 Main St.
P.O. Box 70
Burlington, VT 05402

Virginia Department for Rights of the Disabled
(800) 552-3962 (within Virginia)
101 North 14th St.
Richmond, VA 23219

Virginia Department of Health
AIDS Activity Program
(800) 533-4148 (within Virginia)
109 Governor St., Room 722
Richmond, VA 23219

Vision Foundation, Inc.
(800) 852-3029 (within Massachusetts)
818 Mt. Auburn St.
Watertown, MA 02172

Wake Forest University
Bowman Gray School of Medicine
(800) 642-0500 (within North Carolina)
(Research in epilepsy)
300 S. Hawthorne St.
Winston-Salem, NC 27103

Western NC Poison Control Center
Memorial Mission Hospital
(800) 542-4225
509 Biltmore Ave.
Asheville, NC 28801

Western Ohio Regional Poison and Drug Information Center
Children's Medical Center
(800) 762-0727 (within Ohio)
1 Children's Plaza
Dayton, OH 45404-1815

West Virginia Department of Health
State AIDS Hotline
(800) 624-8244 (within West Virginia)

1422 Washington St. East
South Charleston, WV 25301

West Virginia Poison Center
West Virginia University School of Pharmacy
(800) 642-3625 (within West Virginia)
3110 McCorkle Ave., S.E.
Charleston, WV 25304

West Virginia University
West Virginia Rehabilitation Research Training Center
(800) 624-8284
1 Dunbar Plaza, Suite E
Dunbar, WV 25064

West Virginia University School of Pharmacy
Drug Information Center
(800) 352-2501 (within West Virginia)
Morgantown, WV 26506

Wisconsin Clearinghouse
(800) 262-6243 (outside Wisconsin)
University of Wisconsin
Dean of Students Office
Department K
P.O. Box 1468
Madison, WI 53701

Wisconsin Department of Health and Social Services
AIDS Program
(800) 334-AIDS (within Wisconsin)
1 West Wilson St.
P.O. Box 309
Madison, WI 53701

Women's Sports Foundation
(800) 342-3988
(Physical fitness and sports medicine)
342 Madison Ave., Suite 728
New York, NY 10173

Y-Me Breast Cancer Support Program
(800) 221-2141; (9–5 Central Time)
18220 Harwood Ave.
Homewood, IL 60430

A HEALTH AND HEALTH EDUCATION INTERNET DIRECTORY

Bureau of Labor Statistics
stats.bls.gov

Bureau of the Census
www.census.gov

Cancer Information
www.lib.umich.edu/chdocs/cancer/
cancerguide. html

Centers for Disease Control and Prevention
www.cdc.gov

Department of Education
www.ed.gov

Department of Energy
www.doe.gov

Department of Health and Human Services
www.os.dhhs.gov

Department of Housing and Urban Development
www.hud.gov

Department of the Interior
www.usgs.gov.doi

Department of Justice
www.usdoj.gov

Department of Labor
lcweb.loc.gov/global/executive/labor.html

Department of State
dosfan.lib.uic.edu/dosfan.html

Department of Transportation
www.dot.gov

Diabetes Information
www.biostat.wisc.edu/diaknow/index.html

Environmental Information
www.pacificrim.net/~nature/

Environmental Protection Agency (EPA)
www.epa.gov

Federal Web Locator
www.law.vill.edu/fed-agency/fedwebbloc.html

Food and Drug Administration (FDA)
www.fda.gov

Heart Disease
osler.wustl.edu/~murphy/cardiology/compass.html

Influenza
www.cdc.gov./diseases/viral/html

International Red Cross
www.ifrc.org

Library of Congress
lcweb.loc.gov
www.loc.gov

Men's Health
www.vix.com/pub/men/health/health.html

Mental Health
hpbl.hwc.ca/links/menteng.html

Morbidity and Mortality Weekly Report
(MMWR)
www.crawford.com/cdc/mmwr/mmwr.html

National Center for Health Statistics
www.cdc.gov/nchswww/nchshome.html

National Endowment for the Humanities
nsl.neh.fed.us

National Health Information Center
nhic-nt.health.org

National Institute of Environmental Health
www.niehs.nih.gov

National Institute of Occupational Safety and
Health
www.gov.diseases/niosh.html

National Institutes of Health
www.nih.gov

National Library of Medicine
www.nlm.nih.gov

National Organization of Women (NOW)
now.org/now/home.html

Nutrition Information
hpbl.hwc.ca/datapsb/npu/hpb3.html

Occupational Safety and Health Administration
(OSHA)
www.osha-slc.gov

Peace Corps
www.clark.net/pub/peace/peacecorps.html

Senior Citizens Resources
www.washweb.net/washweb/community/senior

Smithsonian Institute
www.si.sgi.com

Stress Information
www.cts.com/~health/strssbus.html

Substance Abuse Information
www.os.dhhs.gov/0/samhsa/samhsahp.htm

Tuberculosis
www.cdc.gov/diseases/tb.html

Women's Health
hpbl.hwc.ca/links/womeneng.html

World Health Organization (WHO)
who.ch

2003 FEDERAL HEALTH INFORMATION CENTERS AND CLEARINGHOUSES

National Adoption Center
1500 Walnut Street, Suite 701
Philadelphia, PA 19102
(800) 862-3678
(215) 735-9988
(215) 735-9410 (fax)
nac@adopt.org (e-mail)
www.adopt.org/adopt

Mission is to expand adoption opportunities throughout the United States for children with special needs and those from minority cultures. Offers information and referral services. Provides publications on special needs adoption, single parent adoption, open adoption, and searching for birth parents.

National Adoption Information Clearinghouse
330 C Street, S.W.
Washington, DC 20447
(888) 251-0075
(703) 352-3488
(703) 385-3206 (fax)
naic@calib.com (e-mail)
www.calib.com/naic

Provides professionals and the general public with easily accessible information on all aspects of adoption, including infant and intercountry adop-

tion and the adoption of children with special needs. NAIC maintains an adoption literature database, a database of adoption experts, listings of adoption agencies, crisis pregnancy centers, and other adoption-related services, as well as excerpts of state and federal laws on adoption. Ultimately, NAIC's goal is to strengthen adoptive family life. NAIC does not place children for adoption or provide counseling. It does, however, make referrals for such services. NAIC is funded by the Children's Bureau, Administration for Children and Families, U.S. Department of Health and Human Services.

U.S. Administration on Aging
Center for Communication and Consumer Services (CCCS)
330 Independence Avenue, S.W., Room 4656
Washington, DC 20201
(202) 619-7501
(202) 401-7620 (fax)
cccs@aoa.gov (e-mail)
www.aoa.gov/naic

The Center for Communication and Consumer Services (CCCS) serves as a central source for a wide variety of information on aging for older people, their families, and those who work for or on behalf of older persons. The CCCS resources include program and policy-related materials for consumers and practitioners as well as demographic and other statistical data on the health, economic, and social conditions of older Americans. The CCCS public inquiries and Aging Information Resource Library units are the successor to the National Aging Information Center.

National Institute on Aging Information Center
P.O. Box 8057
Gaithersburg, MD 20898-8057
(800) 222-2225
(301) 496-1752
(800) 222-4225 (TTY)
(301) 589-3014 (fax)
niaic@jbs1.com (e-mail)
www.nia.nih.gov

Provides publications on health topics of interest to older adults, doctors, nurses, social activities directors, health educators, and the public.

U.S. Department of Agriculture Extension Service
See the listing in the government section of your telephone book for your local extension office. Provides information on health, nutrition, fitness, and family well-being.

CDC National Prevention Information Network (CDC NPIN)
P.O. Box 6003
Rockville, MD 20849-6003
(800) 458-5231
(800) 243-7012 (TTY)
(888) 282-7681 (fax)
(301) 562-1098 (international)
(301) 588-1589 (international TTY)
info@cdcnpin.org (e-mail)
www.cdcnpin.org

The CDC National Prevention Information Network (NPIN) is the U.S. reference, referral, and distribution service for information on HIV/AIDS, sexually transmitted diseases (STD's), and tuberculosis (TB) sponsored by the Centers for Disease Control and Prevention (CDC). NPIN services are designed to facilitate the sharing of information and resources among people working in HIV, STD, and TB prevention, treatment, and support services. Bilingual staff are available to speak with callers, and all calls are confidential. Hours of operation: 9:00 A.M.–6:00 P.M., Monday–Friday (Eastern Time).

National Clearinghouse for Alcohol and Drug Information
P.O. Box 2345
Rockville, MD 20847-2345
(800) 729-6686
(877) 767-8432 (Spanish)
(301) 468-2600 (local callers)
(800) 487-4889 (TDD)
(301) 468-6433 (fax)
info@health.org (e-mail)
www.health.org

Sponsored by the Center for Substance Abuse Prevention, Substance Abuse and Mental Health Services Administration. Gathers and disseminates information on alcohol and other drug-related subjects, including tobacco. Services include subject searches, provision of statistics and other information, and publications distribution. Operates the Regional Alcohol and Drug Awareness Resource Network, a nationwide linkage of alcohol and other drug information centers. Maintains a library open to the public. The 800 number offers 24-hour voicemail service. Hours of operation: 8:00 A.M.–6:00 P.M., Monday–Friday.

National Institute of Allergy and Infectious Diseases
Office of Communications and Public Liaison
31 Center Drive, MSC 2520
Building 31, Room 7A-50
Bethesda, MD 20892-2520
(301) 496-5717
(301) 402-0120 (fax)
ocpostoffice@niaid.nih.gov (e-mail)
www.niaid.nih.gov

Distributes publications and provides resource information to the public, health professionals, and researchers on HIV/AIDS; allergy and asthma; and bacterial, fungal, immunologic, viral, and parasitic diseases. Provides information on autoimmune disorders and diseases such as malaria, hepatitis, Lyme disease, tuberculosis, and sexually transmitted diseases as well as illness from potential agents of bioterrorism.

National Center for Complementary and
Alternative Medicine
Information Clearinghouse
P.O. Box 7923
Gaithersburg, MD 20898-7923
(888) 644-6226 (toll-free)
(301) 519-3153 (international callers)
(866) 464-3616 (fax)
(866) 464-3615 (TTY)
info@nccam.nih.gov (e-mail)
www.nccam.nih.gov

NCCAM's clearinghouse operates a toll-free telephone service. Information specialists search NCCAM databases for scientific information on CAM therapies or conditions and can answer inquiries in English and Spanish. The fax-on-demand service, with factsheets and other information, is also available through the toll-free number. NCCAM services and materials are provided at no cost. The clearinghouse does not provide medical referrals, medical advice, or recommendations for specific CAM therapies. Hours of operation: 8:30 A.M.–5:00 P.M., Monday–Friday (Eastern Time).

Alzheimer's Disease Education and Referral
Center (ADEAR)
P.O. Box 8250
Silver Spring, MD 20907-8250
(800) 438-4380
(301) 495-3311
(301) 495-3334 (fax)
adear@alzheimers.org (e-mail)
www.alzheimers.org/

Sponsored by the National Institute on Aging, ADEAR provides information and publications on Alzheimer's disease to health and service professionals, patients and their families, caregivers, and the public. Hours of operation: 8:30 A.M.–5:00 P.M. (Eastern Time).

National Institute of Arthritis and
Musculoskeletal and Skin
Diseases Information Clearinghouse
National Institutes of Health
1 AMS Circle
Bethesda, MD 20892-3675
(877) 22-NIAMS
(301) 495-4484
(301) 565-2966 (TTY)
(301) 718-6366 (fax)
niamsinfo@mail.nih.gov (e-mail)
www.niams.nih.gov

Designed to help patients and health professionals identify educational materials concerning arthritis and musculoskeletal and skin diseases. Distributes publications and maintains a file on the Combined Health Information Database (CHID) that indexes publications and audiovisuals. Personal information requests from patients are referred to appropriate organizations for additional information.

National Library Service for the Blind and
Physically Handicapped
Library of Congress
1291 Taylor Street, N.W.
Washington, DC 20542
(800) 424-8567
(202) 707-5100
(202) 707-0744 (TDD)
(202) 707-0712 (fax)
nls@loc.gov (e-mail)
lcweb.loc.gov/nls

A network of 57 regional and 79 subregional libraries that is administered by the National Library Service for the Blind and Physically Handicapped, Library of Congress. Provides free library service to anyone who is unable to read or use standard printed materials because of visual or physical disabilities. Delivers recorded and Braille books and magazines to eligible readers. Specially designed phonographs and cassette players are available for loan. A list of participating libraries is available in print and online. Hours of operation: 8:00 A.M.–4:30 P.M., Monday–Friday.

U.S. Coast Guard Office of Boating Safety
2100 Second Street, S.W., Room 3100
Washington, DC 20593-0001
(800) 368-5647
(202) 267-1077
(800) 689-0816 (TTY)
(703) 313-5910 (BBS)
uscginfoline@gcrm.com (e-mail)
www.uscgboating.org/

Provides safety information to recreational boaters; assists the public in finding boating education classes; answers technical questions; and distributes literature on boating safety, federal laws, and the prevention of recreational boating casualties.

Cancer Information Service
Office of Cancer Communications
National Cancer Institute
31 Center Drive, Room 10A31
Bethesda, MD 20892-2580
(800) 4-CANCER
(800) 332-8615 (TTY)
(800) 624-2511 (fax back)
(301) 402-5874 (fax)
www.cancernet.nci.nih.gov

Provides information about cancer and cancer-related resources to patients, the public, and health professionals. Inquiries are handled by trained information specialists. Spanish-speaking staff members are available. Distributes free publications from the National Cancer Institute. Hours of operation: 9:00 A.M.–4:30 P.M.

National Clearinghouse on Child Abuse and Neglect Information
330 C Street, S.W.
Washington, DC 20447
(800) 394-3366
(703) 385-7565
(703) 385-3206 (fax)
nccanch@calib.com (e-mail)
www.calib.com/nccanch

Serves as a national resource for the acquisition and dissemination of child abuse and neglect and child welfare materials and distributes a free publications catalog upon request. Maintains bibliographic databases of documents, audiovisuals, and national organizations. Services include searches of databases and annotated bibliographies on frequently requested topics.

National Child Care Information Center
243 Church Street, N.W., 2nd Floor
Vienna, VA 22180
(800) 616-2242
(800) 516-2242 (TTY)
(800) 716-2242 (fax)
info@nccic.org (e-mail)
nccic.org

A project of the Child Care Bureau, Administration for Children and Families, U.S. Department of Health and Human Services. A national resource that links information and people to complement, enhance, and promote the child care delivery system, working to ensure that all children and families have access to high-quality comprehensive services.

National Institute of Child Health and Human Development (NICHD)
Information Resource Center
P.O. Box 3006
Rockville, MD 20847
(800) 370-2943
(800) 505-CRIB (2742) "Back to Sleep" campaign
(301) 984-1473 (fax)
NICHDClearinghouse@mail.nih.gov (e-mail)
www.nichd.nih.gov

The National Institute of Child Health and Human Development (NICHD) Information Resource Center provides information on health issues and publications related to NICHD research. The NICHD supports and conducts research on the reproductive, neurobiologic, developmental, and behavioral processes related to the health of children, adults, families, and populations. The NICHD also sponsors the "Back to Sleep" campaign, designed to educate families and care-givers about putting healthy babies on their backs to sleep to reduce the risk of sudden infant death syndrome (SIDS), and the "Milk Matters" calcium education campaign, designed to teach parents, children, and health professionals about the importance of calcium consumption for children and teens. The Information Resource Center offers trained information specialists with access to information and referral services on topics related to the mission of NICHD. Information specialists are available to respond to inquiries Monday–Friday, 8:30 A.M.–5:00 P.M. (Eastern Time).

NIH Consensus Program Information Center
Office of Medical Applications of Research
P.O. Box 2577
Kensington, MD 20891
(888) 644-2667
(301) 593-9485 (fax)
consensus.nih.gov

A service of the Office of Medical Applications of Research, National Institutes of Health. Provides up-to-date information on biomedical technologies to all health care providers. Offers a 24-hour voice mail service to order consensus statements produced by nonfederal panels of experts that evaluate scientific information on biomedical technologies. Information specialists are available 8:30 A.M.–5 P.M. (Eastern Time). Consensus statements can also be ordered by mail, fax, and electronic bulletin board.

U.S. Federal Consumer Information Center
Pueblo, CO 81009
(719) 948-4000 (orders)
catalog.pueblo@gsa.gov (e-mail)
www.pueblo.gsa.gov

Helps federal agencies develop, promote, and distribute consumer information to the public through the Consumer Information Catalog and website. The catalog, available in print and online, lists over 200 free and low-cost federal consumer publications on topics such as product recalls, health, energy conservation, money management, and nutrition. Also offers the Consumer Action

Handbook in print and online and the Lista de Publicaciones Federales en Español Para El Consumidor.

National Institute on Deafness and Other Communication Disorders
Information Clearinghouse
1 Communication Avenue
Bethesda, MD 20892-3456
(800) 241-1044
(800) 241-1055 (TTY)
(301) 907-8830 (fax)
nidcdinfo@nidcd.nih.gov (e-mail)
www.nidcd.nih.gov

Collects and disseminates information on hearing, balance, smell, taste, voice, speech, and language for health professionals, patients, people in industry, and the public. Maintains a database of references to brochures, books, articles, fact sheets, organizations, and educational materials, which is a subfile of the Combined Health Information Database (CHID). Develops publications, including directories, fact sheets, brochures, information packets, and newsletters.

National Diabetes Information Clearinghouse
1 Information Way
Bethesda, MD 20892-3560
(800) 860-8747
(301) 654-3327
(301) 907-8906 (fax)
ndic@info.niddk.nih.gov (e-mail)
www.niddk.nih.gov/health/diabetes/diabetes.htm

The National Diabetes Information Clearinghouse (NDIC) is an information and referral service of the National Institute of Diabetes and Digestive and Kidney Diseases, one of the National Institutes of Health. The clearinghouse responds to written, telephone, and e-mail inquiries; develops and distributes publications about diabetes; and provides referrals to diabetes organizations, including support groups. The NDIC maintains a database of patient and professional education materials from which literature searches are generated. Hours of operation: 8:30 A.M.–5:00 P.M., Monday–Friday (Eastern Time).

National Digestive Diseases Information Clearinghouse
2 Information Way
Bethesda, MD 20892-3570
(800) 891-5389
(301) 654-3810
(301) 907-8906 (fax)
nddic@info.niddk.nih.gov (e-mail)
www.niddk.nih.gov/health/digest/digest.htm

The National Digestive Diseases Information Clearinghouse (NDDIC) is an information and referral service of the National Institute of Diabetes and Digestive and Kidney Diseases, one of the National Institutes of Health. A central information resource on the prevention and management of digestive diseases, the clearinghouse responds to written inquiries, develops and distributes publications about digestive diseases, and provides referrals to digestive disease organizations, including support groups. The NDDIC maintains a database of patient and professional education materials from which literature searches are generated.

National Information Center for Children and Youth with Disabilities
P.O. Box 1492
Washington, DC 20013-1492
(800) 695-0285 (voice/TTY)
(202) 884-8200 (voice/TTY)
(202) 884-8441 (fax)
nichcy@aed.org (e-mail)
www.nichcy.org

Sponsored by the U.S. Department of Education. Assists individuals by providing information in English and Spanish on disabilities and disability-related issues, with a special focus on children and youth with disabilities (birth to age 22). Services include responses to questions, referrals, and technical assistance to parents, educators, caregivers, and advocates. Develops and distributes fact sheets on disability and general information on parent support groups and public advocacy. All information and services are provided free of charge.

OSERS/Communications and Media Support Services (Disabilities, Rehabilitation)
Office of Special Education and Rehabilitative Services (OSERS)
U.S. Department of Education
400 Maryland Ave., S.W.
Washington, DC 20202
(202) 205-5465
customerservice@inet.ed.gov (e-mail)
www.ed.gov/offices/OSERS/

Responds to inquiries on a wide range of topics, especially in the areas of federal funding, legislation, and programs benefiting people with disabling conditions, and also provides referrals.

National Center for Chronic Disease Prevention and Health Promotion (NCCDPHP)
Technical Information and Editorial Services Branch
Centers for Disease Control and Prevention
4770 Buford Highway N.E., MS K13
Atlanta, GA 30341-3724
(770) 488-5080
(770) 488-5969 (fax)
ccdinfo@cdc.gov (e-mail)
www.cdc.gov/nccdphp/index.htm

Provides information and referrals to the public and to professionals. Gathers information on chronic disease prevention and health promotion. Develops the following bibliographic databases focusing on health promotion program information: Health Promotion and Education, Cancer Prevention and Control, Comprehensive School Health with an AIDS school health component, Prenatal Smoking Cessation, and Epilepsy Education and Prevention Activities. Produces bibliographies on topics of interest in chronic disease prevention and health promotion. The NCCDPHP Information Center collections include approximately 400 periodical subscriptions, 4,000 books, and 400 reference books. Visitors may use the collection by appointment. Produces the Chronic Disease Prevention (CDP) File CD-ROM, which includes the mentioned databases and the CDP Directory, a listing of key contacts in public health.

Drug Policy Information Clearinghouse
P.O. Box 6000
Rockville, MD 20849-6000
(800) 666-3332
(301) 519-5212 (fax)
ondcp@ncjrs.org (e-mail)
www.whitehousedrugpolicy.gov/about/
clearingh.html

Supports the White House Office of National Drug Control Policy, National Criminal Justice Reference Service. Staffed by subject matter specialists and serves as a resource for statistics, research data, and referrals useful for developing and implementing drug policy. Disseminates publications; writes and produces documents on drug-related topics; coordinates with federal, state, and local agencies to identify data resources; and maintains a reading room offering a broad range of policy-related materials.

Educational Resources Information Center
(ERIC) Clearinghouse on Teaching and Teacher Education
1307 New York Avenue, N.W., Suite 300
Washington, DC 20005
(800) 822-9229
(202) 293-2450
(202) 457-8095 (fax)
query@aacte.org (e-mail)
www.ericsp.org

Sponsored by the U.S. Department of Education. Acquires, evaluates, abstracts, and indexes literature on the preparation and development of education personnel and on selected aspects of health and physical education, recreation, and dance. Publishes monographs, trends and issues papers, ERIC Digests, and ERIC Recent Resources (annotated bibliographies from the ERIC database). Performs computer searches of the ERIC database and sponsors workshops on searching the ERIC database.

U.S. Environmental Protection Agency
Information Resources Center

West MC: 3404T
1200 Pennsylvania Avenue, N.W.
Washington, DC 20460
(202) 566-0556
(202) 566-0562 (fax)
hq-irc@epa.gov (e-mail)
www.epa.gov

Offers general information about the agency and nontechnical publications on various environmental topics, such as air quality, pesticides, radon, indoor air, drinking water, water quality, and Superfund. Refers inquiries for technical information to the appropriate regional or program office. The public may visit the center 8 A.M.–5 P.M., Monday–Friday (except federal holidays).

National Clearinghouse on Families and Youth
P.O. Box 13505
Silver Spring, MD 20911-3505
(301) 608-8098
(301) 608-8721 (fax)
info@ncfy.com (e-mail)
www.ncfy.com

Links those interested in youth issues with the resources they need to better serve young people, families, and communities. Offers services that can assist in locating answers to questions or in making valuable contacts with other programs.

Federal Information Center (FIC) Program—
National Contact Center
P.O. Box 450
Camby, IN 46113
(800) 688-9889
(800) 326-2996 (TTY)
www.info.gov

Provides information about the federal government's agencies, programs, and services. Information specialists use an automated database, printed reference materials, and other resources to provide answers to inquiries or accurate referrals. Callers who speak Spanish will be assisted. A descriptive brochure on the FIC program is available free from Department 584B at the Consumer Information Center (see listing in this publication). Hours of operation: 9:00 A.M.–8:00 P.M. (Pacific Time), Monday–Friday, except federal holidays.

Food and Drug Administration
5600 Fishers Lane
Rockville, MD 20857
(888) INFO-FDA (463-6332)
webmail@oc.fda.gov (e-mail)
www.fda.gov

Responds to consumer requests for information and publications on foods, drugs, cosmetics, medical devices, radiation-emitting products, and veterinary products. Hours of operation: 10:00 A.M.–4:00 P.M.

Food and Nutrition Information Center
National Agricultural Library, Agricultural Research Service
U.S. Department of Agriculture
10301 Baltimore Avenue, Room 105
Beltsville, MD 20705-2351
(301) 504-5719
(301) 504-6856 (TTY)
(301) 504-6409 (fax)
fnic@nal.usda.gov (e-mail)
www.nal.usda.gov/fnic

One of several information centers located at the National Agricultural Library, part of the U.S. Department of Agriculture's Agricultural Research Service. Provides information on food, human nutrition, and food safety. Resource lists, databases, and many other food- and nutrition-related links available on FNIC website. Collection includes books, manuals, journal articles, and audiovisual materials. Eligible patrons may borrow directly; others may borrow through interlibrary loan. Hours of operation: 8:30 A.M.–4:30 P.M., Monday–Friday.

Agency for Health Care Research and Quality Clearinghouse
P.O. Box 8547
Silver Spring, MD 20907-8547
(800) 358-9295
(410) 381-3150 (outside U.S.)
(410) 290-3841 (fax)

info@ahrq.gov (e-mail)
www.ahrq.gov

Distributes lay and scientific publications produced by the agency, including clinical practice guidelines on a variety of topics, reports from the National Medical Expenditure Survey, and health care technology assessment reports.

National Health Information Center
P.O. Box 1133
Washington, DC 20013-1133
(800) 336-4797
(301) 565-4167
(301) 984-4256 (fax)
info@nhic.org (e-mail)
www.health.gov/nhic

Helps the public and health professionals locate health information through identification of health information resources, an information and referral system, and publications. Uses a database containing descriptions of health-related organizations to refer inquirers to the most appropriate resources. Does not diagnose medical conditions or give medical advice. Prepares and distributes publications and directories on health promotion and disease prevention topics. Hours of operation: 9:00 A.M.–5:30 P.M.

Health Resources and Services Administration (HRSA) Information Center
2070 Chain Bridge Road, Suite 450
Vienna, VA 22182
(888) ASK-HRSA (275-4772)
(703) 821-2098 (fax)
www.ask.hrsa.gov/index.cfm

Provides publications, resources, and referrals on health care services for low-income, uninsured individuals, and those with special health care needs.

National Information Center on Health Services Research and Health Care Technology (NICHSR)
National Library of Medicine
8600 Rockville Pike
Building 38A, Room 4S-410, Mail Stop 20

Bethesda, MD 20894
(301) 496-0176
(301) 402-3193 (fax)
nichsr@nlm.nih.gov (e-mail)
www.nlm.nih.gov/nichsr/nichsr.html

The 1993 NIH Revitalization Act created a National Information Center on Health Services Research and Health Care Technology (NICHSR) at the National Library of Medicine. The center works closely with the Agency for Healthcare Research and Quality (AHRQ), formerly the Agency for Health Care Policy and Research (AHCPR), to improve the dissemination of the results of health services research, with special emphasis on the growing body of evidence reports and technology assessments, which provide organizations with comprehensive, science-based information on common, costly medical conditions and new health care technologies.

National Center for Health Statistics
Data Dissemination Branch
6525 Belcrest Road, Room 1064
Hyattsville, MD 20782
(301) 458-4636
nchsquery@cdc.gov (e-mail)
www.cdc.gov/nchs

The Data Dissemination Branch of the National Center for Health Statistics answers requests for catalogs of publications and electronic data products; disseminates single copies of publications, such as Advance Data reports; provides information for publications and electronic products sold through the Government Printing Office and National Technical Information Service; adds addresses to the mailing list for new publications; and provides specific statistical data collected by the National Center for Health Statistics.

National Heart, Lung, and Blood Institute
(NHLBI) Health Information Center
P.O. Box 30105
Bethesda, MD 20824-0105
(301) 592-8573
(301) 592-8563 (fax)

NHLBIinfo@rover.nhlbi.nih.gov (e-mail)
www.nhlbi.nih.gov

NHLBI serves as a source of information and materials on risk factors for cardiovascular disease. Services include dissemination of public education materials, programmatic and scientific information for health professionals, and materials on worksite health, as well as responses to information requests. Materials on cardiovascular health are available to consumers and professionals. Hours of operation: 8:30 A.M.–5 P.M., Monday–Friday (Eastern Time).

National Highway Traffic Safety Administration
U.S. Department of Transportation
400 Seventh Street, S.W.
Washington, DC 20590
(800) 424-9393 (hotline)
(202) 366-0123 (hotline)
(800) 424-9153 (TTY)
(202) 366-5962 (fax)
www.nhtsa.dot.gov/

Provides information and referral on the effectiveness of occupant protection, such as safety belt use, child safety seats, and automobile recalls. Gives referrals to other government agencies for consumer questions on warranties, service, automobile safety regulations, and reporting safety problems. Works with private organizations to promote safety programs. Provides technical and financial assistance to state and local governments and awards grants for highway safety. Hours of operation: 8:00 A.M.–10:00 P.M.

National Resource Center on Homelessness and Mental Illness
345 Delaware Avenue
Delmar, NY 12054
(800) 444-7415
(518) 439-7415
(518) 439-7612 (fax)
pra@prainc.com (e-mail)
www.nrchmi.com

Collects, synthesizes, and disseminates information on the services, supports, and housing needs of homeless people with serious mental illnesses. Maintains extensive database of published and un-published materials, prepares customized database searches, holds workshops and national conferences, and provides technical assistance.

Housing and Urban Development (HUD) User
P.O. Box 23268
Washington, DC 20026-3268
(800) 245-2691
(202) 708-3178
(800) 927-7589 (TDD)
(202) 708-9981 (fax)
helpdesk@huduser.org (e-mail)
www.huduser.org

Disseminates publications for the U.S. Department of Housing and Urban Development's Office of Policy Development and Research. Offers database searches on housing research. Provides reports on housing safety, housing for elderly and handicapped persons, and lead-based paint.

Indoor Air Quality Information Clearinghouse
P.O. Box 37133
Washington, DC 20013-7133
(800) 438-4318
(703) 356-4020
(703) 356-5386 (fax)
iaqinfo@aol.com (e-mail)
www.epa.gov/iaq

Information specialists provide information, referrals, and publications on indoor air quality. Information is provided about pollutants and sources, health effects, control methods, commercial building operations and maintenance, standards and guidelines, and federal legislation. Hours of operation: 9:00 A.M.–5:00 P.M., Monday–Friday (Eastern Time).

National Injury Information Clearinghouse
U.S. Consumer Product Safety Commission
Washington, DC 20207
(301) 504-0424
(301) 504-0124 (fax)
clearinghouse@cpsc.gov (e-mail)
www.cpsc.gov/about/clrnghse.html

Sponsored by the U.S. Consumer Product Safety Commission (CPSC). The clearinghouse collects and disseminates information on the causes and prevention of death, injury, and illness associated with consumer products. Compiles data obtained from accident reports, consumer complaints, death certificates, news clips, and the National Electronic Injury Surveillance System operated by the CPSC. Publications include statistical analyses of data and hazard and accident patterns.

National Kidney and Urologic Diseases
Information Clearinghouse
3 Information Way
Bethesda, MD 20892-3580
(800) 891-5390
(301) 654-4415
(301) 907-8906 (fax)
nkudic@info.niddk.nih.gov (e-mail)
www.niddk.nih.gov/health/kidney/
nkudic.htm

The National Kidney and Urologic Diseases Information Clearinghouse (NKUDIC) is an information and referral service of the National Institute of Diabetes and Digestive and Kidney Diseases, one of the National Institutes of Health. The clearinghouse responds to written inquiries, e-mail, and telephone requests, develops and distributes publications about kidney and urologic diseases, and provides referrals to kidney and urologic disease organizations, including support groups. The NKUDIC maintains a database of patient and professional education materials from which literature searches are generated.

National Lead Information Center (NLIC)
801 Roeder Road, Suite 600
Silver Spring, MD 20910
(800) 424-LEAD (5323)
(301) 588-8495 (fax)
www.epa.gov/lead/nlic.htm

The National Lead Information Center (NLIC) is sponsored by the Environmental Protection Agency. NLIC provides information on lead poisoning and children, lead-based paint, a list of local and state contacts who can help, and other lead-related questions.

Maternal and Child Health Information Resource Center (MCHIRC)
1200 18th Street, N.W., Suite 700
Washington, DC 20036
(202) 842-2000
(202) 728-9469 (fax)
mchirc@hsrnet.com (e-mail)
www.mchirc.net

The Maternal and Child Health Information Resource Center (MCHIRC) is dedicated to the goal of helping MCH practitioners on the federal, state, and local levels to improve their capacity to gather, analyze, and use data for planning and policymaking. MCHIRC is funded by Health Resources and Services Administration, Maternal and Child Health Bureau's Office of Data and Information Management.

National Institute of Mental Health (NIMH)
Information Resources and Inquiries Branch
6001 Executive Boulevard
Room 8184, MSC 9663
Bethesda, MD 20892-9663
(301) 443-4513
(301) 443-8431 (TTY)
(301) 443-5158 (MENTAL HEALTH FAX4U — fax information system)
(888) 8-ANXIETY (publications on anxiety disorders)
(800) 421-4211 (publications on depression)
nimhinfo@nih.gov (e-mail)
www.nimh.nih.gov

The National Institute of Mental Health (NIMH), a component of the National Institutes of Health, conducts and supports research that seeks to understand, treat, and prevent mental illness. The institute's public inquiries line is staffed with trained information specialists who respond to information requests from the lay public, clinicians, and the scientific community with a variety of publications. These include printed materials on such

subjects as basic behavioral research, neuroscience of mental health, and rural mental health; children's mental disorders, schizophrenia, depression, and bipolar disorder; attention deficit hyperactivity disorder; Alzheimer's disease; and panic, obsessive–compulsive, and posttraumatic stress disorder and other anxiety disorders. Information and publications on NIMH-sponsored educational programs on depressive and anxiety disorders, their symptoms, and treatments are also available. A list of NIMH publications, including several in Spanish, is available upon request. Information on NIMH-sponsored meetings, workshops, and symposia is available on the institute's website.

SAMHSA's National Mental Health Information Center
P.O. Box 42490
Washington, DC 20015
(800) 789-2647
(866) 889-2647 (TDD)
(301) 984-8796 (fax)
8:30 A.M.–5:00 P.M., Monday–Friday (Eastern Time)
ken@mentalhealth.org (e-mail)
www.mentalhealth.samhsa.gov/

The Substance Abuse and Mental Health Services Administration's (SAMHSA) National Mental Health Information Center provides information about mental health, including more than 200 publications. The National Mental Health Information Center was developed for users of mental health services and their families, the general public, policy makers, providers, and the media. Information center staff members are skilled at listening and responding to questions from the public and professionals. The staff quickly directs callers to federal, state, and local organizations dedicated to treating and preventing mental illness. The information center also has information on federal grants, conferences, and other events.

Office of Minority Health Resource Center
5515 Security Lane, Suite 101
Rockville, MD 20852

(800) 444-6472
(301) 230-7874
(301) 230-7199 (TDD)
(301) 230-7198 (fax)
info@omhrc.gov (e-mail)
www.omhrc.gov

Responds to information requests from health professionals and consumers on minority health issues and locates sources of technical assistance. Provides referrals to relevant organizations and distributes materials. Spanish-speaking operators are available. Hours of operation: 9:00 A.M.–5:00 P.M., Monday–Friday (Eastern Time).

Clearinghouse for Occupational Safety and Health Information
National Institute for Occupational Safety and Health
4676 Columbia Parkway
Cincinnati, OH 45226-1998
(800) 356-4674
(513) 533-8328
(513) 533-8573 (fax)
(888) 232-3299 (fax-on-demand)
pubstaff@cdc.gov (e-mail)
www.cdc.gov/niosh

Provides technical information support for the National Institute for Occupational Safety and Health (NIOSH) research programs and disseminates information to others on request. Services include reference and referral, and information about NIOSH studies. Distributes a publications list of NIOSH materials. Maintains an automated database covering the field of occupational safety and health.

National Oral Health Information Clearinghouse
1 NOHIC Way
Bethesda, MD 20892-3500
(301) 402-7364
(301) 907-8830 (fax)
nohic@nidcr.nih.gov (e-mail)
www.nohic.nidcr.nih.gov

A service of the National Institute of Dental and Craniofacial Research. Focuses on the oral health concerns of special care patients, including people with genetic disorders or systemic diseases that compromise oral health, people whose medical treatment causes oral problems, and people with mental or physical disabilities that make good oral hygiene practices and dental care difficult. Develops and distributes information and educational materials on special care topics, maintains a bibliographic database on oral health information and materials, and provides information services with trained staff to respond to specific interests and questions. Hours of operation: 8:30 A.M.–5:00 P.M., Monday–Friday (Eastern Time).

NIH Osteoporosis and Related Bone Diseases National Resource Center
1232 22nd Street, N.W.
Washington, DC 20037-1292
(800) 624-BONE
(202) 466-4315 (TTY)
(202) 293-2356 (fax)
orbdnrc@nof.org (e-mail)
www.osteo.org

Sponsored by the National Institute of Arthritis and Musculoskeletal and Skin Diseases, National Institute of Child Health and Human Development, National Institute of Dental and Craniofacial Research, National Institute of Environmental Health Sciences, NIH Office of Research on Women's Health, HHS Office on Women's Health, and National Institute on Aging. Provides resources and information to patients, health professionals, and the public on metabolic bone diseases such as osteoporosis, Paget's disease of the bone, osteogenesis imperfecta, and primary hyperparathyroidism. Specific populations include the elderly, men, women, and adolescents. Hours of operation: 8:30 A.M.–5:00 P.M., Monday–Friday (Eastern Time).

President's Council on Physical Fitness and Sports
Hubert H. Humphrey Building, Room 738-H
200 Independence Avenue, S.W.
Washington, DC 20201
(202) 690-9000

(202) 690-5211 (fax)
www.fitness.gov

The President's Council on Physical Fitness and Sports promotes, encourages, and motivates the development of physical fitness and sports participation for Americans of all ages through its work with partners in government and the private sector. Offers recognition and incentive programs for individuals and organizations. Materials on fitness and physical activity for all ages are available. Hours of operation: 7:30 A.M.–4:30 P.M. (Eastern Time).

Policy Information Center (PIC)
Office of the Assistant Secretary for Planning and Evaluation
U.S. Department of Health and Human Services
Hubert H. Humphrey Building, Room 438-F
200 Independence Avenue, S.W.
Washington, DC 20201
(202) 690-6445
pic@osaspe.dhhs.gov (e-mail)
aspe.dhhs.gov/pic/

A centralized repository of evaluations, short-term evaluative research reports and program inspections/audits relevant to the department's operations, programs, and policies. It includes relevant reports from the General Accounting Office, Congressional Budget Office, and the Institute of Medicine and the National Research Council's Committee on National Statistics, both part of the National Academy of Sciences. Reports are also available from the Departments of Agriculture, Labor, and Education, as well as the private sector. Final reports and executive summaries are available for review at the facility, or final reports may be purchased from the National Technical Information Service. In addition, the PIC online database of evaluation abstracts is accessible through HHS home page, http://www.hhs.gov. The database includes over 6,000 project descriptions of both in-process and completed studies. *PIC Highlights,* a quarterly publication, features articles of recently completed studies.

Office of Population Affairs (OPA) Clearinghouse
P.O. Box 30686
Bethesda, MD 20824-0686
(301) 654-6190
(301) 215-7731 (fax)
opa@osophs.dhhs.gov (e-mail)
opa.osophs.dhhs.gov/clearinghouse.html

Sponsored by the Office of Population Affairs. Provides information and distributes publications to health professionals and the public in the areas of family planning, adolescent pregnancy, and adoption. Makes referrals to other information centers in related subject areas.

National Clearinghouse for Primary Care Information
2070 Chain Bridge Road, Suite 450
Vienna, VA 22182
(703) 821-8955 ext. 248
(703) 821-2098 (fax)
www.bphc.hrsa.dhhs.gov

Sponsored by the Bureau of Primary Health Care (BPHC), Health Resources and Services Administration. Provides information services to support the planning, development, and delivery of ambulatory health care to urban and rural areas that have shortages of medical personnel and services. A primary role of the clearinghouse is to identify, obtain, and disseminate information to community and migrant health centers. Distributes publications focusing on ambulatory care, financial management, primary health care, and health services administration of special interest to professionals working in primary care centers funded by BPHC. Materials are available on health education, governing boards, financial management, administrative management, and clinical care. Bilingual medical phrase books, a directory of federally funded health centers, and an annotated bibliography are available also.

U.S. Consumer Product Safety Commission Hotline (CPSC)
Washington, DC 20207
(800) 638-2772 (Toll-Free Hotline)
(800) 638-8270 (TTY)

info@cpsc.gov (e-mail)
cpsc.gov/

Maintains the National Injury Information Clearinghouse, conducts investigations of alleged unsafe or defective products, and establishes product safety standards. Assists consumers in evaluating the comparative safety of products and conducts education programs to increase consumer awareness. Operates the National Electronic Injury Surveillance System, which monitors a statistical sample of hospital emergency rooms for injuries associated with consumer products. Maintains free hotline to provide information about recalls and to receive reports on unsafe products and product-related injuries. Publications describe hazards associated with electrical products and children's toys. Spanish-speaking operator available through the toll-free number listed.

National Rehabilitation Information Center
4200 Forbes Boulevard, Suite 202
Lanham, MD 20706
(800) 346-2742
(301) 459-5900
(301) 459-4263 (TTY/fax)
naricinfo@heitechservices.com (e-mail)
www.naric.com

The National Rehabilitation Center (NARIC) is a library and information center on disability and rehabilitation. Funded by the National Institute on Disability and Rehabilitation Research, NARIC collects and disseminates the results of federally funded research projects. The collection, which also includes books, journal articles, and audiovisuals, grows at a rate of about 300 documents per month.

National Center on Sleep Disorders Research
2 Rockledge Center, Suite 10038
6701 Rockledge Drive, MSC 7920
Bethesda, MD 20892-7920
(301) 435-0199
(301) 480-3451 (fax)
ncsdr@nih.gov (e-mail)
www.nhlbi.nih.gov/sleep

Promotes basic, clinical, and applied research on sleep and sleep disorders by strengthening existing sleep research programs, training new investigators, and creating new programs aimed at addressing important gaps and opportunities in sleep and sleep disorders. Sponsors workshops, conferences, and programs to educate health care professionals about sleep disorders and sleep-related research findings.

Office on Smoking and Health
Centers for Disease Control and Prevention
National Center for Chronic Disease Prevention and Health Promotion
Mail Stop K-50, 4770 Buford Highway, N.E.
Atlanta, GA 30341-3724
(800) CDC-1311
(770) 488-5705
(770) 488-5939 (fax)
tobaccoinfo@cdc.gov (e-mail)
www.cdc.gov/tobacco

Develops and distributes the annual Surgeon General's Report on Smoking and Health, coordinates a national public information and education program on tobacco use and health, and coordinates tobacco education and research efforts within the Department of Health and Human Services and throughout both federal and state governments. Maintains the Smoking and Health database, consisting of approximately 60,000 records available on CD-ROM (CDP File) through the Government Printing Office (Superintendent of Documents, Government Printing Office, Washington, DC 20402). Provides information on smoking cessation, environmental tobacco smoke/passive smoking, pregnancy/infants, professional/technical information, and a publications list upon request.

National Sudden Infant Death Syndrome
Resource Center (NSRC)
2070 Chain Bridge Road, Suite 450
Vienna, VA 22182
(866) 866-7437
(703) 821-2098 (fax)

sids@circlesolutions.com (e-mail)
www.sidscenter.org

Sponsored by the Maternal and Child Health Bureau, Health Resources and Services Administration. Provides information and educational materials on sudden infant death syndrome (SIDS), apnea, and other related topics. Responds to information requests from parents, professionals, and the public. Maintains a library/database of public awareness and medical research materials on SIDS and related topics and conducts customized searches of this database and MEDLINE in response to users' requests. Maintains and updates mailing lists of state programs, groups, and individuals concerned with SIDS. Also develops fact sheets, catalogs, and bibliographies on topics of special interest to the SIDS community.

National Technical Information Service
U.S. Department of Commerce
5285 Port Royal Road
Springfield, VA 22161
(800) 553-6847
(703) 605-6900 (fax)
info@ntis.gov (e-mail)
www.ntis.gov

Sells more than 9,000 federally produced audiovisual programs. Provides catalogs at no cost. Several catalogs cover health-related topics, including alcohol and other drug abuse, emergency fire services, industrial safety, and occupational health.

National Women's Health Information Center
8850 Arlington Boulevard, Suite 300
Fairfax, VA 22310
(800) 994-9662
(888) 220-5446 (TDD)
4woman@soza.com (e-mail)
www.4woman.gov

NWHIC is a health information and federal publication referral service that provides a gateway to women's health information from other government agencies, public and private organizations, and consumer and health care professional groups.

National Youth Violence Prevention Resource Center (NYVPRC)
P.O. Box 6003
Rockville, MD 20849-6003
(866) 723-3968
(800) 243-7012 (TTY)
(301) 562-1001 (fax)
NYVP@safeyouth.org (e-mail)
www.safeyouth.org

NYVPRC is a central source of information on prevention and intervention programs, publications, research, and statistics on violence committed by and against children and teens. The resource center is a collaboration between the Centers for Disease Control and Prevention and the Federal Working Group on Youth Violence, which includes representatives from the Department of Health and Human Services; the Departments of Agriculture, Education, Housing and Urban Development, Labor, and Justice; and the Health Resources and Services Administration. Hours of operation: 8:00 A.M.–6:00 P.M. (Eastern Time).

Federal Health Information Centers and Clearinghouses

Agency for Healthcare Research and Quality Clearinghouse
(800) 358-9295
(410) 381-3150 (outside U.S.)
(410) 290-3841 (fax)
info@ahrq.gov (e-mail)
www.ahrq.gov

Alzheimer's Disease Education and Referral Center (ADEAR)
(800) 438-4380
(301) 495-3311
(301) 495-3334 (fax)
adear@alzheimers.org (e-mail)
www.alzheimers.org/

Cancer Information Service
(800) 4-CANCER

(800) 435-3848
(800) 332-8615 (TTY)
(800) 624-2511 (fax back)
(301) 402-5874 (fax)
www.cancernet.nci.nih.gov

CDC National Prevention Information Network
(CDC NPIN)
(800) 458-5231
(800) 243-7012 (TTY)
(888) 282-7681 (fax)
(301) 562-1098 (international)
(301) 588-1589 (international TTY)
info@cdcnpin.org (e-mail)
www.cdcnpin.org

Clearinghouse for Occupational Safety and
Health Information
(800) 356-4674
(513) 533-8328
(513) 533-8573 (fax)
(888) 232-3299 (fax-on-demand)
pubstaft@cdc.gov (e-mail)
www.cdc.gov/niosh

Drug Policy Information Clearinghouse
(800) 666-3332
(301) 519-5212 (fax)
ondcp@ncjrs.org (e-mail)
www.whitehousedrugpolicy.gov/about/
clearingh.html

Educational Resources Information Center
(ERIC) Clearinghouse on Teaching and Teacher
Education
(800) 822-9229
(202) 293-2450
(202) 457-8095 (fax)
query@aacte.org (e-mail)
www.ericsp.org

Federal Information Center (FIC) Program–
National Contact Center
(800) 688-9889
(800) 326-2996 (TTY)
www.info.gov

Food and Drug Administration
(888) INFO-FDA (463-6332)

webmail@oc.fda.gov (e-mail)
www.fda.gov

Food and Nutrition Information Center
(301) 504-5719
(301) 504-6856 (TTY)
(301) 504-6409 (fax)
fnic@nal.usda.gov (e-mail)
www.nal.usda.gov/fnic

Housing and Urban Development (HUD) User
(800) 245-2691
(202) 708-3178
(800) 927-7589 (TDD)
(202) 708-9981 (fax)
helpdesk@huduser.org (e-mail)
www.huduser.org

Indoor Air Quality Information Clearinghouse
(800) 438-4318
(703) 356-4020
(703) 356-5386 (fax)
iaqinfo@aol.com (e-mail)
www.epa.gov/iaq

Maternal and Child Health Information Resource
Center (MCHIRC)
(202) 842-2000
(202) 728-9469 (fax)
mchirc@hsrnet.com (e-mail)
www.mchirc.net

National Adoption Center
(800) 862-3678
(215) 735-9988
(215) 735-9410 (fax)
nac@adopt.org (e-mail)
www.adopt.org/adopt

National Adoption Information Clearinghouse
(888) 251-0075
(703) 352-3488
(703) 385-3206 (fax)
naic@calib.com (e-mail)
www.calib.com/naic

National Center for Chronic Disease Prevention
and Health Promotion (NCCDPHP)
(770) 488-5080

(770) 488-5969 (fax)
ccdinfo@cdc.gov (e-mail)
www.cdc.gov/nccdphp/index.htm

National Center for Complementary and
Alternative Medicine Information Clearinghouse
(888) 644-6226
(301) 519-3153 International callers
(866) 464-3616 (fax)
(866) 464-3615 (TTY)
info@nccam.nih.gov (e-mail)
www.nccam.nih.gov

National Center for Health Statistics
(301) 458-4636
nchsquery@cdc.gov (e-mail)
www.cdc.gov/nchs

National Center on Sleep Disorders Research
(301) 435-0199
(301) 480-3451 (fax)
ncsdr@nih.gov (e-mail)
www.nhlbi.nih.gov/sleep

National Child Care Information Center
(800) 616-2242
(800) 516-2242 (TTY)
(800) 716-2242 (fax)
info@nccic.org (e-mail)
nccic.org

National Clearinghouse for Alcohol and Drug
Information
(800) 729-6686
(877) 767-8432 (Spanish)
(301) 468-2600 (local callers)
(800) 487-4889 (TDD)
(301) 468-6433 (fax)
info@health.org (e-mail)
www.health.org

National Clearinghouse for Primary Care
Information
(703) 821-8955 ext. 248
(703) 821-2098 (fax)
www.bphc.hrsa.dhhs.gov

National Clearinghouse on Child Abuse and
Neglect Information
(800) 394-3366
(703) 385-7565
(703) 385-3206 (fax)
nccanch@calib.com (e-mail)
www.calib.com/nccanch

National Clearinghouse on Families and Youth
(301) 608-8098
(301) 608-8721 (fax)
info@ncfy.com (e-mail)
www.ncfy.com

National Diabetes Information Clearinghouse
(800) 860-8747
(301) 654-3327
(301) 907-8906 (fax)
ndic@info.niddk.nih.gov (e-mail)
www.niddk.nih.gov/health/diabetes/
diabetes.htm

National Digestive Diseases Information
Clearinghouse
(800) 891-5389
(301) 654-3810
(301) 907-8906 (fax)
nddic@info.niddk.nih.gov (e-mail)
www.niddk.nih.gov/health/digest/digest.htm

National Health Information Center
(800) 336-4797
(301) 565-4167
(301) 984-4256 (fax)
info@nhic.org (e-mail)
www.health.gov/nhic

National Heart, Lung, and Blood Institute
(NHLBI) Health Information Center
(301) 592-8573
(301) 592-8563 (fax)
NHLBIinfo@rover.nhlbi.nih.gov (e-mail)
www.nhlbi.nih.gov

National Highway Traffic Safety Administration
(800) 424-9393 (Hotline)
(202) 366-0123 (Hotline)

(800) 424-9153 (TTY)
(202) 366-5962 (fax)
www.nhtsa.dot.gov

National Information Center for Children and Youth With Disabilities
(800) 695-0285 (voice/TTY)
(202) 884-8200 (voice/TTY)
(202) 884-8441 (fax)
nichcy@aed.org (e-mail)
www.nichcy.org

National Injury Information Clearinghouse
(301) 504-0424
(301) 504-0124 (fax)
clearinghouse@cpsc.gov (e-mail)
www.cpsc.gov/about/clrnghse.html

National Institute of Allergy and Infectious Diseases
(301) 496-5717
(301) 402-0120 (fax)
ocpostoffice@niaid.nih.gov (e-mail)
www.niaid.nih.gov

National Institute of Arthritis and Musculoskeletal and Skin Diseases Information Clearinghouse
(877) 22-NIAMS
(301) 495-4484
(301) 565-2966 (TTY)
(301) 718-6366 (fax)
niamsinfo@mail.nih.gov (e-mail)
www.niams.nih.gov

National Institute of Child Health and Human Development (NICHD)
Information Resource Center
P.O. Box 3006
Rockville, MD 20847
(800) 370-2943
(800) 505-CRIB (2742) "Back to Sleep" campaign
(301) 984-1473 (fax)
NICHDClearinghouse@mail.nih.gov (e-mail)
www.nichd.nih.gov

National Institute of Mental Health (NIMH)
Information Resources and Inquiries Branch

(301) 443-4513
(301) 443-8431 (TTY)
(301) 443-5158 (MENTAL HEALTH FAX4U– fax information system)
(888) 8-ANXIETY (publications on anxiety disorders)
(800) 421-4211 (publications on depression)
nimhinfo@nih.gov (e-mail)
www.nimh.nih.gov

National Institute on Aging Information Center
(800) 222-2225
(301) 496-1752
(800) 222-4225 (TTY)
(301) 589-3014 (fax)
niaic@jbs1.com (e-mail)
www.nia.nih.gov

National Institute on Deafness and Other Communication Disorders Information Clearinghouse
(800) 241-1044
(800) 241-1055 (TTY)
(301) 907-8830 (fax)
nidcdinfo@nidcd.nih.gov (e-mail)
www.nidcd.nih.gov

National Kidney and Urologic Diseases Information Clearinghouse
(800) 891-5390
(301) 654-4415
(301) 907-8906 (fax)
nkudic@info.niddk.nih.gov (e-mail)
www.niddk.nih.gov/health/kidney/nkudic.htm

National Lead Information Center (NLIC)
(800) 424-LEAD (5323)
(301) 588-8495 (fax)
www.epa.gov/lead/nlic.htm

National Library Service for the Blind and Physically Handicapped
(800) 424-8567
(202) 707-5100
(202) 707-0744 (TDD)
(202) 707-0712 (fax)

nls@loc.gov (e-mail)
lcweb.loc.gov/nls

National Oral Health Information Clearinghouse
(301) 402-7364
(301) 907-8830 (fax)
nohic@nidcr.nih.gov (e-mail)
www.nohic.nidcr.nih.gov

National Rehabilitation Information Center
(800) 346-2742
(301) 459-5900
(301) 459-4263 (TTY/fax)
naricinfo@heitechservices.com (e-mail)
www.naric.com

National Resource Center on Homelessness and
Mental Illness
(800) 444-7415
(518) 439-7415
(518) 439-7612 (fax)
pra@prainc.com (e-mail)
www.nrchmi.com

National Sudden Infant Death Syndrome
Resource Center (NSRC)
(866) 866-7437
(703) 821-2098 (fax)
sids@circlesolutions.com (e-mail)
www.sidscenter.org

National Technical Information Service
(800) 553-6847
(703) 605-6900 (fax)
info@ntis.gov (e-mail)
www.ntis.gov

National Women's Health Information Center
(800) 994-9662
(888) 220-5446 (TDD)
4woman@soza.com (e-mail)
www.4woman.gov

National Youth Violence Prevention Resource
Center (NYVPRC)
(866) 723-3968
(800) 243-7012 (TTY)

(301) 562-1001 (fax)
NYVP@safeyouth.org (e-mail)
www.safeyouth.org

NIH Consensus Program Information Center
(888) 644-2667
(301) 593-9485 (fax)
consensus.nih.gov

NIH Osteoporosis and Related Bone Diseases
National Resource Center
(800) 624-BONE
(202) 466-4315 (TTY)
(202) 293-2356 (fax)
orbdnrc@nof.org (e-mail)
www.osteo.org

Office of Minority Health Resource Center
(800) 444-6472
(301) 230-7874
(301) 230-7199 (TDD)
(301) 230-7198 (fax)
info@omhrc.gov (e-mail)
www.omhrc.gov

Office of Population Affairs (OPA)
Clearinghouse
(301) 654-6190
(301) 215-7731 (fax)
opa@osophs.dhhs.gov (e-mail)
opa.osophs.dhhs.gov/clearinghouse.html

Office on Smoking and Health
(800) CDC-1311
(770) 488-5705
(770) 488-5939 (fax)
tobaccoinfo@cdc.gov (e-mail)
www.cdc.gov/tobacco

OSERS/Communications and Media Support
Services (Disabilities, Rehabilitation)
(202) 205-5465
customerservice@inet.ed.gov (e-mail)
www.ed.gov/offices/OSERS

Policy Information Center (PIC)
(202) 690-6445

pic@osaspe.dhhs.gov (e-mail)
aspe.dhhs.gov/pic

President's Council on Physical Fitness and
Sports
(202) 690-9000
(202) 690-5211 (fax)
www.fitness.gov

U.S. Administration on Aging, Center for
Communication and Consumer Services (CCCS)
(202) 619-7501
(202) 401-7620 (fax)
cccs@aoa.gov (e-mail)
www.aoa.gov/naic

U.S. Coast Guard Office of Boating Safety
(800) 368-5647
(202) 267-1077
(800) 689-0816 (TTY)
(703) 313-5910 (BBS)
uscginfoline@gcrm.com (e-mail)
www.uscgboating.org

U.S. Consumer Product Safety Commission
Hotline (CPSC)
(800) 638-2772 (toll-free hotline)
(800) 638-8270 (TTY)
info@cpsc.gov (e-mail)
cpsc.gov

U.S. Environmental Protection Agency
Information Resources Center
(202) 566-0556
(202) 566-0562 (fax)
hq-irc@epa.gov (e-mail)
www.epa.gov

U.S. Federal Consumer Information Center
Pueblo, CO 81009
(719) 948-4000 (orders)
catalog.pueblo@gsa.gov (e-mail)
www.pueblo.gsa.gov

HEALTH EDUCATION STANDARDS

Health Education Standard 1:

Students will comprehend concepts related to health promotion and disease prevention.

Rationale

Basic to health education is a foundation of knowledge about the interrelationship of behavior and health, interactions within the human body, and the prevention of diseases and other health problems. Experiencing physical, mental, emotional, and social changes as one grows and develops provides a self-contained "learning laboratory." Comprehension of health promotion strategies and disease prevention concepts enables students to become health-literate, self-directed learners, which establishes a foundation for leading healthy and productive lives.

PERFORMANCE INDICATORS

As a result of health instruction in Grades K–4, students will

1. Describe relationships between personal health behaviors and individual well being.

2. Identify indicators of mental, emotional, social, and physical health during childhood.

As a result of health instruction in Grades 5–8, students will

1. Explain the relationship between positive health behaviors and the prevention of injury, illness, disease, and premature death.

2. Describe the interrelationship of mental, emotional, social, and physical health during adolescence.

As a result of health instruction in Grades 9–11, students will

1. Analyze how behavior can impact health maintenance and disease prevention.

2. Describe the interrelationships of mental, emotional, social, and physical health throughout adulthood.

This information is reprinted with permission from the *Journal of Health Education*. The *Journal of Health Education* is a publication of the American Alliance for Health, Physical Education, Recreation and Dance, 1900 Association Drive, Reston, Virginia 22091.

As a result of health instruction in Grades K–4, students will

3. Describe the basic structure and functions of the human body systems.

4. Describe how the family influences personal health.

5. Describe how physical, social, and emotional environments influence personal health.

6. Identify common health problems of children.

7. Identify health problems that should be detected and treated early.

8. Explain how childhood injuries and illnesses can be prevented or treated.

As a result of health instruction in Grades 5–8, students will

3. Explain how health is influenced by the interaction of body systems.

4. Describe how family and peers influence the health of adolescents.

5. Analyze how environment and personal health are interrelated.

6. Describe ways to reduce risks related to adolescent health problems.

7. Explain how appropriate health care can prevent premature death and disability.

8. Describe how lifestyle, pathogens, family history, and other risk factors are related to the cause or prevention of disease and other health problems.

As a result of health instruction in Grades 9–11, students will

3. Explain the impact of personal health behaviors on the functioning of body systems.

4. Analyze how the family, peers, and community influence the health of individuals.

5. Analyze how the environment influences the health of the community.

6. Describe how to delay onset and reduce risks of potential health problems during adulthood.

7. Analyze how public health policies and government regulations influence health promotion and disease prevention.

8. Analyze how the prevention and control of health problems are influenced by research and medical advances.

Health Education Standard 2:

Students will demonstrate the ability to access valid health information and health-promoting products and services.

Rationale

Accessing valid health information and health-promoting products and services is important in the prevention, early detection, and treatment of most health problems. Critical thinking involves the ability to identify valid health information and to analyze, select, and access health-promoting services and products. Applying skills of information analysis, organization, comparison, synthesis, and evaluation to health issues provides a foundation for individuals to move toward becoming health literate and responsible, productive citizens.

PERFORMANCE INDICATORS

As a result of health instruction in Grades K–4, students will

1. Identify characteristics of valid health information and health-promoting products and services.

2. Demonstrate the ability to locate resources from home, school, and community that provide valid health information.

3. Explain how media influence the selection of health information, products, and services.

4. Demonstrate the ability to locate school and community health helpers.

As a result of health instruction in Grades 5–8, students will

1. Analyze the validity of health information, products, and services.

2. Demonstrate the ability to utilize resources from home, school, and community that provide valid health information.

3. Analyze how media influence the selection of health information and products.

4. Demonstrate the ability to locate health products and services.

5. Compare the costs and validity of health products.

6. Describe situations requiring professional health services.

As a result of health instruction in Grades 9–11, students will

1. Evaluate the validity of health information, products, and services.

2. Demonstrate the ability to evaluate resources from home, school, and community that provide valid health information.

3. Evaluate factors that influence personal selection of health products and services.

4. Demonstrate the ability to access school and community health services for self and others.

5. Analyze the cost and accessibility of health care services.

6. Analyze situations requiring professional health services.

Health Education Standard 3:

Students will demonstrate the ability to practice health-enhancing behaviors and reduce health risks.

Rationale

Research confirms that many diseases and injuries can be prevented by reducing harmful and risk-taking behaviors. More importantly, recognizing and practicing health-enhancing behaviors can contribute to a positive quality of life. Strategies used to maintain and improve positive health behaviors will utilize knowledge and skills that help students become critical thinkers and problem solvers. By accepting responsibility for personal health, students will have a foundation for living a healthy, productive life.

PERFORMANCE INDICATORS

As a result of health instruction in Grades K–4, students will

1. Identify responsible health behaviors.

2. Identify personal health needs.

3. Compare behaviors that are safe to those that are risky or harmful.

4. Demonstrate strategies to improve or maintain personal health.

5. Develop injury prevention and management strategies for personal health.

6. Demonstrate ways to avoid and reduce threatening situations.

7. Apply skills to manage stress.

As a result of health instruction in Grades 5–8, students will

1. Explain the importance of assuming responsibility for personal health behaviors.

2. Analyze a personal health assessment to determine health strengths and risks.

3. Distinguish between safe and risky or harmful behaviors in relationships.

4. Demonstrate strategies to improve or maintain personal and family health.

5. Develop injury prevention and management strategies for personal and family health.

6. Demonstrate ways to avoid and reduce threatening situations.

7. Demonstrate strategies to manage stress.

As a result of health instruction in Grades 9–11, students will

1. Analyze the role of individual responsibility for enhancing health.

2. Evaluate a personal health assessment to determine strategies for health enhancement and risk reduction.

3. Analyze the short-term and long-term consequences of safe, risky, and harmful behaviors.

4. Develop strategies to improve or maintain personal, family, and community health.

5. Develop injury prevention and management strategies for personal, family, and community health.

6. Demonstrate ways to avoid and reduce threatening situations.

7. Evaluate strategies to manage stress.

Health Education Standard 4:

Students will analyze the influence of culture, media, technology, and other factors on health.

Rationale

Health is influenced by a variety of factors that coexist within society. These include the cultural context as well as media and technology. A critical thinker and problem solver is able to analyze, evaluate, and interpret the influence of these factors on health. The health-literate, responsible, and productive citizen draws upon the contributions of culture, media, technology, and other factors to strengthen individual, family, and community health.

PERFORMANCE INDICATORS

As a result of health instruction in Grades K–4, students will

1. Describe how culture influences personal health behaviors.

2. Explain how media influences thoughts, feelings, and health behaviors.

3. Describe ways technology can influence personal health.

4. Explain how information from school and family influences health.

As a result of health instruction in Grades 5–8, students will

1. Describe the influence of cultural beliefs on health behaviors and the use of health services.

2. Analyze how messages from media and other sources influence health behaviors.

3. Analyze the influence of technology on personal and family health.

4. Analyze how information from peers influences health.

As a result of health instruction in Grades 9–11, students will

1. Analyze how cultural diversity enriches and challenges health behaviors.

2. Evaluate the effect of media and other factors on personal, family, and community health.

3. Evaluate the impact of technology on personal, family, and community health.

4. Analyze how information from the community influences health.

Health Education Standard 5:

Students will demonstrate the ability to use interpersonal communication skills to enhance health.

Rationale

Personal, family, and community health are enhanced through effective communication. A responsible individual will use verbal and nonverbal skills in developing and maintaining healthy personal relationships. Ability to organize and to convey information, beliefs, opinions, and feelings are skills that strengthen interactions and can reduce or avoid conflict. When communicating, individuals who are health literate demonstrate care, consideration, and respect of self and others.

PERFORMANCE INDICATORS

As a result of health instruction in Grades K–4, students will

1. Distinguish between verbal and nonverbal communication.

As a result of health instruction in Grades 5–8, students will

1. Demonstrate effective verbal and nonverbal communication skills to enhance health.

As a result of health instruction in Grades 9–11, students will

1. Demonstrate skills for communicating effectively with family, peers, and others.

As a result of health instruction in Grades K–4, students will	*As a result of health instruction in Grades 5–8, students will*	*As a result of health instruction in Grades 9–11, students will*
2. Describe characteristics needed to be a responsible friend and family member.	2. Describe how the behavior of family and peers affects interpersonal communication.	2. Analyze how interpersonal communication affects relationships.
3. Demonstrate healthy ways to express needs, wants, and feelings.	3. Demonstrate healthy ways to express needs, wants, and feelings.	3. Demonstrate healthy ways to express needs, wants, and feelings.
4. Demonstrate ways to communicate care, consideration, and respect of self and others.	4. Demonstrate ways to communicate care, consideration, and respect of self and others.	4. Demonstrate ways to communicate care, consideration, and respect of self and others.
5. Demonstrate attentive listening skills to build and maintain healthy relationships.	5. Demonstrate communication skills to build and maintain healthy relationships.	5. Demonstrate strategies for solving interpersonal conflicts without harming self or others.
6. Demonstrate refusal skills to enhance health.	6. Demonstrate refusal and negotiation skills to enhance health.	6. Demonstrate refusal, negotiation, and collaboration skills to avoid potentially harmful situations.
7. Differentiate between negative and positive behaviors used in conflict situations.	7. Analyze the possible causes of conflict among youth in school and communities.	7. Analyze the possible causes of conflict in schools, families, and communities.
8. Demonstrate nonviolent strategies to resolve conflicts.	8. Demonstrate strategies to manage conflict in healthy ways.	8. Demonstrate strategies used to prevent conflict.

Health Education Standard 6:

Students will demonstrate the ability to use goal-setting and decision-making skills to enhance health.

Rationale

Decision making and goal setting are essential lifelong skills needed in order to implement and sustain health-enhancing behaviors. These skills make it possible for individuals to transfer health knowledge into healthful lifestyles. When applied to health issues, decision-making and goal-setting skills will enable individuals to collaborate with others to improve the quality of life in their families, schools, and communities.

PERFORMANCE INDICATORS

As a result of health instruction in Grades K–4, students will

1. Demonstrate the ability to apply a decision-making process to health issues and problems.

2. Explain when to ask for assistance in making health-related decisions and setting health goals.

3. Predict outcomes of positive health decisions.

4. Set a personal health goal and track progress toward its achievement.

As a result of health instruction in Grades 5–8, students will

1. Demonstrate the ability to apply a decision-making process to health issues and problems individually and collaboratively.

2. Analyze how health-related decisions are influenced by individuals, family, and community values.

3. Predict how decisions regarding health behaviors have consequences for self and others.

4. Apply strategies and skills needed to attain personal health goals.

5. Describe how personal health goals are influenced by changing information, abilities, priorities, and responsibilities.

6. Develop a plan that addresses personal strengths, needs, and health risks.

As a result of health instruction in Grades 9–11, students will

1. Demonstrate the ability to utilize various strategies when making decisions related to health needs and risks of young adults.

2. Analyze health concerns that require collaborative decision making.

3. Predict immediate and long-term impact of health decisions on the individual, family, and community.

4. Implement a plan for attaining a personal health goal.

5. Evaluate progress toward achieving personal health goals.

6. Formulate an effective plan for lifelong health.

Health Education Standard 7:

Students will demonstrate the ability to advocate for personal, family, and community health.

Rationale

Quality of life depends on an environment that protects and promotes the health of individuals, families, and communities. Responsible citizens, who are health literate, are characterized by advocating and communicating for positive health in their communities. A variety of health advocacy skills are critical to these activities.

PERFORMANCE INDICATORS

As a result of health instruction in Grades K–4, students will

1. Describe a variety of methods to convey accurate health information and ideas.

2. Express information and opinions about health issues.

3. Identify community agencies that advocate for healthy individuals, families, and communities.

4. Demonstrate the ability to influence and support others in making positive health choices.

As a result of health instruction in Grades 5–8, students will

1. Analyze various communication methods to accurately express health information and ideas.

2. Express information and opinions about health issues.

3. Identify barriers to effective communication of information, ideas, feelings, and opinions about health issues.

4. Demonstrate the ability to influence and support others in making positive health choices.

5. Demonstrate the ability to work cooperatively when advocating for healthy individuals, families, and schools.

As a result of health instruction in Grades 9–11, students will

1. Evaluate the effectiveness of communication methods for accurately expressing health information and ideas.

2. Express information and opinions about health issues.

3. Utilize strategies to overcome barriers when communicating information, ideas, feelings, and opinions about health issues.

4. Demonstrate the ability to influence and support others in making positive health choices.

5. Demonstrate the ability to work cooperatively when advocating for healthy communities.

6. Demonstrate the ability to adapt health messages and communication techniques to the characteristics of a particular audience.

2003 NATIONAL
HEALTH OBSERVANCES

January

National Volunteer Blood Donor Month
American Association of Blood Banks
8101 Glenbrook Road
Bethesda, MD 20814
(301) 215-6526
aabb@aabb.org
www.aabb.org
Materials available
Contact: Jennifer Garfinkel

Cervical Health Awareness Month
National Cervical Cancer Coalition
16501 Sherman Way Avenue, Suite 110
Van Nuys, CA 91406
(818) 909-3849
(818) 780-8199 (fax)
ncccak@nccc-online.org
www.nccc-online.org
Materials available
Contact: none available

National Birth Defects Prevention Month
March of Dimes Birth Defects Foundation
1275 Mamaroneck Avenue
White Plains, NY 10605

(888) M-O-DIMES
askus@marchofdimes.com
www.marchofdimes.com
Materials available
Contact: Pregnancy and Newborn Health
Education Center

National Glaucoma Awareness Month
Prevent Blindness America
500 East Remington Road
Schaumburg, IL 60173-5611
(800) 331-2020
info@preventblindness.org
www.preventblindness.org
Materials available
Contact: Center for Sight

19–25
Healthy Weight Week
Healthy Weight Network
402 South 14th Street
Hettinger, ND 58639
(701) 567-2646
hwj@healthyweight.net
www.healthyweight.net
Materials available
Contact: none available

Source: U.S. Department of Health and Human Services, Office of Disease Prevention and Health Promotion.

February

American Heart Month
American Heart Association
7272 Greenville Avenue
Dallas, TX 75231
(800) 242-8721
inquire@americanheart.org
www.americanheart.org
Materials available
Contact: program departments or local chapters

AMD/Low Vision Awareness Month
Prevent Blindness America
500 East Remington Road
Schaumburg, IL 60173
(800) 331-2020
info@preventblindness.org
www.preventblindness.org
Materials available
Contact: Center for Sight

National Children's Dental Health Month
American Dental Association
211 E. Chicago Avenue
Chicago, IL 60611
(312) 440-2593
publicinfo@ada.org
www.ada.org
Contact: Department of Public Information

Wise Health Consumer Month
American Institute for Preventive Medicine
30445 Northwestern Highway, Suite 350
Farmington Hills, MI 48334
(800) 345-2476
(248) 539-1800 x247
aipm@healthylife.com
www.healthylife.com
Materials available
Contact: Customer Care Department

Kids E.N.T. (Ears, Nose, Throat) Month
American Academy of Otolaryngology, Head and
Neck Surgery, Inc.
One Prince Street
Alexandria, VA 22314-3357
703-836-4444
www.entnet.org
Contact: Jennifer Felsher

2–8
National Burn Awareness Week
Shriners Burns Hospital
3229 Burnet Avenue
Cincinnati, OH 45229
(513) 872-6000
Lhoelker@shrinenet.org
www.shrinershq.org/shc/cincinnati/index.html
Materials available
Contact: Pat Harrison

5
National Girls and Women in Sports Day
Women's Sports Foundation
Eisenhower Park
East Meadow, NY 11554
(800) 227-3988
wosport@aol.com
www.womenssportsfoundation.org
Materials available
Contact: Colleen Horan

9–15
National Children of Alcoholics Week
National Association for Children of Alcoholics
11426 Rockville Pike, Suite 100
Rockville, MD 20852
(888) 554-2627
nacoa@nacoa.org
www.nacoa.org
Materials available
Contact: none available

9–15
National Child Passenger Safety Awareness Week
Office of Occupant Protection, National Highway
Traffic Safety Administration
U.S. Department of Transportation
400 Seventh Street, S.W.
Washington, DC 20590
(888) DASH-2-DOT
(202) 366-9550

none available
www.nhtsa.dot.gov
Materials available
Contact: none available

10–14
Cardiac Rehabilitation Week
American Association of Cardiovascular and Pulmonary Rehabilitation
401 North Michigan Ave., Suite 2200
Chicago, IL 60611
(312) 321-5146
aacvpr@sba.com
www.aacvpr.org
Materials available
Contact: Dana Fennewalb

14
National Condom Day
American Social Health Association
P.O. Box 13827
Research Triangle Park, NC 27709
(919) 361-8400
Traada@ashastd.org
www.ashastd.org
Materials available
Contact: public relations assistant

21
Give Kids A Smile Day
American Dental Association
211 East Chicago Avenue
Chicago, IL 60611
(312) 440-2500
www.ada.org
Contact: Jane Forsberg Jasek

23–28
National Eating Disorders Awareness Week
National Eating Disorders Association
603 Stewart Street, Suite 803
Seattle, WA 98101
(206) 382-3587 x19
(206) 829-8501 (fax)
info@nationaleatingdisorders.org
www.nationaleatingdisorders.org
Materials available
Contact: Kari Augustyn

March

Save Your Vision Month
American Optometric Association
243 North Lindbergh Boulevard
St. Louis, MO 63141
(314) 991-4100
(314) 991-4101 (fax)
slthomas@aoa.org
www.aoa.org
Materials available
Contact: Susan Thomas and Julie M. Mahoney

Mental Retardation Awareness Month
The ARC of the United States
1010 Wayne Avenue, Suite 650
Silver Spring, MD 20910
(301) 565-3842
info@thearc.org
www.thearc.org
Materials available
Contact: Chris Privette

National Chronic Fatigue Syndrome Awareness Month
National Chronic Fatigue Syndrome and
Fibromyalgia Association
P.O. Box 18426
Kansas City, MO 64133
(816) 313-2000
none available
Materials available
Contact: Public Information

National Colorectal Cancer Awareness Month
Cancer Research and Prevention Foundation
1600 Duke Street
Alexandria, VA 22314
(800) 227-2732
(703) 836-4412
Enica.Lewis@preventcancer.org
www.preventcancer.org/colorectal/
Materials available
Contact: Enica Lewis

National Eye Donor Month
Eye Bank Association of America
1015 18th Street, N.W., Suite 1010

Washington, DC 20036
(202) 775-4999
sightebaa@aol.com
www.restoresight.org
Materials available
Contact: administrative manager

National Kidney Month
National Kidney Foundation
30 East 33rd Street, Suite 1100
New York, NY 10016
(800) 622-9010
(212) 689-9261 (fax)
info@kidney.org
www.kidney.org
Materials available
Contact: Ellie Schlam

National Nutrition Month
American Dietetic Association
216 West Jackson Boulevard, Suite 800
Chicago, IL 60606-6995
(800) 877-1600
(800) 546-6180 Orders Only
info@eatright.org
www.eatright.org/
Materials available
Contact: Communications department

Workplace Eye Health and Safety Month
Prevent Blindness America
500 East Remington Road
Schaumburg, IL 60173
(800) 331-2020
info@preventblindness.org
www.preventblindness.org
Materials available
Contact: Center for Sight

American Red Cross Month
American Red Cross
431 18th Street, N.W.
Washington, DC 20006
(202) 639-3520
info@redcross.org
www.redcross.org
Materials available
Contact: none available

3–7

National School Breakfast Week
American School Food Service Association
700 South Washington Street, Suite 300
Alexandria, VA 22314-4287
(800) 877-8822
(703) 739-3915 (fax)
servicecenter@asfsa.org
www.asfsa.org
Materials available
Contact: Linda Ross

9–15

National Patient Safety Awareness Week
National Patient Safety Foundation
515 North State Street
Chicago, IL 60610
(312) 464-4848
(312) 464-4154 (fax)
info@npsf.org
www.npsf.org
Materials available
Contact: none available

10–16

Brain Awareness Week
Dana Alliance for Brain Initiatives
745 Fifth Avenue, Suite 900
New York, NY 10151
(212) 401-1680
bawinfo@dana.org
www.dana.org/brainweek
Materials available
Contact: Kathleen Roina

16–22

National Inhalants and Poisons Awareness Week
National Inhalant Prevention Coalition
2904 Kerby Lane
Austin, TX 78703
(800) 269-4237
nipc@io.com
www.inhalants.org
Materials available
Contact: Harvey Weiss

16–22
National Poison Prevention Week
Poison Prevention Week Council
P.O. Box 1543
Washington, DC 20013
(800) 638-2772
kgiles@cpsc.org
www.poisonprevention.org
Materials available
Contact: Ken Giles

17–21
Pulmonary Rehabilitation Week
American Association of Cardiovascular and
Pulmonary Rehabilitation
401 North Michigan Ave., Suite 2200
Chicago, IL 60611
(312) 321-5146
aacvpr@sba.com
www.aacvpr.org
Materials available
Contact: Dana Fennewalb

24
World Tuberculosis Day
American Association for World Health
1825 K Street, N.W.,
Suite 1208
Washington, DC 20006
(202) 466-5883
staff@aawhworldhealth.org
www.aawhworldhealth.org
Contact: none available

25
American Diabetes Alert Day
American Diabetes Association
1701 North Beauregard Street
Alexandria, VA 22311
(800) DIABETES
none available
www.diabetes.org
Materials available
Contact: local affiliates

31–6
National Sleep Awareness Week
National Sleep Foundation

1522 K Street, N.W., #500
Washington, DC 20005
(202) 347-3471 ext. 205
(202) 347-3472 (fax)
nsf@sleepfoundation.org
www.sleepfoundation.org
Materials available
Contact: Public Relations

April

Alcohol Awareness Month
National Council on Alcoholism and Drug
Dependence, Inc.
20 Exchange Place, Suite 2902
New York, NY 10005
(212) 269-7797
(800) NCA-CALL (24-hr. hopeline)
(212) 269-7510 (fax)
national@ncadd.org
www.ncadd.org
Materials available
Contact: Public Information Department

Cancer Control Month
American Cancer Society
1599 Clifton Road, N.E.
Atlanta, GA 30329
(800) ACS-2345
(404) 320-3333
none available
www.cancer.org
Materials available
Contact: local chapters

Counseling Awareness Month
American Counseling Association
5999 Stevenson Avenue
Alexandria, VA 22304-3300
(800) 347-6647
(703) 823-9800
aca@counseling.org
www.counseling.org
Materials available
Contact: Christie Lunn

IBS (Irritable Bowel Syndrome) Awareness Month
International Foundation for Functional Gastrointestinal Disorders (IFFGD)
P.O. Box 170864
Milwaukee, WI 53217
(888) 964-2001 8:30 A.M.–5 P.M. CST
(414) 964-1799
iffgd@iffgd.org
www.aboutibs.org
Materials available
Contact: Nancy Norton

National Autism Awareness Month
Autism Society of America
7910 Woodmont Avenue, Suite 300
Bethesda, MD 20814-3015
(800) 3-AUTISM
(301) 657-0881 x150
none available
www.autism-society.org
Materials available
Contact: none available

National Child Abuse Prevention Month
National Clearinghouse on Child Abuse and Neglect Information
330 C Street, S.W.
Washington, DC 20447
(800) 394-3366
(703) 385-7565
none available
www.calib.com/nccanch
Materials available
Contact: Public Awareness Department

National Occupational Therapy Month
The American Occupational Therapy Association, Inc.
4720 Montgomery Lane
P.O. Box 31220
Bethesda, MD 20824-1220
(301) 652-2682
(800) 377-8555 (TDD)
(800) 701-7735 (fax)
praota@aota.org
www.aota.org

Materials available
Contact: Communications Group

National STD Awareness Month
American Social Health Association
P.O. Box 13827
Research Triangle Park, NC 27709
(919) 361-8400
Traada@ashastd.org
www.ashastd.org
Materials available
Contact: Tracey Adams

National Youth Sports Safety Month
National Youth Sports Safety Foundation
333 Longwood Avenue, Suite 202
Boston, MA 02115
(617) 277-1171
nyssf@aol.com
www.nyssf.org
Materials available
Contact: Rita Glassman

Women's Eye Health and Safety Month
Prevent Blindness America
500 East Remington Road
Schaumburg, IL 60173-5611
(800) 331-2020
info@preventblindness.org
www.preventblindness.org
Materials available
Contact: Center for Sight

Foot Health Awareness Month
American Podiatric Medical Association
9312 Old Georgetown Road
Bethesda, MD 20814
(800) FOOTCARE
(301) 530-2752 (fax)
ajbrewer@apma.org
www.apma.org/footmouth02.htm
Materials available
Contact: Allison Brewer

Sexual Assault Awareness Month
National Sexual Violence Resource Center
123 N. Enola Drive
Enola, PA 17025

(877) 739-3895
(717) 909-0714 (fax)
resources@nsvrc.org
www.nsvrc.org
Materials available
Contact: Resource Center

Sports Eye Safety Month
American Academy of Ophthalmology
P.O. Box 7424
San Francisco, CA 94120
(415) 561-8525
(415) 561-8533 (fax)
eyemd@aao.org
www.aao.org
Materials available
Contact: Annamarie Harris

2
Kick Butts Day
Campaign for Tobacco-Free Kids
1707 L Street, N.W., Suite 800
Washington, DC 20036
(800) 803-7178
(202) 296-5469
info@tobaccofreekids.org
www.kickbuttsday.org
Materials available
Contact: none available

4–6
Alcohol-Free Weekend
National Council on Alcoholism and Drug
Dependence, Inc.
20 Exchange Place, Suite 2902
New York, NY 10005
(212) 269-7797
(800) NCA-CALL (24-hr. helpline)
(212) 269-7510 (fax)
national@ncadd.org
www.ncadd.org
Materials available
Contact: none available

5
YMCA Healthy Kids Day
YMCA of the USA
101 North Wacker Drive

Chicago, IL 60606
(312) 977-0031
(888) 333-YMCA
none available
www.ymca.net
Materials available
Contact: Angela Franta

7–13
National Public Health Week
American Public Health Association
800 I Street, N.W.
Washington, DC 20001-3710
(202) 777-APHA
(202) 770-2500 TTY
comments@apha.org
www.apha.org
Materials available
Contact: Sharon Hammon

7
World Health Day
American Association for World Health
1825 K Street, N.W., Suite 1208
Washington, DC 20006
(202) 466-5883
staff@aawhworldhealth.org
www.aawhworldhealth.org
Materials available
Contact: none available

10
National Alcohol Screening Day
Screening for Mental Health
One Washington Street, Suite 304
Wellesly Hills, MA 02481
(781) 239-0071
nasd@mentalhealthscreening.org
www.mentalhealthscreening.org
Contact: Anne Keliher, Program Manager

13–19
National Infants Immunization Week
Centers for Disease Control and Prevention:
National Immunization Program
1600 Clifton Road Mail Stop E-05
Atlanta, GA 30333
(800) 232-2522 (English)

(800) 232-0233 (Spanish)
(888) CDC-FAXX (free fax-back)
none available
www.cdc.gov/nip
Contact: Community Outreach and Planning Branch

20–26
National Organ and Tissue Donor Awareness Week
Coalition on Donation
1100 Boulders Parkway, Suite 700
Richmond, VA 23225-8770
(804) 330-8620
coalition@shareyourlife.org
www.shareyourlife.org
Materials available
Contact: coalition@shareyourlife.org

20–26
National Minority Cancer Awareness Week
National Cancer Institute
Center to Reduce Cancer Health Disparities
6116 Executive Boulevard, Suite 602
Rockville, MD 20852
(301) 402-5557
none available
www.cancer.gov
Materials available
Contact: none available

26–27
2003 WalkAmerica
March of Dimes Birth Defects Foundation
1275 Mamaroneck Avenue
White Plains, NY 10605
(888) M-O-DIMES
(800) 525-WALK
(914) 997-4617
walkamerica@modimes.org
www.walkamerica.org
Materials available
Contact: Angela Hill

26
Candlelight Vigil for Eating Disorders Awareness
National Association of Anorexia Nervosa and Associated Disorders

Box 7
Highland Park, IL 60035
(847) 831-4348
anad20@aol.com
www.anad.org
Materials available
Contact: Millie Plotkin

27–3
National Volunteer Week
Points of Light Foundation
The Volunteer Centers National Network
1400 I Street, N.W., Suite 800
Washington, DC 20005
(202) 729-8168
(202) 729-8100 (fax)
volunteerweek@pointsoflight.org
www.pointsoflight.org/programs/programs_nvwintroa.htm
Materials available
Contact: none available

May

Asthma and Allergy Awareness Month
Asthma and Allergy Foundation of America
1233 20th Street, N.W., Suite 402
Washington, DC 20036
(800) 7-ASTHMA
info@aafa.org
www.aafa.org
Materials available
Contact: Colleen Horn

Better Hearing and Speech Month
American Speech-Language-Hearing Association
10801 Rockville Pike
Rockville, MD 20852
(800) 498-2071
(301) 897-5700 TTY
actioncenter@asha.org
www.asha.org
Materials available
Contact: Action Center

Better Sleep Month
Better Sleep Council

501 Wythe Street
Alexandria, VA 22314
(703) 683-8371
bsc@sleepproducts.org
www.bettersleep.org
Materials available
Contact: Nancy L. Blatt

Correct Posture Month
American Chiropractic Association
1701 Clarendon Boulevard
Arlington, VA 22209
(800) 986-4636
(703) 276-8800
Amerchiro@aol.com
www.amerchiro.org
Materials available
Contact: Omar Malik

Hepatitis Awareness Month
Hepatitis Foundation International
30 Sunrise Terrace
Cedar Grove, NJ 07009
(800) 891-0707
(973) 239-1035
mail@hepfi.org
www.hepfi.org
Materials available
Contact: Thelma King Thiel

Huntington's Disease Awareness Month
Huntington's Disease Society of America, Inc.
158 West 29th Street, 7th Floor
New York, NY 10001
(800) 345-4372
hdsinfo@hdsa.org
www.hdsa.org
Materials available
Contact: local chapters or national office

National Arthritis Month and Annual Arthritis Walk
Arthritis Foundation
1330 West Peachtree Street
Atlanta, GA 30309
(800) 283-7800
www.arthritis.org

Materials available
Contact: Public Relations Department

National Digestive Diseases Awareness Month
Digestive Disease National Coalition
507 Capitol Court, N.E., Suite 200
Washington, DC 20002
(202) 544-7497
none available
none available
Materials available
Contact: Dale Dirks

National High Blood Pressure Education Month
National Heart, Lung, and Blood Institute
(NHLBI) Health Information Center
P.O. Box 30105
Bethesda, MD 20824-0105
(301) 592-8573
(301) 592-8563 (fax)
nhlbiinfo@rover.nhlbi.nih.gov
www.nhlbi.nih.gov
Materials available
Contact: information specialist

National Melanoma/Skin Cancer Detection and Prevention Month
American Academy of Dermatology
930 North Meacham Road
Schaumburg, IL 60173
(888) 462-DERM
(847) 330-0230 x343
none available
www.aad.org
Materials available
Contact: Donna Stein

Mental Health Month
National Mental Health Association and National Council for Community Behavioral Healthcare
2001 North Beauregard Street
Alexandria, VA 22311
(800) 969-6642
none available
www.nmha.org
Materials available
Contact: Kristin Battista-Frazee

National Physical Fitness and Sports Month
President's Council on Physical Fitness and
Sports
Department W
200 Independence Ave., S.W., Room 738-H
Washington, DC 20201-0004
(202) 690-9000
(202) 690-5211 (fax)
PCPFS@OSOPHS.DHHS.GOV
www.fitness.gov/getmovingamerica.html
Materials available
Contact: none available

Clean Air Month
American Lung Association
1740 Broadway
New York, NY 10019-4374
(800) LUNG-USA
info@lungusa.org
www.lungusa.org
Contact: Communications Department

National Neurofibromatosis Month
National Neurofibromatosis Foundation
95 Pine Street, 16th Floor
New York, NY 10005
(800) 323-7938
nnff@nf.org
www.nf.org
Materials available
Contact: John Radziejewski

**National Osteoporosis Awareness and
Prevention Month**
National Osteoporosis Foundation
1232 22nd Street, N.W.
Washington, DC 20037
(202) 223-2226
none available
www.nof.org
Materials available
Contact: campaign coordinator

National Stroke Awareness Month
National Stroke Association
9707 East Easter Lane
Englewood, CO 80112-3747
(800) STROKES

info@stroke.org
www.stroke.org
Contact: Rachelle Trujillo

National Teen Pregnancy Prevention Month
Advocates for Youth
1025 Vermont Avenue, N.W., Suite 200
Washington, DC 20005
(202) 347-5700
info@advocatesforyouth.org
www.advocatesforyouth.org
Materials available
Contact: Laura Davis

National Trauma Awareness Month
American Trauma Society
8903 Presidential Parkway, Suite 512
Upper Marlboro, MD 20772-2656
(800) 556-7890
info@amtrauma.org
www.amtrauma.org
Materials available
Contact: public relations coordinator

Older Americans Month
Administration on Aging
330 Independence Avenue, S.W.
Washington, DC 20201
(202) 619-2617
none available
www.aoa.gov
Materials available
Contact: Carol Crecy

Skin Cancer Awareness Month
American Cancer Society
1599 Clifton Road, N.E.
Atlanta, GA 30329
(800) ACS-2345
none available
www.cancer.org
Contact: national office

Lyme Disease Awareness Month
Lyme Disease Foundation
One Financial Plaza
Hartford, CT 06103-2610
(800) 886-5963

(860) 525-2000
lymefnd@aol.com
www.lyme.org
Materials available
Contact: Karen Forschner

National Sight-Saving Month: Ultraviolet Awareness & Home Eye Safety
Prevent Blindness America
500 East Remington Road
Schaumburg, IL 60173
(800) 331-2020
info@preventblindness.org
www.preventblindness.org
Materials available
Contact: Center for Sight

Tuberous Sclerosis Awareness Month
Tuberous Sclerosis Alliance
801 Roeder Road, Suite 750
Silver Spring, MD 20910
(800) 225-6872
(301) 562-9890
info@tsalliance.org
www.tsalliance.org
Materials available
Contact: Mary Beth Leongini

Healthy Vision Month
National Eye Institute
2020 Vision Place
Bethesda, MD 20892-3655
(301) 770-5800 x5815
jmcinerney@shs.net
www.healthyvision2010.org/hvm2003/
Materials available
Contact: John McInerney

3–10
National SAFE KIDS Week
National SAFE KIDS Campaign
1301 Pennsylvania Avenue, N.W., Suite 1000
Washington, DC 20004-1707
(202) 662-0600
lbos@safekids.org
www.safekids.org
Contact: Laura Bos

4–10
National Mental Health Counseling Week
American Mental Health Counselors Association
801 North Fairfax Street, Suite 304
Alexandria, VA 22314
(800) 326-2642
vmoore@amhca.org
www.amhca.org
Contact: none available

4–10
Children's Mental Health Week
Federation of Families for Children's Mental Health
1101 King Street, Suite 420
Alexandria, VA 22314
(703) 684-7710
ffcmh@ffcmh.org
www.ffcmh.org
Materials available
Contact: none available

4–10
Brain Tumor Action Week
North American Brain Tumor Coalition
274 Madison Avenue, Suite 1301
New York, NY 10016
(212) 448-9494
(212) 448-1022 (fax)
info@cbtf.org
www.nabraintumor.org/events.html
Materials available
Contact: Jeremy Shatan

4–10
North American Occupational Safety and Health Week (NAOSH)
American Society of Safety Engineers (ASSE)
Canadian Society of Safety Engineering (CSSE)
ASSE Public Relations Department
1800 East Oakton Street
Des Plaines, IL 60018 -2187
(847) 699-2929
dhurns@asse.org
www.asse.org
Materials available
Contact: Diane Hurns

4
Mother's Day Comes Early for Too Many of Our Nation's Teens
National Organization on Adolescent Pregnancy, Parenting and Prevention
2401 Pennsylvania Avenue, N.W., Suite 408
Washington, DC 20037
(202) 293-8370
noappp@noappp.org
www.noappp.org
Materials available
Contact: none available

6–12
National Suicide Awareness Week
American Association of Suicidology
4201 Connecticut Avenue N.W., Suite 310
Washington, DC 20008
(202) 237-2280
info@suicidology.org
www.suicidology.org
Contact: Amy Kulp

6
Childhood Depression Awareness Day
National Mental Health Association
2001 North Beauregard Street
Alexandria, VA 22311
(800) 969-6642 x4787
none available
www.nmha.org
Materials available
Contact: Kristin Battista-Frazee

7
National Anxiety Disorders Screening Day
Freedom From Fear
308 Seaview Avenue
Staten Island, NY 10305
(718) 351-1717
contactfff@aol.com
www.freedomfromfear.org
Contact: Jeanine Christiana

11–17
Food Allergy Awareness Week
Food Allergy and Anaphylaxis Network

10400 Eaton Place, Suite 107
Fairfax, VA 22030-2208
(800) 929-4040
faan@foodallergy.org
www.foodallergy.org
Materials available
Contact: Traci Tavares

11–17
National Women's Health Week
Office on Women's Health
Department of Health and Human Services
200 Independence Avenue, S.W.
Room 730B
Washington, DC 20201
(800) 994-9662
4woman@soza.com
www.4woman.gov
Materials available
Contact: National Women's Health Information Center

11–17
National Running and Fitness Week
American Running Association and American Medical Athletic Association
4405 East-West Highway, Suite 405
Bethesda, MD 20814
(800) 776-2732
(301) 913-9517
(301) 913-9520 (fax)
run@americanrunning.org
www.americanrunning.org
Materials available
Contact: Barbara Baldwin

12–18
National Alcohol-and Other Drug-Related Birth Defects Week
National Council on Alcoholism and Drug Dependence, Inc.
20 Exchange Place, Suite 2902
New York, NY 10005
(212) 269-7797
(800) NCA-CALL (24-hour helpline)
(212) 269-7510 (fax)
national@ncadd.org

www.ncadd.org
Materials available
Contact: none available

12–18
National Stuttering Awareness Week
Stuttering Foundation of America
3100 Walnut Grove Road, Suite 603
P.O. Box 11749
Memphis, TN 38111
(800) 992-9392
(901) 452-3931 (fax)
stutter@stutteringhelp.org
www.stutteringhelp.org
Materials available
Contact: Laura Beauchamp

12
International Chronic Fatigue Syndrome (CFIDS/ME) Awareness Day
The CFIDS Association of America
P.O. Box 220398
Charlotte, NC 28222-0398
(704) 365-2343
(704) 364-3729 (fax)
info@cfids.org
www.cfids.org
Materials available
Contact: Vicki Walker

18–24
National Emergency Medical Services Week
American College of Emergency Physicians
1125 Executive Circle
Irving, TX 75038-2522
(800) 798-1822
dfechner@acep.org
www.acep.org/emsweek
Materials available
Contact: Denise Fechner

19–26
Buckle Up America! Week
Office of Occupant Protection, National Highway
Transportation Safety Administration
U.S. Department of Transportation
400 Seventh Street, S.W.

Washington, DC 20590
(202) 366-9550
none available
www.nhtsa.dot.gov
Materials available
Contact: Tina Fowley

21
National Employee Health and Fitness Day
National Association for Health and Fitness
401 West Michigan Street
Indianapolis, IN 46202
(317) 955-0957
info@physicalfitness.org
www.physicalfitness.org/nehf.html
Materials available
Contact: Sara Utley

24
National Schizophrenia Awareness Day
National Schizophrenia Foundation
403 Seymour Street, Suite 202
Lansing, MI 48933
(517) 485-7168 x105
(517) 485-7180 (fax)
harwin@NSFoundation.org
www.NSFoundation.org
Materials available
Contact: Laura Harwin

25–31
Older Americans' Mental Health Week
Older Women's League
666 11th Street., N.W., Suite 700
Washington, DC 20001
(800) 825-3695
owlinfo@owl-national.org
www.owl-national.org
Materials available
Contact: Laura Harwin

25
National Missing Children's Day
Child Find of America, Inc.
Box 277
New Paltz, NY 12561
(800) I-AM-LOST

childfindamerica@aol.com
www.childfindofamerica.org
Materials available
Contact: Carol Robins

28

National Senior Health and Fitness Day
Mature Market Resource Center
1850 West Winchester, Suite 213
Libertyville, IL 60048-5355
(800) 828-8225
fitnessday@aol.com
www.fitnessday.com
Materials available
Contact: Tina Godin

31

World "No Tobacco" Day
American Association for World Health
1825 K Street, N.W., Suite 1208
Washington, DC 20006
(202) 466-5883
(202) 466-5896 (fax)
staff@aaworldhealth.org
www.aaworldhealth.org
Contact: none available

June

1–4

Fireworks Safety Month (through July 4)
Prevent Blindness America
500 East Remington Road
Schaumburg, IL 60173
(800) 331-2020
info@preventblindness.org
www.preventblindness.org
Materials available
Contact: Center for Sight

National Scleroderma Awareness Month
Scleroderma Foundation
12 Kent Way, Suite 101
Byfield, MA 01922
(800) 722-HOPE
sfinfo@scleroderma.org
www.scleroderma.org

Materials available
Contact: local chapters or national office

National Aphasia Awareness Month
National Aphasia Association
156 Fifth Avenue, Suite 707
New York, NY 10010
(800) 922-4622
naa@aphasia.org
www.aphasia.org
Contact: none available

Vision Research Month
Prevent Blindness America
500 East Remington Road
Schaumburg, IL 60173-5611
(800) 331-2020
info@preventblindness.org
www.preventblindness.org
Materials available
Contact: Center for Sight

Myasthenia Gravis Awareness Month
The Myasthenia Gravis Foundation of America, Inc.
5841 Cedar Lake Road, Suite 204
Minneapolis, MN 55416
(800) 541-5454
(952) 646-2028 (fax)
myasthenia@myasthenia.org
www.myasthenia.org
Materials available
Contact: none available

1–7

National Headache Awareness Week
National Headache Foundation
820 N. Orleans, Suite 217
Chicago, IL 60610
(888) NHF-5552
info@headaches.org
www.headaches.org
Materials available
Contact: Suzanne E. Simons

1

National Cancer Survivors Day
American Cancer Society

1599 Clifton Road, N.E.
Atlanta, GA 30329
(800) ACS-2345
(404) 320-3333
none available
www.cancer.org
Materials available
Contact: local chapters

9–15
National Men's Health Week
National Men's Health Network
P.O. Box 75972
Washington, DC 20013
(202) 543-MHN-1 (6461)
(202) 543-2727 (fax)
info@menshealthweek.org
www.menshealthweek.org.
Materials available
Contact: none available

22–28
Helen Keller Deaf–Blind Awareness Week
Helen Keller National Center for Deaf-Blind
Youth and Adults
111 Middle Neck Road
Sands Point, NY 11050
(516) 944-8900 x325
(516) 944-8637 TTY
(516) 944-7302 (fax)
HKncpr@aol.com
www.helenkeller.org
Materials available
Contact: Development Department

27–5
Eye Safety Awareness Week
United States Eye Injury Registry
1201 11th Avenue South, Suite 300
Birmingham, AL 35205
(205) 933-0064
(205) 933-1341 (fax)
loretta@useironline.org
www.useironline.org
Contact: Loretta Mann

July

Hemochromatosis Screening Awareness Month
Hemochromatosis Foundation
P.O. Box 8569
Albany, NY 12208
(518) 489-0972
none available
www.hemochromatosis.org
Materials available
Contact: Margit A. Krikker, M.D.

Light the Night for Sight
Prevent Blindness America
500 East Remington Road
Schaumburg, IL 60173-5611
(800) 331-2020
info@preventblindness.org
www.preventblindness.org
Materials available
Contact: Center for Sight

International Group B Strep Awareness Month
The Jesse Cause — Saving the Babies from
Group B Strep
567 West Channel Islands Blvd., #235
Port Hueneme, CA 93041
(877) HALT-GBS
(805) 984-7933
thejessecause@iolwest.com
www.groupbstrep.com
Materials available
Contact: Marti Perhach

Eye Injury Prevention Month
American Academy of Ophthalmology
P.O. Box 7424
San Francisco, CA 94120
(415) 561-8525
(415) 561-8533 (fax)
eyemd@aao.org
www.aao.org
Materials available
Contact: Annamarie Harris

14–18
National Therapeutic Recreation Week
National Therapeutic Recreation Society
National Recreation and Park Association
22377 Belmont Ridge Road
Ashburn, VA 20148
(703) 858-0784
spotts@nrpa.org
www.nrpa.org/index.cfm?publicationid=21
Materials available
Contact: Susan Potts

August

Amblyopia Awareness
Prevent Blindness America
500 East Remington Road
Schaumburg, IL 60173
(800) 331-2020
info@preventblindness.org
www.preventblindness.org
Materials available
Contact: Center for Sight

Cataract Awareness Month
American Academy of Ophthalmology
P.O. Box 7424
San Francisco, CA 94120
(415) 561-8525
(415) 561-8533 (fax)
eyemd@aao.org
www.aao.org
Materials available
Contact: Annamarie Harris

National Immunization Awareness Month
(NIAM)
National Partnership for Immunization
121 North Washington St., Suite 300
Alexandria, VA 22314
(703) 836-6110
dwichans@hmhb
www.partnersforimmunization.org
Materials available
Contact: Denna Penner

Psoriasis Awareness Month
National Psoriasis Foundation
6600 SW 92nd Ave., Suite 300
Portland, OR 97223-7195
(800) 723-9166
(503) 546-8369
(503) 245-0626 (fax)
molly@npfusa.org
www.psoriasis.org
Materials available
Contact: Molly Marshall

Spinal Muscular Atrophy Awareness Month
Families of Spinal Muscular Atrophy
P.O. Box 196
Libertyville, IL 60048-0196
(800) 886-1762
sma@fsma.org
www.fsma.org
Materials available
Contact: Audrey N. Lewis

1–7
World Breastfeeding Week
World Alliance for Breastfeeding Action and La
Leche League International
1400 North Meacham Road
Schaumburg, IL 60173-4840
(847) 519-7730 x286
PRAssociate@llli.org
www.lalecheleague.org
Materials available
Contact: Mary Hurt

1
National Minority Donor Awareness Day
(NMDAD)
National Minority Organ Tissue Transplant
Education Program
2041 Georgia Avenue, N.W.
Ambulatory Care Center, Suite 3100
Washington, DC 20060
(800) 393-2839
(202) 865-4888
(202) 865-4880 (fax)
gmaddox@nationalmottep.org

www.nationalmottep.org
Materials available
Contact: Gwendolyn Maddox

September

Baby Safety Month
Juvenile Products Manufacturers Association
17000 Commerce Parkway, Suite C
Mt. Laurel, NJ 08054
none available
jszwalek@ahint.com
www.jpma.org
Materials available
Contact: none available

Children's Eye Health Safety Month
Prevent Blindness America
500 East Remington Road
Schaumburg, IL 60173
(800) 331-2020
info@preventblindness.org
www.preventblindness.org
Materials available
Contact: Center for Sight

Cold and Flu Campaign
American Lung Association
1740 Broadway
New York, NY 10019-4374
(800) LUNG-USA
(212) 315-8700
info@lungusa.org
www.lungusa.org
Contact: Nancy Cease

Gynecologic Cancer Awareness Month
Gynecologic Cancer Foundation
401 North Michigan Avenue
Chicago, IL 60611
(800) 444-4441
(312) 644-6610
gcf@sba.com
www.wcn.org
Materials available
Contact: Karen Carlson

Healthy Aging Month
Educational Television Network, Inc.
P.O. Box 442
Unionville, PA 19375
(610) 793-0979
(610) 793-0978 (fax)
etnet@discovernet.net
www.healthyaging.net
Contact: Carolyn Worthington

Leukemia & Lymphoma Awareness Month
The Leukemia & Lymphoma Society
1311 Mamaroneck Avenue
White Plains, NY 10605
(800) 955-4572
(914) 821-8806
(914) 821-3607 (fax)
infocenter@leukemia-lymphoma.org
www.leukemia-lymphoma.org
Materials available
Contact: Resource Center

National Cholesterol Education Month
National Heart, Lung, and Blood Institute Health
Information Center
P.O. Box 30105
Bethesda, MD 20824-0105
(301) 592-8573
nhlbiinfo@rover.nhlbi.nih.gov
www.nhlbi.nih.gov
Materials available
Contact: information specialist

National Food Safety Education Month
International Food Safety Council
National Restaurant Association Education
Foundation
175 West Jackson, Suite 1500
Chicago, IL 60604
(317) 261-5329
Bsirt@foodtrain.org
www.nraef.org/index.asp
Materials available
Contact: Bethany Sirt

National Sickle Cell Month
Sickle Cell Disease Association of America, Inc.
200 Corporate Pointe, Suite 495

Culver City, CA 90230-8727
(800) 421-8453
scdaa@sicklecelldisease.org
www.SickleCellDisease.org
Materials available
Contact: Ralph D. Sutton

Ovarian Cancer Awareness Month
The National Ovarian Cancer Coalition
500 N.E. Spanish River Boulevard, Suite 14
Boca Raton, FL 33431
(888) OVARIAN
(561) 393-0005
nocc@ovarian.org
www.ovarian.org
Materials available
Contact: Maxine Stein

Prostate Cancer Awareness Month
National Prostate Cancer Coalition
1154 15th Street
Washington, DC 20005
(888) 245-9455
info@pcacoalition.org
www.pcacoalition.org
Materials available
Contact: community liaison

National Pediculosis Prevention Month/Head Lice Prevention Month
National Pediculosis Association, Inc.
50 Kearney Rd.
Neetham, MA 02494
(781) 499-NITS
(781) 499-8129 (fax)
npa@headlice.org
www.headlice.org
Materials available
Contact: Jane Cotter

National Alcohol and Drug Addiction Recovery Month
Substance Abuse and Mental Health Services Administration
Center for Substance Abuse Treatment (CSAT)
5600 Fishers Lane
Rockville, MD 20857
(301) 443-5052

www.recoverymonth.gov
Materials available
Contact: CSAT

14–20
Prostate Cancer Awareness Week
American Cancer Society
1599 Clifton Road, N.E.
Atlanta, GA 30329
(800) ACS-2345
(404) 320-3333
www.cancer.org
Materials available
Contact: local chapters

14–20
National Rehabilitation Week
National Rehabilitation Awareness Foundation
475 Morgan Highway
P.O. Box 71
Scranton, PA 18501-0071
(800) 943-NRAF
(570) 341-4637
jbrogn@allied-services.org
www.nraf-rehabnet.org
Materials available
Contact: James Brogna

21–27
National 5 A Day Week
National Cancer Institute/Produce for Better Health Foundation
6130 Executive Boulevard EPN 4050
Bethesda, MD 20892
(800) 4-CANCER
(301) 496-8520
(800) 332-8615 TTY
none available
www.5aday.gov
Materials available
Contact: NCI 5-A-Day Program Office

21–27
National Reye's Syndrome Week
National Reye's Syndrome Foundation
P.O. Box 829
Bryan, OH 43506-0829
(800) 233-7393

(419) 636-2679
nrsf@reyessyndrome.org
www.reyessyndrome.org
Materials available
Contact: Susan Landversicht

24
National Women's Health and Fitness Day
Health Information Resource Center
1850 West Winchester, Suite 213
Libertyville, IL 60048
(800) 828-8225
(847) 816-8662 (fax)
healthprograms@aol.com
www.fitnessday.com
Materials available
Contact: Carrie Farella

27
Family Health and Fitness Days USA
Health Information Resource Center
1850 West Winchester, Suite 213
Libertyville, IL 60048
(800) 828-8225
(847) 816-8662 (fax)
healthprograms@aol.com
www.fitnessday.com
Materials available
Contact: Pat Henze

October

Auto Battery Safety Month
Prevent Blindness America
500 East Remington Road
Schaumburg, IL 60173
(800) 331-2020
info@preventblindness.org
www.preventblindness.org
Materials available
Contact: Center for Sight

Celiac Sprue Awareness Month
Celiac Sprue Association/USA
P.O. Box 31700
Omaha, NE 68131-0700

(402) 558-0600
celiacs@csaceliacs.org
www.csaceliacs.org
Materials available
Contact: Mary Schluckebier

Domestic Violence Awareness Month
National Coalition Against Domestic Violence
P.O. Box 18749
Denver, CO 80218-0749
(303) 839-1852
none available
www.ncadv.org
Materials available
Contact: none available

Family Health Month
American Academy of Family Physicians
11400 Tomahawk Creek Parkway
Leawood, KS 66211
(800) 274-2237
fp@aafp.org
www.familyhealth.org
Materials available
Contact: none available

Healthy Lung Month
American Lung Association
1740 Broadway
New York, NY 10019-4374
(800) LUNG-USA
info@lungusa.org
www.lungusa.org
Contact: communications department

National Breast Cancer Awareness Month
National Breast Cancer Awareness Month Board
of Sponsors
233 N. Michigan Avenue, Suite 1400
Chicago, IL 60601
none available
none available
www.nbcam.org
Materials available
Contact: Susan Nathanson

National Dental Hygiene Month
American Dental Hygienists' Association

444 North Michigan Avenue, Suite 3400
Chicago, IL 60611
(312) 440-8900
ndhm@adha.net
www.adha.org
Materials available
Contact: Rosetta Gervasi

National Family Sexuality Education Month
Planned Parenthood Federation of America
810 Seventh Avenue
New York, NY 10019
(212) 541-7800
education@ppfa.org
www.plannedparenthood.org
Materials available
Contact: Estelle Raboni

National Lupus Awareness Month
Lupus Foundation of America, Inc.
1300 Piccard Drive, Suite 200
Rockville, MD 20850-4303
(888) 38-LUPUS
(301) 670-9292
info@lupus.org
www.lupus.org
Materials available
Contact: Dorothy Howe

National Physical Therapy Month
American Physical Therapy Association
1111 North Fairfax Street
Alexandria, VA 22314-1488
(703) 684-2782 ext. 3248
public-relations@apta.org
www.apta.org
Materials available
Contact: public relations department

National Spina Bifida Awareness Month
Spina Bifida Association of America
4590 MacArthur Boulevard, N.W., Suite 250
Washington, DC 20007-4226
(800) 621-3141
(202) 944-3285
sbaa@sbaa.org
www.sbaa.org

Materials available
Contact: National Resource Center

National Spinal Health Month
American Chiropractic Association
1701 Clarendon Boulevard
Arlington, VA 22209
(800) 986-4636
AmerChiro@aol.com
none available
Materials available
Contact: Omar Malik

Rett Syndrome Awareness Month
International Rett Syndrome Association
9121 Piscataway Road, Suite 2B
Clinton, MD 20735
(800) 818-RETT
irsa@rettsyndrome.org
www.rettsyndrome.org
Materials available
Contact: Kathy Hunter

Sudden Infant Death Syndrome (SIDS) Awareness Month
SIDS Alliance
1314 Bedford Avenue, Suite 210
Baltimore, MD 21208
(800) 221-SIDS
sidshq@charm.net
www.sidsalliance.org
Materials available
Contact: Public Affairs

"Talk About Prescriptions" Month
National Council on Patient Information and Education
4915 St. Elmo Avenue, Suite 505
Bethesda, MD 20814-6082
(301) 656-8565
ncpie@erols.com
www.talkaboutrx.org
Materials available
Contact: information specialist

National Liver Awareness Month
American Liver Foundation
75 Maiden Lane, Suite 603

New York, NY 10038-4810
(800) GO-LIVER
webmail@liverfoundation.org
www.liverfoundation.org
Materials available
Contact: information distribution center

National Medical Librarians Month
Medical Library Association
65 East Wacker Place, Suite 1900
Chicago, IL 60602
(312) 419-9094 x11
(312) 419-8950 (fax)
info@mlahq.org
www.mlanet.org/press/nml-month/index.html
Materials available
Contact: Tomi Gunn

Health Literacy Month
Health Literacy Consulting
31 Highland Street, Suite 201
Natick, MA 01760
(508) 653-1199
(508) 650-9492 (fax)
helen@healthliteracy.com
www.healthliteracymonth.com
Contact: Helen Osborne

National Brain Injury Awareness Month
Brain Injury Association of America
105 N. Alfred Street
Alexandria, VA 22314
(703) 236-6000
publicrelations@biausa.org
www.biausa.org
Materials available
Contact: communications coordinator

World Blindness Awareness Month
American Academy of Ophthalmology
P.O. Box 7424
San Francisco, CA 94120
(415) 561-8525
(415) 561-8533 (fax)
eyemd@aao.org
www.aao.org

Materials available
Contact: Annamarie Harris

5–11
National Fire Prevention Week
National Fire Protection Association
1 Batterymarch Park
P.O. Box 9101
Quincy, MA 02269
(800) 344-3555 orders only
custserv@NFPA.org
www.nfpa.org
Materials available
Contact: Peg O'Brian

5–11
Mental Illness Awareness Week
American Psychiatric Association
1400 K Street, N.W.
Washington, DC 20005
(888) 357-7924
(202) 682-6122
apa@psych.org
www.psych.org
Materials available
Contact: Cecilia Arradaza

6–10
Drive Safely Work Week
Network of Employers for Traffic Safety
8150 Lessburg Pike, Suite 410
Vienna, VA 22182
(888) 221-0045
(703) 891-6005
(703) 891-6010 (fax)
nets@trafficsafety.org
www.trafficsafety.org
Materials available
Contact: Kathryn Lusby-Treber

6
National Child Health Day
Maternal and Child Health Bureau
Health Resources and Services Administration
U.S. Department of Health and Human Services
Parklawn Building, Room 18-20

5600 Fishers Lane
Rockville, MD 20857
(301) 443-2170
pbandyck@hrsa.gov
www.mchb.hrsa.gov
Contact: Cynthia Tibbs

7–14
Ulcer Awareness Week
Centers for Disease Control and Prevention
1600 Clifton Road, N.E.
MS C09
Atlanta, GA 30333
(404) 371-5375
ulcers@cdc.gov
www.cdc.gov
Materials available
Contact: none available

9
National Depression Screening Day
Screening for Mental Health, Inc.
1 Washington Street, Suite 304
Wellesly Hills, MA 02481
(781) 239-0071
info@mentalhealthscreening.org
www.mentalhealthscreening.org
Materials available
Contact: Mary Brant

12–18
National Adult Immunization Awareness Week
National Coalition for Adult Immunization
4733 Bethesda Avenue, Suite 750
Bethesda, MD 20814-5228
(301) 656-0003
ncai@nfid.org
www.nfid.org/ncai
Materials available
Contact: David A. Neumann, Ph.D.

13–17
National School Lunch Week
American School Food Service Association
700 South Washington Street, Suite 300
Alexandria, VA 22314-4287

(800) 728-0728 (catalog)
(800) 877-8822
asfsa@asfsa.org
www.asfsa.org
Materials available
Contact: Emporium

16
World Food Day
U.S. National Committee for World Food Day
2175 K Street, N.W., Suite 300
Washington, DC 20437
(202) 653-2404
none available
www.worldfooddayusa.org
Materials available
Contact: Patricia Young

17
National Mammography Day
American Cancer Society
1599 Clifton Road, N.E.
Atlanta, GA 30329
(800) ACS-2345
none available
www.cancer.org
Contact: none available

19–25
National Childhood Lead Poisoning Prevention Week
National Lead Information Center
801 Roeder Road, Suite 600
Silver Spring, MD 20910
(800) 424-LEAD
www.epa.gov/lead/nlicdocs.htm
Materials available
Contact: National Lead Information Center

19–25
National Radon Action Week
U.S. Environmental Protection Agency
Ariel Rios Building
1200 Pennsylvania Avenue, N.W.
6609J
Washington, DC 20460

(800) SOS-RADON
(202) 564-9370
(202) 260-5922
public-access@epamail.epa.gov
www.epa.gov
Materials available
Contact: Dennis Hellberg

20–26
National Health Education Week
National Center for Health Education
242 W. 30th Street, 10th Floor
New York, NY 10001
(212) 463-4050
nche@nche.org
www.nche.org
Materials available
Contact: Roz Coralle

23–31
National Red Ribbon Celebration
(Campaign to keep kids off drugs)
National Family Partnership
Informed Family Education Center
2490 Coral Way
Miami, FL 33145
(800) 705-8997
info@informedfamilies.org
www.nfp.org
Materials available
Contact: Molly Osendorf

November

National American Indian and Alaska Native Heritage Month
Indian Health Service
The Reyes Building
801 Thompson Avenue, Suite 400
Rockville, MD 20852
(301) 443-3593
Heritage@hqe.ihs.gov
www.ihs.gov/Heritage/
Contact: public affairs

Diabetic Eye Disease Month
Prevent Blindness America
500 East Remington Road
Schaumburg, IL 60173
(800) 331-2020
info@preventblindness.org
www.preventblindness.org
Materials available
Contact: Center for Sight

National Alzheimer's Disease Awareness Month
Alzheimer's Disease and Related Disorders Association
919 North Michigan Avenue, Suite 1100
Chicago, IL 60611-1676
(800) 272-3900
(312) 335-8882 (TDD)
info@alz.org
www.alz.org
Materials available
Contact: local chapters or national office

American Diabetes Month
American Diabetes Association
1701 North Beauregard Street
Alexandria, VA 22314
(800) 232-3472
none available
www.diabetes.org
Materials available
Contact: local chapters or national office

National Epilepsy Month
Epilepsy Foundation
4351 Garden City Drive
Landover, MD 20785
(800) EFA-1000
(800) 213-5821 (publications)
postmaster@efa.org
www.epilepsyfoundation.org
Materials available
Contact: Marc Rutledge

National Marrow Awareness Month
National Marrow Donor Program®

3001 Broadway Street, N.E., Suite 500
Minneapolis, MN 55413
(800) 627-7692
(800) MARROW2
rpinder@nmdp.org
www.marrow.org
Materials available
Contact: Robert Pinderhughes

Pancreatic Cancer Awareness Month
Pancreatic Cancer Action Network
2221 Rosecrans Avenue, Suite 131
El Segundo, CA 90245
(877) 272-6226
(310) 725-0025
(310) 725-0029 (fax)
information@pancan.org
www.pancan.org
Materials available
Contact: none available

Lung Cancer Awareness Month
Alliance for Lung Cancer Advocacy, Support,
and Education
500 W. 8th Street
Vancouver, WA 98660
(800) 298-2436
(360) 696-2436
(360) 735-1305 (fax)
info@alcase.org
www.alcase.org
Materials available
Contact: customer service

National Hospice Month
National Hospice and Palliative Care Organization
1700 Diagonal Road, Suite 625
Alexandria, VA 22314
(703) 837-1500
info@nhpco.org
www.nhpco.org
Contact: Pam Bouchard

16–22
National Adoption Week
National Council for Adoption

225 North Washington Street
Alexandria, VA 22314
(703) 299-6633
info@ncfa-usa.org
www.ncfa-usa.org
Materials available
Contact: Laura Elliot

20
Great American Smokeout
American Cancer Society
1599 Clifton Road, N.E.
Atlanta, GA 30329
(800) ACS-2345
Information Specialist
www.cancer.org
Materials available
Contact: national office

23–29
GERD Awareness Week
(gastroesophageal reflux disease)
International Foundation for Functional
Gastrointestinal Disorders (IFFGD)
P.O. Box 170864
Milwaukee, WI 53217
(414) 964-1799
(888) 964-2001 8:30 A.M.–5:00 P.M. CST
iffgd@iffgd.org
www.aboutgerd.org
Materials available
Contact: Nancy Norton

December

National Drunk and Drugged Driving (3D)
Prevention Month
3D Prevention Month Coalition
1900 L Street, N.W., Suite 705
Washington, DC 20036
(202) 452-6004
none available
www.3dmonth.org
Contact: John Moulden

Safe Toys and Gifts Month
Prevent Blindness America
500 East Remington Road
Schaumburg, IL 60173-5611
(800) 331-2020
info@preventblindness.org
www.preventblindness.org
Materials available
Contact: Center for Sight

1–7
National Aplastic Anemia Awareness Week
Aplastic Anemia and MDS International
Foundation
P.O. Box 613
Annapolis, MD 21404
(800) 747-2820
help@aamds.org
www.aamds.org
Materials available
Contact: Marilyn Baker

1
World AIDS Day
American Association for World Health
1825 K Street, N.W., Suite 1208
Washington, DC 20006
(202) 466-5883
staff@aawhworldhealth.org
www.aawhworldhealth.org
Materials available
Contact: any staff person

7–13
National Hand Washing Awareness Week
Henry the Hand Foundation
11714 U.S. Route 42
Cincinnati, OH 45241
(513) 769-3660
dr.will@henrythehand.com
www.henrythehand.com
Materials available
Contact: Dr. Will Sawyer

SELECTED PROFESSIONAL HEALTH EDUCATION ORGANIZATIONS

American College Health Association (ACHA)
P.O. Box 28937
Baltimore, MD 21240-8937 (410) 859-1500

American Public Health Association
800 I Street, N.W.
Washington, DC 20001-3710 (202) 777-2742

American School Health Association (ASHA)
P.O. Box 708
Kent, OH 44240 (216) 678-1601

Association for the Advancement of Health Education (AAHE)
1900 Association Drive
Reston, VA 22091 (703) 476-3400

National Commission for Health Education Credentialing, Inc.
944 Marcon Boulevard
Suite 310
Allentown, PA 18103 (610) 264-8200

Society of Behavioral Medicine (SBM)
7600 Terrace Avenue
Middleton, WI 53562 (608) 827-7267

Society for Public Health Education (SOPHE)
750 First Street
Suite 910
Washington, DC 20002-4242
(202) 408-9804

BIBLIOGRAPHY

Abt Associates, Inc. *School Health Education Evaluation.*
Supported by the Centers for Disease Control, Contract
No. 200-81-060, 1985.

Adair, Nancy. "A Rationale for Sex Education in the
Schools." Master's degree project, State University of
New York at Buffalo, 1974.

Aldana, Steven G. "Financial Impact of Health Promotion
Programs: A Comprehensive Review of the Literature."
American Journal of Health Promotion
15(2001):296–320.

Alliance for Service-Learning in Education Reform. *Standards
of Quality for School-Based Service-Learning.* Undated.

American Heart Association. *RISKO.* Dallas: American Heart
Association, 1981.

Anderson, D.; R. Whitmer; R. Geotzel; et al. "The Relation-
ship between Modifiable Risk and Group-Level Health
Care Expenditures." *American Journal of Health
Promotion* 18(2000):42–52.

"Anorexia: The Starving-Disease Epidemic." *U.S. News and
World Report,* August 30, 1982, 47–48.

Apple, R. W. Jr. "Limits on Abortion Seen Less Likely
(New York Times/CBS News Poll)." *The New York Times,*
September 29, 1989.

Arloc, S. *Wasting America's Future: The Children's Defense
Fund Report on the Costs of Child Poverty.* Boston:
Beacon Press, 1994.

Association for the Advancement of Health Education. *A
Code of Ethics for Health Educators.* Reston, VA: Association for the Advancement of Health Education, 1994.

Association for the Study of Abortion. "Abortion and Health."
Pamphlet, n.d.

Astin, A. W. *Student Involvement in Community Service:
Institutional Commitment and the Campus Compact.* Paper
presented at a meeting of the California Campus Compact,
Royce Hall, UCLA Campus, December 6, 1990.

Bassuk, E., and L. Rosenberg. "Psychosocial Characteristics
of Homeless Children and Children with Homes."
Pediatrics 85 (1990):257–61.

Bennett, William J. *What Works: Schools Without Drugs.*
Washington, D.C.: United States Department of
Education, 1986.

Benson, Herbert. *The Relaxation Response.* New York:
Avon, 1975.

Benson, Herbert; and Miriam Z. Klipper. *The Relaxation
Response.* New York: William Morrow, 2000.

"The Binge–Purge Syndrome." *Newsweek,* November 2,
1982, 68–69.

Black Community Crusade for Children. *Progress and Peril:
Black Children in America.* Washington, DC: Children's
Defense Fund, 1993.

Boss, J. A. "The Effects of Community Service Work on the
Moral Development of College Ethics Students." *Journal
of Moral Education* 23(1994):183–98.

Breckon, Donald J.; John R. Harvey; and R. Brick Lancaster.
Community Health Education: Settings, Roles, and Skills.
Rockville, MD: Aspen, 1985.

Briggs, Kenneth A. "Aging: A Need for Sensitivity." *Health
Education* 8(1977):37–38.

Brouha, Lucien. "The Step Test: A Simple Method of
Measuring Physical Fitness for Muscular Work in
Young Men." *Research Quarterly* 14(1943):31.

Burnett, Kim Y. "HIV/AIDS Facts Millionaire Game."
American Journal of Health Education
33(2002):125–28.

Calabrese, R., and H. Schumer. "The Effects of Service
Activities on Adolescent Alienation." *Adolescence*
21(1986):675–87.

Castillo, Gloria A. *Left-Handed Teaching: Lessons in
Affective Education.* New York: Praeger, 1974.

Chavent, Georgia. "Students Design Innovative Food
Products to Learn Nutrition Labeling." *American
Journal of Health Education* 33(2002):58–60.

Checkley, Kathy. "The First Seven . . . and the Eighth:
A Conversation with Howard Gardner." *Educational
Leadership* 55(1997):1–8.

Chernin, K. "The Politics of Small." *Tikkun* 8(1993):15.

Children's Defense Fund. *The State of America's Children:
Yearbook 1994.* Washington, DC: Children's Defense
Fund, 1994.

———. *The State of America's Children: Yearbook 1999.*
Washington, DC: Children's Defense Fund, 1999.

Cognetta, P. V., and N. A. Sprinthall. "Students as Teachers:
Role Taking as a Means of Promoting Psychological and
Ethical Development during Adolescence." In *Value
Development as the Aim of Education,* edited by N. A.
Sprinthall and R. L. Mosher, 53–68. Schenectady, NY:
Character Research Press, 1978.

Connell, David B.; Ralph R. Turner; and Elaine F. Mason.
"Summary of Findings of the School Health Education
Evaluation: Health Promotion Effectiveness,

Implementation, and Costs." *Journal of School Health* 55(1985):316–21.

Conrad, D., and D. Hedin. "The Impact of Experiential Education on Adolescent Development." *Child & Youth Services* 4(1982):57–76.

———. "School-Based Community Service: What We Know from Research and Theory." *Phi Delta Kappan* 72(1991):743–49.

Collins, Janet et al. "School Health Education." *Journal of School Health* 65(1995):302–11.

Cooper, Theodore. "Keynote Address." In *Program Summary of a Conference on Worksite Health Promotion and Human Resources: A Hard Look at the Data,* 12–16. Washington, DC: U.S. Government Printing Office, 1984.

Cost, Patricia A, and Jennifer M. Turley. "Teaching the Food Guide Pyramid Using Multiple Intelligence Learning Centers." *Journal of Health Education* 31(2000):111–12.

CRM Books. *Instructor's Guide to Life and Health.* New York: Random House, 1972.

Cureton, T. K. *Physical Fitness Workbook.* Urbana, IL: Stipes Publishing Co., 1944.

Dalis, Gus T., and Ben B. Strasser. *Teaching Strategies for Values Awareness and Decision Making in Health Education.* Columbus, OH: Charles B. Merrill, 1977.

Deitch, C. "Ideology and Opposition to Abortion: Trends in Public Opinion, 1972–1980." *Alternative Lifestyles* 6(1983):6–26.

Dever, G. E. Alan. *Community Health Analysis: A Holistic Approach.* Germantown, MD: Aspen Systems, 1980.

Dewey, John. *Democracy and Education.* New York: Macmillan, 1916.

Dintiman, George B., and Jerrold S. Greenberg. *Health through Discovery.* 2d ed. Reading, MA: Addison-Wesley, 1983.

———. *Health through Discovery.* 3d ed. New York: Random House, 1986.

———. *Health through Discovery.* 4th ed. New York: Random House, 1989.

Dintiman, G. B., and J. S. Greenberg. *Exploring Health.* Englewood Cliffs, NJ: Prentice-Hall, 1992.

Dumont, Richard, and Dennis Foss. *The American View of Death: Acceptance or Denial?* Cambridge, MA: Schenkman, 1972.

Dunn, Patricia C. "Teaching Strategy for Choosing a Contraceptive." *American Journal of Health Education* 32(2001):246–47.

Dusek, Dorothy E., and Daniel A. Girdano. *Drugs: A Factual Account.* New York: Random House, 1987.

Eberst, Richard. "Defining Health: A Multidimensional Model." *Journal of School Health* 54(1985):99–104.

Ehrenreich, Barbara; Elizabeth Hess; and Gloria Jacobs. *Re-Making Love: The Feminization of Sex.* New York: Doubleday, 1986.

Engs, Ruth; Eugene Barnes; and Molly Wantz. *Health Games Students Play.* Dubuque, IA: Kendall/Hunt, 1975.

Eta Sigma Gamma. *A National Directory of College and University Health Education Programs and Faculty.* 10th ed. Muncie, IN: Eta Sigma Gamma, 1986.

Everly, George S., and Robert H. L. Feldman. *Occupational Health Promotion: Health Behavior in the Workplace.* New York: John Wiley, 1985.

Federal Interagency Forum on Child and Family Statistics. *America's Children: Key National Indicators of Well Being, 2001.* Washington, DC: Federal Interagency Forum on Child and Family Statistics.

Fetro, Joyce V. "Perspectives on Death and Dying: Reflections in Music and the Arts." *American Journal of Health Education* 32(2001):371–73.

Fodor, John T., and Gus T. Dalis. *Health Instruction: Theory and Application.* Philadelphia: Lea & Febiger, 1966.

Fors, Stuart W., and Mildred E. Doster. "Implications of Results: Factors for Success." *Journal of School Health* 55(1985):332–34.

Geiger, Brian F. "Learning about Stress through Interviews." *American Journal of Health Education* 32(2001):313–14.

Gerhard, Victor J. "Sorry Charlie . . ." *Phi Delta Kappan* 53(1972):536.

Giles, D. E., and J. Eyler. "The Impact of a College Community Service Laboratory on Students' Personal, Social, and Cognitive Outcomes." *Journal of Adolescence* 17(1994):327–39.

Girdano, Daniel A. *Occupational Health Promotion: A Practical Guide to Program Development.* New York: Macmillan, 1986.

Golaszewski, Thomas. "Shining Lights: Studies That Have Most Influenced the Understanding of Health Promotion's Financial Impact." *American Journal of Health Promotion* 15(2001):332–40

Goldman, Karen Denard. "12 Angry Men: A Health Educator's Tool for Group Dynamics Training." *The Health Educator* (Spring 2000):9–13.

Granberg, D., and B. Granberg. "Abortion Attitudes, 1965–1980." *Family Planning Perspectives* 12(1980):250–61.

Green, Lawrence W., and C. L. Anderson. *Community Health.* 4th ed. St. Louis: C. V. Mosby, 1982.

Green, Lawrence W., and Marshall W. Kreuter. *Health Promotion Planning: An Educational and Environmental Approach.* 2d ed. Mountain View, CA: Mayfield, 1991.

———. *Health Promotion Planning: An Educational and Ecological Approach.* 3rd ed. Palo Alto, CA: Mayfield, 1999.

Green, Lawrence W.; Marshall W. Kreuter; Sigrid G. Deeds; and Kay B. Partridge. *Health Education Planning: A Diagnostic Approach.* Palo Alto, CA: Mayfield, 1980.

Green, Lawrence W., and Frances Marcus Lewis. *Measurement and Evaluation in Health Education and Health Promotion.* Palo Alto, CA: Mayfield, 1986.

Greenberg, Jerrold S. "Health Education as Freeing." *Health Education* 9(1978):20–21.

————. *Student-Centered Health Instruction: A Humanistic Approach.* Reading, MA: Addison-Wesley, 1978.

————. "Health and Wellness: A Conceptual Differentiation." *Journal of School Health* 55(1985):403–6.

————. "Iatrogenic Health Education Disease." *Health Education* 16(1985):4–6.

————. *Comprehensive Stress Management.* 2d ed. Dubuque, IA: Wm. C. Brown, 1987.

————. *Comprehensive Stress Management.* 3d ed. Dubuque, IA: Wm. C. Brown, 1990.

————. *Comprehensive Stress Management.* 5th ed. Dubuque, IA: Brown and Benchmark, 1996.

————. *Comprehensive Stress Management.* 7th ed. New York: McGraw-Hill, 2002.

————. *The Code of Ethics for the Health Education Profession: A Case Study Book.* Boston: Jones and Bartlett, 2001.

Greenberg, Jerrold S.; Clint E. Bruess; and Debra W. Haffner. *Exploring the Dimensions of Human Sexuality.* Boston: Jones and Bartlett, 2002.

Greenberg, Jerrold S.; Clint E. Bruess; and Doris W. Sands. *Sexuality: Insights and Issues.* Dubuque, IA: Wm. C. Brown, 1987.

Greenberg, Jerrold S., and David Pargman. *Physical Fitness: A Wellness Approach.* Englewood Cliffs, NJ: Prentice-Hall, 1986.

————. *Physical Fitness: A Wellness Approach.* 2d ed. Englewood Cliffs, NJ: Prentice-Hall, 1990.

Greenberg, J. S.; G. B. Dintiman; and B. M. Oakes. *Physical Fitness and Wellness.* Boston, MA: Allyn and Bacon, 1995.

————. *Physical Fitness and Wellness.* 2nd ed. Boston, MA: Allyn and Bacon, 1998.

Greenberg, Jerrold S.; Sheila Ramsey; and Janet Fraser Hale. "Development, Implementation, and Evaluation of a Portable, Self-Instructional Stress Management Program for College Students." Paper presented at the annual meeting of the American School Health Association, Denver, October 10, 1986.

Greene, Walter H. "The Search for a Meaningful Definition of Health." In *New Directions in Health Education: Some Contemporary Issues for the Emerging Age,* edited by Donald A. Read. New York: Macmillan, 1971.

Greene, Walter H., and Bruce G. Simons-Morton. *Introduction to Health Education.* New York: Macmillan, 1984.

Halnen, Andrew; Antoinette Powers; and Karen Christaldi. *Environmental Awareness Sampler.* Wellesley, MA: Wellesley Public School District, 1971.

"Health Education and Credentialing: The Role Delineation Project." *Focal Points,* July 1980, 6.

Hedin, D. "Students as Teachers: A Tool for Improving School Climate and Productivity." *Social Policy* 17(1987):42–47.

————. "The Power of Community Service." *Proceedings of the Academy of Political Science* 37(1989):201–13.

Henshaw, S., et al. "A Portrait of American Women Who Obtain Abortions." *Family Planning Perspectives* 17(1985):90–96.

Hiltz Publishing Company. *Did You Know?* Pamphlet, n.d.

Hobday, Jennifer R. "Innovative Education—Tobacco Roulette." *Journal of Health Education* 31(2000):171–72.

Horowitz, L. "The Self-Care Motivational Model: Theory and Practice in Healthy Human Development." *Journal of School Health* 55(1985):57–61.

Howe, L. W., and M. M. Howe. *Personalizing Education: Values Clarification and Beyond.* New York: Hart, 1975.

Ivancevich, John M.; Michael T. Matteson; and Edward P. Richards. "Who's Liable for Stress on the Job." *Harvard Business Review,* March–April 1985, 6.

Jacobson, Edmund. *Progressive Relaxation.* Chicago: University of Chicago Press, 1938.

————. *Teaching and Learning: New Methods for Old Arts.* Chicago: National Foundation for Progressive Relaxation, 1973.

Jee, S.; M. O'Donnell; I. Suh; and I. Kim. "The Relationship between Modifiable Health Risks and Future Health Care Expenditures." *American Journal of Health Promotion* 15(2001):244–55.

Joint Committee on National Health Education Standards. *National Health Education Standards: Achieving Health Literacy.* New York: American Cancer Society, 1995.

Joyce, Theodore J., and Mocan, Naci H. "The Impact of Legalized Abortion on Adolescent Childbearing in New York City." *American Journal of Public Health* 80(1990):273–78.

Kirby, Douglas; Judith Alter; and Peter Scales. *An Analysis of U.S. Sex Education Programs and Evaluation Methods.* Washington, DC: Department of Health Education and Welfare, 1979.

Koop, C. Everett. *Surgeon General's Report on Acquired Immune Deficiency Syndrome.* Washington, DC: U.S. Public Health Service, October 1986.

Krauthammer, Charles. "The Hired Incubator." *Washington Post,* January 16, 1987, 23.

Levy, Norman. "The Use of Drugs by Teenagers for the Sanctuary and Illusion." *New York State Narcotics Addiction Control Commission Reprints* 3(n.d.):4.

Luchs, K. P. *Selected Changes in Urban High School Students after Participation in Community-Based Learning and Service Activities.* Ph.D. diss., University of Maryland, 1981.

Mager, Robert F. *Preparing Instructional Objectives.* Palo Alto, CA: Fearon, 1962.

Malamud, Daniel I., and Solomon Machover. *Toward Self-Understanding: Group Techniques in Confrontation.* Springfield, IL: Charles C. Thomas, 1965.

Malfetti, James L., and Elizabeth Eidlitz, eds. *Perspectives on Sexuality: A Literary Collection.* New York: Holt, Rinehart, and Winston, 1972.

Markus, G. B.; J. P. F. Howard; and D. C. King. "Integrating Community Service and Classroom Instruction Enhances Learning: Results from an Experiment." *Educational Evaluation and Policy Analysis* 15(1993):410–19.

Masters, William, and Virginia Johnson. *Human Sexual Response.* Boston: Little, Brown, 1966.

Mathews, Jay. "Antisodomy Laws Targeted for Repeal after High Court Ruling." *Washington Post,* February 4, 1987, A16.

Mayshark, Cyrus, and Roy Foster. *Methods in Health Education: A Workbook Using the Critical Incident Technique.* St. Louis: C. V. Mosby, 1966.

McDermott, Robert J., and Paul Sarvela. *Health Education Evaluation and Measurement.* 2nd ed. New York: McGraw-Hill, 1999.

Meichenbaum, Donald. *Stress Inoculation Training.* New York: Pergamon Press, 1985.

Metcalf, L. E., ed. *Values Education: Rationale, Strategies, and Procedures, Forty-First Yearbook.* Washington, DC: National Council for the Social Studies, 1971.

Metropolitan Life Foundation. *Healthy Me: 1985 School Health Education Survey.* New York: Metropolitan Life Foundation, 1985.

Michigan Department of Education. *Patterns and Features of School Health Education in Michigan Public Schools.* Michigan: Department of Education, 1969.

Morrison, Eleanor, and Mila Underhill. *Values in Sexuality.* New York: Hart, 1974.

National Academy of Sciences. *Homelessness, Health and Human Needs.* Washington, DC: National Academy Press, 1988.

National Association for Repeal of Abortion Laws. *50 Physicians Evaluate Legal Abortion in New York.* Pamphlet, n.d.

National Center for Health Statistics. *Health, United States, 1994.* Hyattsville, MD: Public Health Service, 1995.

———. *Health, United States, 2000.* Hyattsville, MD: National Center for Health Statistics, 2000.

———. "Induced Termination of Pregnancy: Reporting States, 1987." *Monthly Vital Statistics Report* 38 (January 5, 1990).

National Center for Service Learning in Early Adolescence. *Reflection: The Key to Service Learning.* New York: National Helpers Network, 1991.

National Institute of Drug Abuse. *Frequently Prescribed and Abused Drugs.* Washington, DC: National Institute of Drug Abuse, 1980.

———. *Theories on Drug Abuse: Selected Contemporary Perspectives.* Washington, DC: National Institute of Drug Abuse, 1980.

———. *National Directory of Drug Abuse and Alcoholism Treatment and Prevention Programs.* Washington, DC: National Institute of Drug Abuse, 1982.

———. *Highlights from Drugs and American High School Students: 1975–1983.* Washington, DC: National Institute of Drug Abuse, 1984.

———. *Etiology of Drug Abuse: Implications for Prevention.* Washington, DC: National Institute of Drug Abuse, 1985.

New York State Urban Development Corporation. *Audobon: Plan Digest.* Getzville, NY: New York State Urban Development Corporation, n.d.

O'Donnell, Michael P. "Health Impact of Workplace Health Promotion Programs and Methodological Quality of the Research Literature." *The Art of Health Promotion* 1(1997):1–7.

Osman, Jack. "Teaching Nutrition with a Focus on Values." *Nutrition News* 36(1973):5.

Perry, Portia E. "Behavior Modification and Social Learning Theory: Application in the School." *Journal of Education* 53(1971):20.

Peterman, T. A., and J. W. Curran. "Sexual Transmission of Human Immunodeficiency Virus." *JAMA* 256(1986):2222–26.

Pew Health Professions Commission. *Critical Challenges: Revitalizing the Health Professions for the Twenty-First Century.* San Francisco, CA: Pew Health Professions Commission, 1995.

Pfeiffer, J. William, and John E. Jones, eds. *A Handbook of Structured Experiences for Human Relations Training.* Vol. 2. Iowa City, IA: University Associates Press, 1970.

Pine, Patricia. *Critical Issues Report: Promoting Health Education in Schools.* Arlington, VA: American Association of School Administrators, 1985.

Popham, W. James. "The Instructional Objectives Exchange: New Support for Criterion-Referenced Instruction." *Phi Delta Kappan* 1970, 174–75.

Pronk, N. P.; M. J. Goodman; P. J. O'Connor; and B. C. Martinson. "Relationship Between Modifiable Health Risks and Short-Term Health Care Charges." *Journal of the American Medical Association* 282(1999):2235–39.

Putnam, Robert D. "Bowling Alone: America's Declining Social Capital." *Journal of Democracy* 6(1995):65–78.

———. *Bowling Alone: The Collapse and Revival of American Community.* New York: Simon and Schuster, 2000.

Raths, Louis; Merrill Harmin; and Sidney Simon. *Values and Teaching: Working with Values in the Classroom.* Columbus, OH: Charles E. Merrill, 1966.

Read, Donald A. *Looking In: Exploring One's Personal Health Values.* Englewood Cliffs, NJ: Prentice-Hall, 1977.

Read, Donald A., and Sidney B. Simon. *Humanistic Education Sourcebook.* Englewood Cliffs, NJ: Prentice-Hall, 1976.

Redican, Kerry J.; Larry K. Olsen; and Charles R. Baffi. *Organization of School Health Programs.* New York: Macmillan, 1986.

"Report of the 2000 Joint Committee on Health Education and Promotion Terminology." *American Journal of Health Education* 32(2001):89–98.

Roszak, Betty, and Theodore Roszak, ed. *Masculine/ Feminine: Readings in Sexual Mythology and the Liberation of Women.* New York: Harper & Row, 1969.

Rubinson, Laurna, and Wesley F. Alles. *Health Education: Foundations for the Future.* St. Louis: C. V. Mosby, 1984.

Rubinson, Laurna, and James J. Neutens. *Research Techniques for the Health Sciences.* New York: Macmillan, 1987.

Schlatt, Richard G., and Peter T. Shannon. *Drugs of Choice: Current Perspectives on Drug Use.* Englewood Cliffs, NJ: Prentice-Hall, 1990.

Schmitt, Raymond H. "Sleep: An Instructional Unit." April 1976.

Seffrin, John. "The Comprehensive School Health Curriculum: Closing the Gap between State-of-the-Art and State-of-the-Practice." *Journal of School Health* 60(1990):151–56.

Shirreffs, Janet H. *Community Health: Contemporary Perspectives.* Englewood Cliffs, NJ: Prentice-Hall, 1982.

Simon, Sidney B.; Leland W. Howe; and Howard Kirschenbaum. *Values Clarification: A Handbook of Practical Strategies for Teachers and Students.* New York: Hart, 1972.

Smith, Roger B. "Remarks." In *Program Summary of a Conference on Worksite Health Promotion and Human Resources: A Hard Look at the Data,* 3–5. Washington, DC: U.S. Government Printing Office, 1984.

Smolensky, Jack. *Principles of Community Health.* Philadelphia: Saunders, 1982.

Society for Public Health Education Task Force on Ethics. *Code of Ethics.* San Francisco: Society for Public Health Education, Inc., 1976.

"Standards for the Preparation of Graduate Level Health Educators." *Journal of Health Education* 28(1997):69–73.

Strong, Bryan; Christine DeVault; Barbara W. Sayad; and William L. Yarber. *Human Sexuality: Diversity in Contemporary America.* 4th ed. New York: McGraw-Hill, 2002.

Squyres, Wendy D. *Patient Education and Health Promotion in Medical Care.* Palo Alto, CA: Mayfield, 1985.

Stark, Elizabeth. "Young, Innocent, and Pregnant." *Psychology Today,* October 1986, 28–35.

"Teenage Pregnancy, Birth and Abortion." *SIECUS Reports* 30(2002):39–43.

U.S. Census Bureau. *Statistical Abstracts of the United States: 2001* (121st edition). Washington, DC: U.S. Government Printing Office, 2001.

United States Conference of Mayors. *A Status Report on Hunger and Homelessness in America's Cities: 1993, A 26-City Survey.* Washington, DC: United States Conference of Mayors, 1993.

U.S. Department of Health and Human Services. *Healthy People: The Surgeon General's Report on Health Promotion and Disease Prevention.* Washington, DC: U.S. Government Printing Office, 1979.

———. *Healthy People 2010: Understanding and Improving Health.* 2nd ed. Washington, DC: U.S. Government Printing Office, November 2000.

———. *Promoting Health/Preventing Disease: Objectives for the Nation.* Washington, DC: U.S. Government Printing Office, 1981.

———. *Proceedings of Prospects for a Healthier America: Achieving the Nation's Health Promotion Objectives.* Washington, DC: U.S. Department of Health and Human Services, 1984.

———. *Program Summary of a Conference on Worksite Health Promotion and Human Resources: A Hard Look at the Data.* Washington, DC: U.S. Government Printing Office, 1984.

———. *Prevention 84/85.* Washington, DC: U.S. Government Printing Office, 1985.

———. *Promoting Health/Preventing Disease: Year 2000 Objectives for the Nation—Draft for Public Review and Comment.* Washington, DC: U.S. Government Printing Office, 1989.

Wilson, Thomas C. *An Alternative Community-Based School Education Program and Student Political Development.* Ph.D. dissertation, University of Southern California, 1974.

Windsor, Richard A.; Thomas Baranowski; Noreen Clark; and Gary Cutter. *Evaluation of Health Promotion and Education Programs.* Palo Alto, CA: Mayfield, 1984.

Windsor, Richard; Thomas Baranowski; and Gary Cutter. *Evaluation of Health Promotion, Health Education, and Disease Prevention Programs,* 2nd ed. New York: McGraw-Hill, 1994.

Wittner, Dale. "Life or Death." *Today's Health,* March 1974, 48–49.

Wood, Ralph J., and Daniel B. Hollander. "In Search of Spirit: Strategies for the Development of Wholeness, Health, and Spirit." *American Journal of Health Education* 33(2002):186–88.

Yates, Su. "U.S. Far Exceeds Other Nations in Teen Pregnancy." *Health Link* 2(1986):45–46.